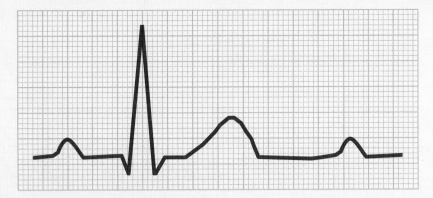

ECG Cases
for EMS

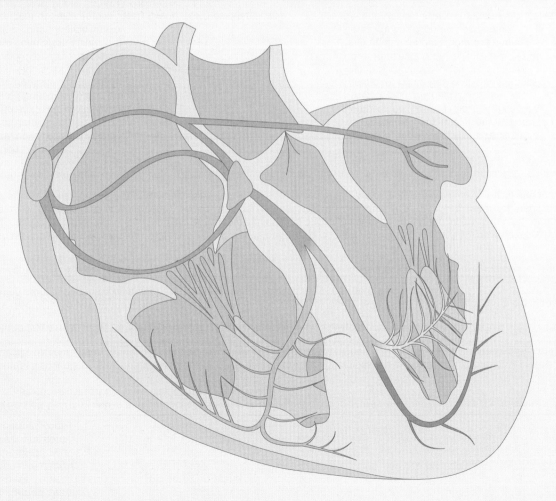

Benjamin Lawner
DO, EMT-P, FAAEM

Christopher Touzeau
MS, NREMT-P, RN

Amal Mattu
MD, FAAEM, FACEP

JONES & BA
LEARN

World Headquarters
Jones & Bartlett Learning
5 Wall Street
Burlington, MA 01803
978-443-5000
info@jblearning.com
www.jblearning.com

Jones & Bartlett Learning books and products are available through most bookstores and online booksellers. To contact Jones & Bartlett Learning directly, call 800-832-0034, fax 978-443-8000, or visit our website, www.jblearning.com.

Production Credits
Chief Executive Officer: Ty Field
President: James Homer
SVP, Editor-in-Chief: Michael Johnson
SVP, Chief Marketing Officer: Alison M. Pendergast
Executive Publisher: Kimberly Brophy
Executive Acquisitions Editor—EMS: Christine Emerton
Managing Editor: Carol B. Guerrero
Associate Editor: Ron Elliott
Production Editor: Marcia Murray
Vice President of Sales, Public Safety Group: Matthew Maniscalco
Director of Sales, Public Safety Group: Patricia Einstein

Director of Marketing: Alisha Weisman
V.P., Manufacturing and Inventory Control: Therese Connell
Composition: Cenveo Publisher Services
Cover Design: Michael O'Donnell
Director of Photo Research and Permissions: Amy Wrynn
Rights & Photo Research Assistant: Miranda Rivers
Cover Image: © Nataliia Natykach/ShutterStock, Inc.
Printing and Binding: Courier Companies
Cover Printing: Courier Companies
Section Opener Images (bottom) © Nataliia Natykach/ShutterStock, Inc.

Library of Congress Cataloging-in-Publication Data
Lawner, Benjamin.
  ECG cases for EMS / contributing authors, Benjamin Lawner, Christopher Touzeau, Amal Mattu.—1st ed.
    p. ; cm.
  ISBN 978-1-4496-0918-4
  I. Touzeau, Christopher.   II. Mattu, Amal.   III. Title.
  [DNLM: 1. Electrocardiography—Case Reports.   2. Emergencies—Case Reports.   3. Heart Diseases—diagnosis—Case Reports. WG 140]
  616.1'207547—dc23
                        2012025533

6048

Printed in the United States of America
16 15 14 13 12   10 9 8 7 6 5 4 3 2 1

CONTENTS

ACKNOWLEDGMENTS

Jones & Bartlett Learning and the authors would like to thank the following people for their help in developing this text.

CONTRIBUTORS

Adam Brenner, MD
University of Maryland Medical System
Baltimore, Maryland

Adam Friedlander, MD
Northside Emergency Associates
Atlanta, Georgia

Linda J. Kesselring, MS, ELS
University of Maryland School of Medicine
Baltimore, Maryland

REVIEWERS

Robert Jay Alley, EMT-P, BS
Blue Ridge Community College
Flat Rock, North Carolina

Anthony Caliguire, AS, REMT-P
Hudson Valley Community College
Jordan, New York

Keith H. Carter, BS, NREMT-P, CCEMT-P, LP, FP-C
Pafford EMS/AIR ONE
Ruston, Louisiana

Christopher L. Carver, BA, LP
Austin Community College
Austin, Texas

Scott Corcoran, BS, EMT-P
Erie Community College
Batavia, New York

Alexander Fein, BA, EMT-P
Penn Medicine Clinical Simulation Center
Philadelphia, Pennsylvania

David Glendenning, EMT-P
New Hanover Regional EMS
Wilmington, North Carolina

Gary Green, EMT-P, EMS-I
Mid-East Career and Technology Center
Zanesville, Ohio

Thomas Herron, AAS, NREMT-P
Cape Fear Community College
Castle Hayne, North Carolina

Chris Jackson, AA, NREMT-P
Colorado Mountain College
Glenwood Springs, Colorado

Phil Klein, BA, NREMT-P
Chattahoochee Technical College
Jasper, Georgia

Keith A. Monosky, PhD, MPM, EMT-P
Central Washington University
Ellensburg, Washington

Tamera Nailen, AAS, NREMT-P
Hinds Community College
Jackson, Mississippi

Melissa J. Osborne, NREMT-P, CCEMT-P, EMS-I
Ashford, Connecticut

Brian C. Saso, MS
Benedictine University
Lisle, Illinois

Sean G. Smith, RN, NREMT-P, BSN, FP-C, C-NPT, CCRN-CMC-CSC, CEN, CFRN
Critical Care Professionals International
Durham, North Carolina

Troy Stauter, BA, NREMT-P
Blue Ridge Community College
Flat Rock, North Carolina

Charles F. Swearingen, BS, NREMT-P, FP-C
Oklahoma City Community College
Oklahoma City, Oklahoma

David Tauber, NREMT-P, CCEMT-P, FP-C, NCEE, I/C
New Haven Sponsor Hospital
New Haven, Connecticut

Michael L. Wallace, MPA, EMT-P, CCEMT
Central Jackson County Fire Protection District
Blue Springs, Missouri

FOREWORD

Interpretation of the electrocardiogram (ECG) requires a scientific *and* an artistic approach. The authors of this book believe that the skills needed to successfully interpret the ECG are best acquired through constant repetition and the use of "real world" scenarios. This resource is not intended to replace formal ECG interpretation education but rather to supplement initial training. Ideally, providers will hone their skills and explore the boundaries of their own ECG knowledge base. Each scenario depicts a real patient encounter and enables the reader to become engrossed in the material. Additionally, the use of actual prehospital ECGs maximizes the students' exposure to what they will encounter in the field.

Each case starts off with the presentation of a chief complaint and a brief description of the current illness. Vital signs, physical exam findings, pertinent medical history, and an ECG are also provided. The interpretation for each ECG trace can be found in the second half of the text. Clinical pearls that are designed to summarize and reinforce key concepts are included at the end of each case.

The authors acknowledge that many "rules" exist for ECG interpretation, and the following criteria should be kept in mind when reviewing these cases: Myocardial ischemia can result in a number of electrocardiographic changes including ST depression; T wave inversion; ST elevation; and peaked, hyperacute, symmetrical, and broad-based T wave changes (see the appendix "Types of Ischemic Change"). The authors use the terms *ischemia*, *injury*, and *ST elevation myocardial infarction (STEMI)* interchangeably throughout the text when referring to the ECG changes associated with a lack of adequate myocardial tissue perfusion. This inclusive definition of ischemia assists providers with the recognition of significant electrocardiographic findings.

Many cases included in this text feature ECGs that illustrate STEMI. The diagnosis of STEMI is made using the following criteria: 1) ST elevation ≥1 mm in two or more contiguous limb leads, 2) ST elevation ≥2 mm in two or more contiguous precordial leads*. Patients with STEMI require rapid reperfusion and should be transported to a facility capable of performing cardiac catheterization or administering fibrinolytic therapy.

Localization of myocardial ischemia, injury, and infarction can be accomplished through the use of lead groups (see the appendix "ECG Localization of Ischemic Change"). The following lead groups are used to describe the location of ischemic changes on the ECG:

INFERIOR WALL:	Leads II, III, aVF
LATERAL WALL:	Leads I, aVL, and Leads V_5 through V_6
ANTERIOR WALL:	Leads V_1 through V_5
SEPTAL WALL:	Leads V_1 through V_2
RIGHT VENTRICLE:	Lead V_4R

It is important to note that, although lead groups can be used to localize ischemic myocardium, determination of the culprit artery can only be accomplished during cardiac angiography. Indeed, there may be significant anatomic overlap with respect to ECG findings. An anterior wall myocardial infarction, for example, might involve ST segment abnormalities in leads V_1 through V_6. Although the ECG can provide clues to the actual anatomic location of a ruptured plaque or active infarction, the electrocardiogram cannot definitively localize a lesion to one geographic region versus another.

Note: Most ECGs in this text are presented at real-life size. However, some have been reduced in size for publishing purposes. For the purposes of interpretation, readers should assume that each small grid box equals 1 mm × 1 mm (or 40 ms of time and 0.1 mV of amplitude), and that each large grid box equals 5 mm × 5 mm (or 200 ms of time and 0.5 mV of amplitude).

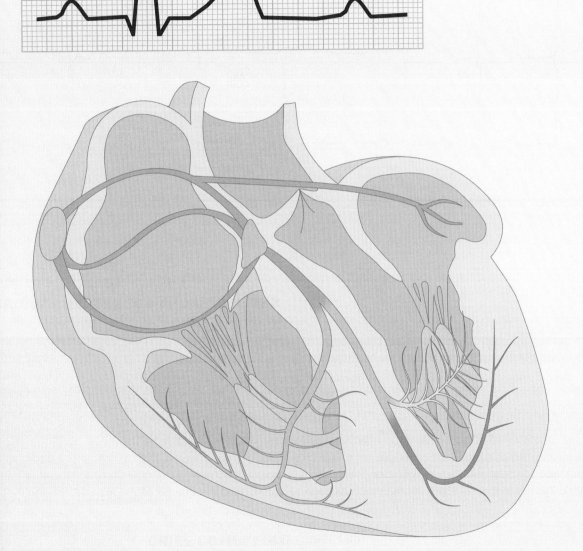

Test ECGs

CASE 1   CHIEF COMPLAINT: Chest pain

HISTORY OF PRESENT ILLNESS	You are assessing a 74-year-old woman in the triage area. She reports "crushing" pain in her chest and describes it as an 8 on a 10-point scale. The pain has lasted approximately 40 minutes. The pain radiates to both shoulders. She reports mild associated shortness of breath. The patient states that she is nauseated but has not vomited.
PAST MEDICAL HISTORY	Coronary artery disease, hypertension, diabetes mellitus, shingles
MEDICATIONS	Aspirin, lisinopril, metoprolol
ALLERGIES	Erythromycin
VITAL SIGNS	BP: 180/100 mm Hg, P: 56 beats/min., R: 14 breaths/min., SpO$_2$: 95%
EXAM	Patient appears ill and is in mild distress. She is alert and oriented. Heart sounds are normal. Lungs have crackles at the bases. No chest wall retractions are noted. Abdomen is soft and nontender. Extremity exam reveals no edema; symmetric 2+ radial pulses.

CLINICAL CHALLENGES AND QUESTIONS

1. What does this 12-lead ECG show?

2. How would you treat this patient?

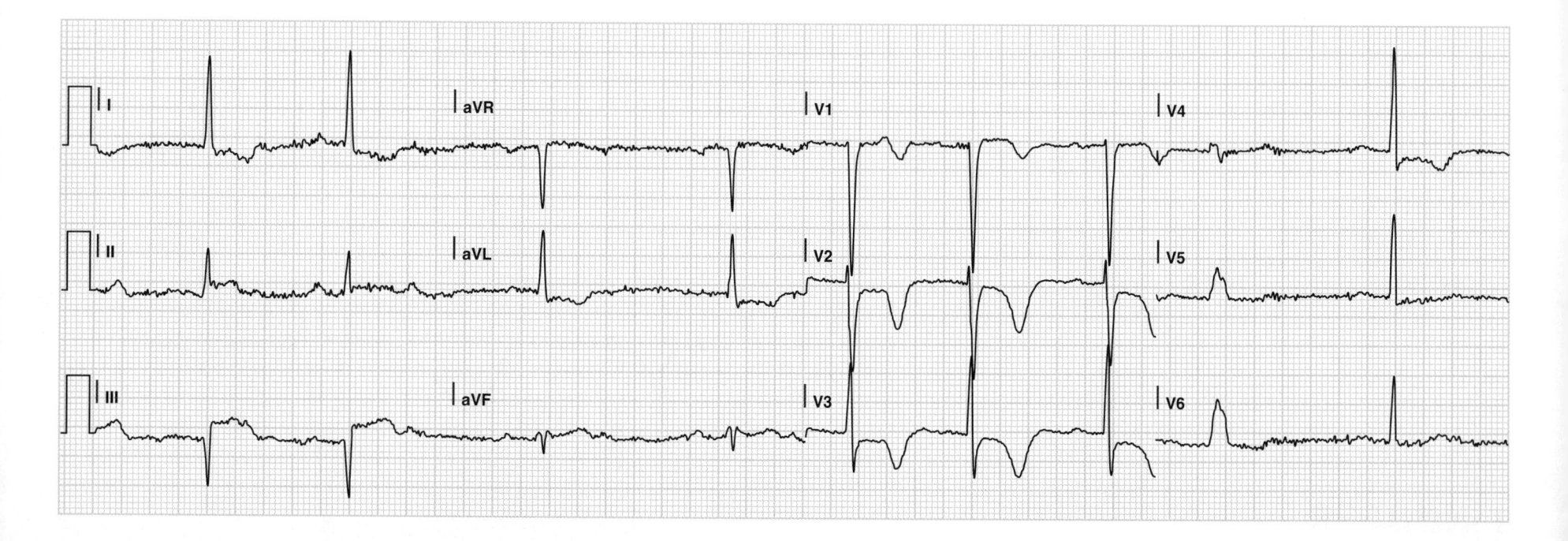

CHIEF COMPLAINT: Weakness

HISTORY OF PRESENT ILLNESS	You arrive on the scene of an 89-year-old male who has experienced progressive weakness over the last couple of days.
PAST MEDICAL HISTORY	Recent pneumonia, myocardial infarction
MEDICATIONS	Atenolol, aspirin, atorvastatin
ALLERGIES	None
VITAL SIGNS	BP: 106/58 mm Hg, P: 60s, R: 26 breaths/min., SpO$_2$: 92%
EXAM	The patient appears frail and emaciated. He is awake and alert. Heart sounds are regular and normal. Lung sounds are diminished in the right lower and middle lobes. The abdomen is soft. Pulses are 1+ bilaterally. Muscle strength is decreased in the upper and lower extremities.

CLINICAL CHALLENGES AND QUESTIONS

1. What does this 12-lead ECG show?

2. How would you treat this patient?

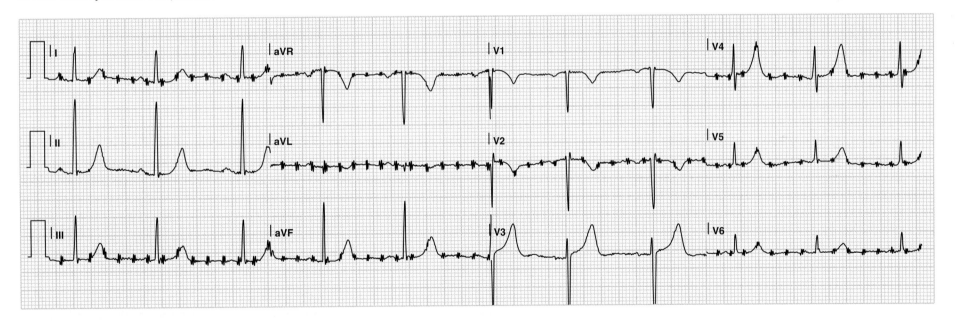

CASE 3

CHIEF COMPLAINT: Unresponsiveness

HISTORY OF PRESENT ILLNESS	You are dispatched to the scene of an elderly homeless man on a park bench. He is partially covered in blankets but is extremely cold. He arouses to painful stimuli and withdraws from such stimuli. The patient does not cooperate with your examination and does not follow commands. There is no further information about the call; the patient offers no historical information.
PAST MEDICAL HISTORY	Unknown
MEDICATIONS	Unknown
ALLERGIES	Unknown
VITAL SIGNS	BP: 90 mm Hg (by palpation), P: 42 beats/min., R: 9 breaths/min., SpO$_2$: unobtainable
EXAM	Elderly male in lateral recumbency. The patient withdraws from pain. Heart sounds are bradycardic. Lung fields are clear bilaterally. Abdomen is soft and not distended. Extremities are cool; 1+ radial pulses are present bilaterally. There are no obvious signs of trauma, bruising, or bleeding. Skin is cool to the touch and has a mottled appearance. Capillary refill is delayed.

CLINICAL CHALLENGES AND QUESTIONS

1. What does this 12-lead ECG show?

2. How would you treat this patient?

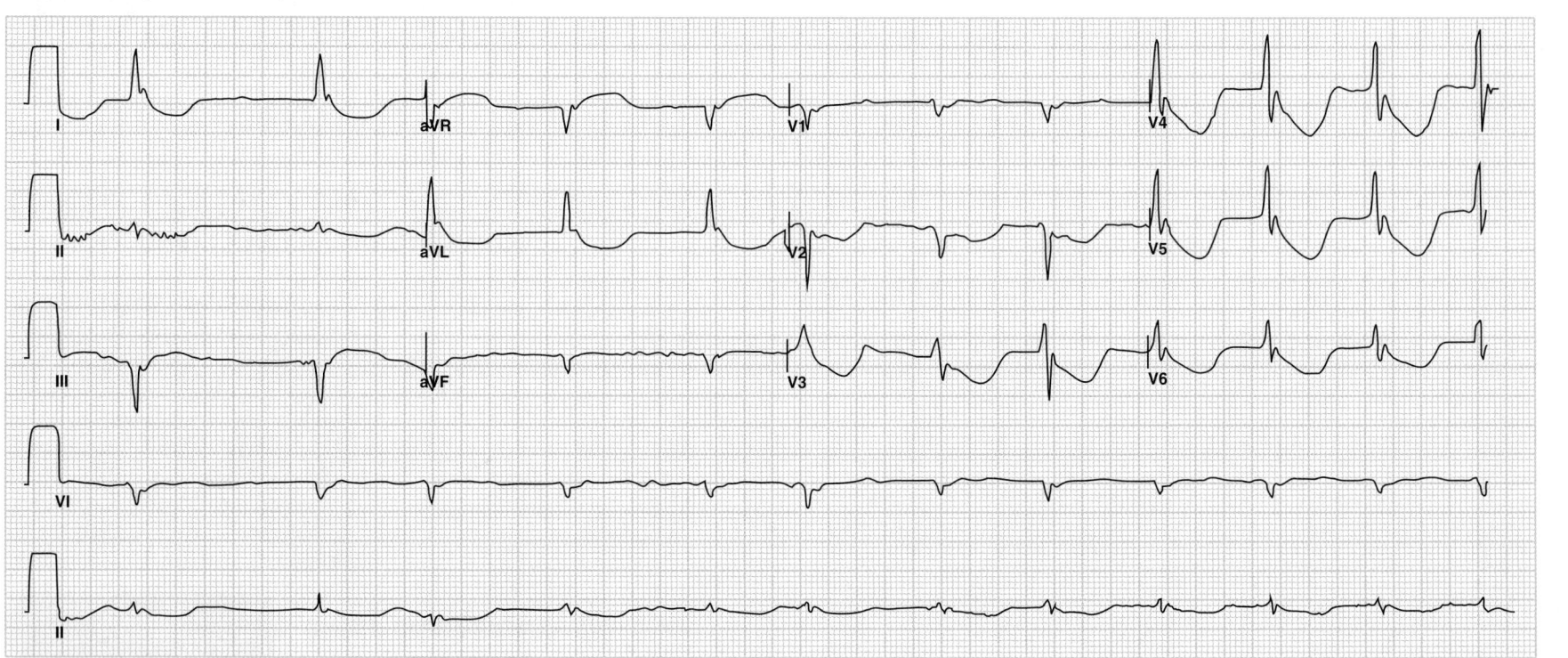

CHIEF COMPLAINT: Chest pressure

HISTORY OF PRESENT ILLNESS	In the triage area, you are assessing a 40-year-old man who experienced the onset of chest pressure, nausea, and perspiration 30 minutes after eating dinner. He rates the intensity of the pressure as 5 on a 10-point scale. The patient is clearly anxious and states that he is in "excellent health." The onset of symptoms alarmed him, so he decided to come to the local ED for evaluation.
PAST MEDICAL HISTORY	Denies
ALLERGIES	Denies
MEDICATIONS	Herbal "vitamins"
VITAL SIGNS	BP: 134/70 mm Hg, P: 70 beats/min. and strong, R: 22 breaths/min.
EXAM	Patient is in mild distress—anxious but cooperative. Heart sounds are normal. Lung sounds are clear. Abdomen is soft and nontender. Extremities are cool with strong peripheral pulses and normal capillary refill. Skin is warm and dry.

CLINICAL CHALLENGES AND QUESTIONS

1. What does this 12-lead ECG show?

2. How would you treat this patient?

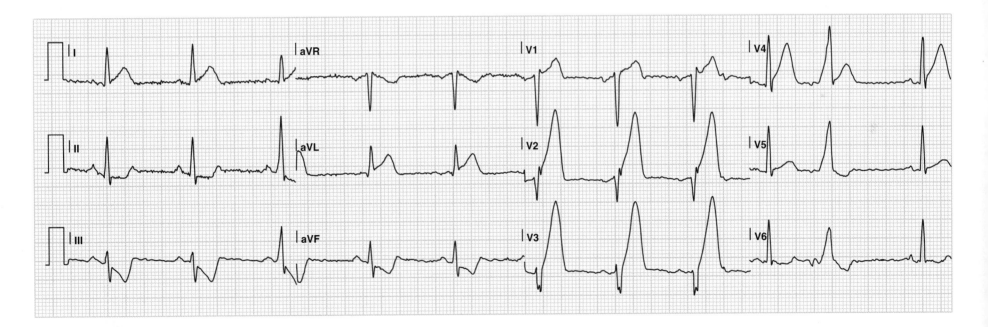

CASE 5   **CHIEF COMPLAINT:** Syncope

HISTORY OF PRESENT ILLNESS	You are transporting a 70-year-old woman with a history of coronary artery disease. She experienced a syncopal episode prior to arrival at a rural freestanding ED. Cardiac enzyme measurements have been negative, and other pertinent lab studies were unremarkable. You are told that the patient is pain free but is experiencing nausea and associated weakness. Your crew is also advised that the patient's ECG showed sinus rhythm with a right bundle branch block. A chest film was clear. Estimated drive time to the referral center is 30 minutes. Before you depart for the referral center, you ask the ED nurse for the most recent ECG and a repeat set of vital signs.
PAST MEDICAL HISTORY	Coronary artery disease, coronary stents, hypertension, diabetes mellitus
MEDICATIONS	Labetalol, aspirin, clopidogrel, glucophage, captopril, amlodipine
ALLERGIES	None
VITAL SIGNS	BP: 110/60 mm Hg, P: 70 beats/min., regular, R: 18 breaths/min., SpO$_2$: 95%
EXAM	An elderly woman is seated on an ED stretcher. She is now slightly diaphoretic but remains awake, alert, and oriented. Heart sounds are regular. Examination of her lungs reveals crackles at the bases. Abdomen is soft and nontender to palpation. Her extremities show no pitting edema; 2+ radial pulses are present bilaterally. Skin is cool and slightly wet.

(Continued)

CLINICAL CHALLENGES AND QUESTIONS

1. What does this 12-lead ECG show?

2. How would you treat this patient?

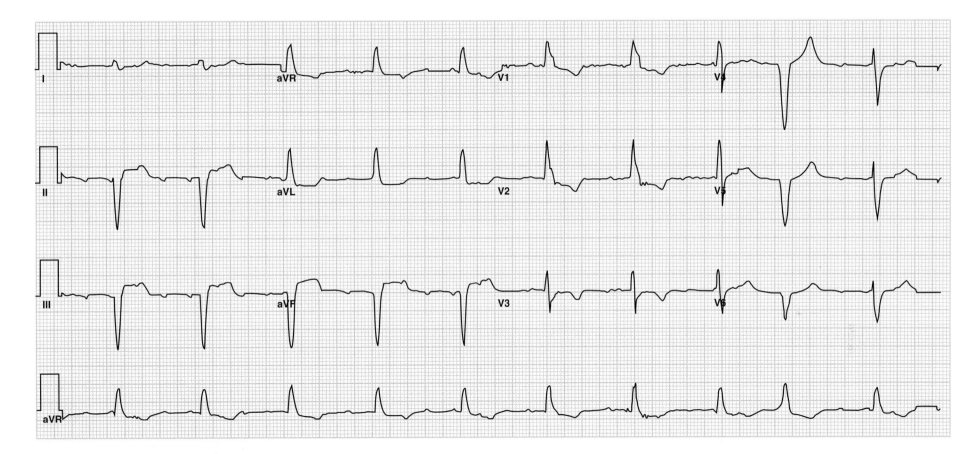

CASE 6   CHIEF COMPLAINT: Dizziness

HISTORY OF PRESENT ILLNESS	Advanced providers respond to a call regarding an 85-year-old man who reports dizziness. The dizziness was sudden in onset, and it is worsened by changes in position or physical activity. It is associated with nausea but no vomiting. The patient denies chest pain, shortness of breath, weakness, or syncope.
PAST MEDICAL HISTORY	Myocardial infarction, pacemaker insertion
MEDICATIONS	Daily aspirin, atorvastatin
ALLERGIES	None
VITAL SIGNS	BP: 130/70 mm Hg, P: 80 beats/min., R: 12 breaths/min., SpO$_2$: 98%
EXAM	The patient is an elderly male with an unsteady gate. He appears in mild distress and is awake, alert, and oriented. Horizontal nystagmus is observed. Heart sounds are normal. The lungs are clear to auscultation. The patient has an unremarkable abdominal examination. Extremities are warm and well perfused. Distal pulses are 2+ and symmetric. Skin is warm and dry.

CLINICAL CHALLENGES AND QUESTIONS

1. What does this 12-lead ECG show?

2. How would you treat this patient?

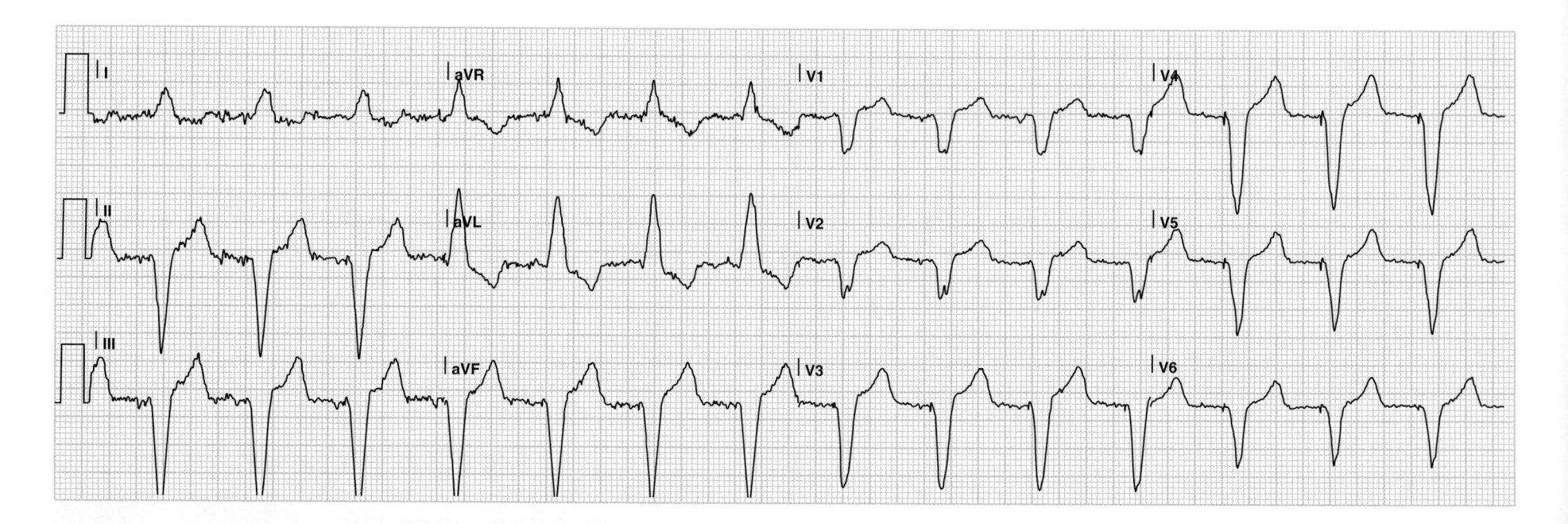

CHIEF COMPLAINT: Syncope

HISTORY OF PRESENT ILLNESS	You respond to a call regarding a 32-year-old man who experienced a syncopal episode while playing basketball. The patient is alert, and he denies chest pain, shortness of breath, nausea, or vomiting. He also denies a history of similar events.
PAST MEDICAL HISTORY	None
MEDICATIONS	None
ALLERGIES	None
VITAL SIGNS	BP: 118/62 mm Hg; P: 60 beats/min., R: 18 breaths/min., SpO$_2$: 99%
EXAM	The patient is an athletic adult male in no obvious distress. He is awake, alert, and oriented. Heart sounds are normal. Lungs are clear to auscultation bilaterally. The abdomen is soft and nontender. Extremities are warm and well perfused. No edema. Peripheral pulses are strong, and the skin is warm and dry.

(Continued)

CASE 7　　CHIEF COMPLAINT: Syncope

CLINICAL CHALLENGES AND QUESTIONS

1. What does this 12-lead ECG show?

2. How would you treat this patient?

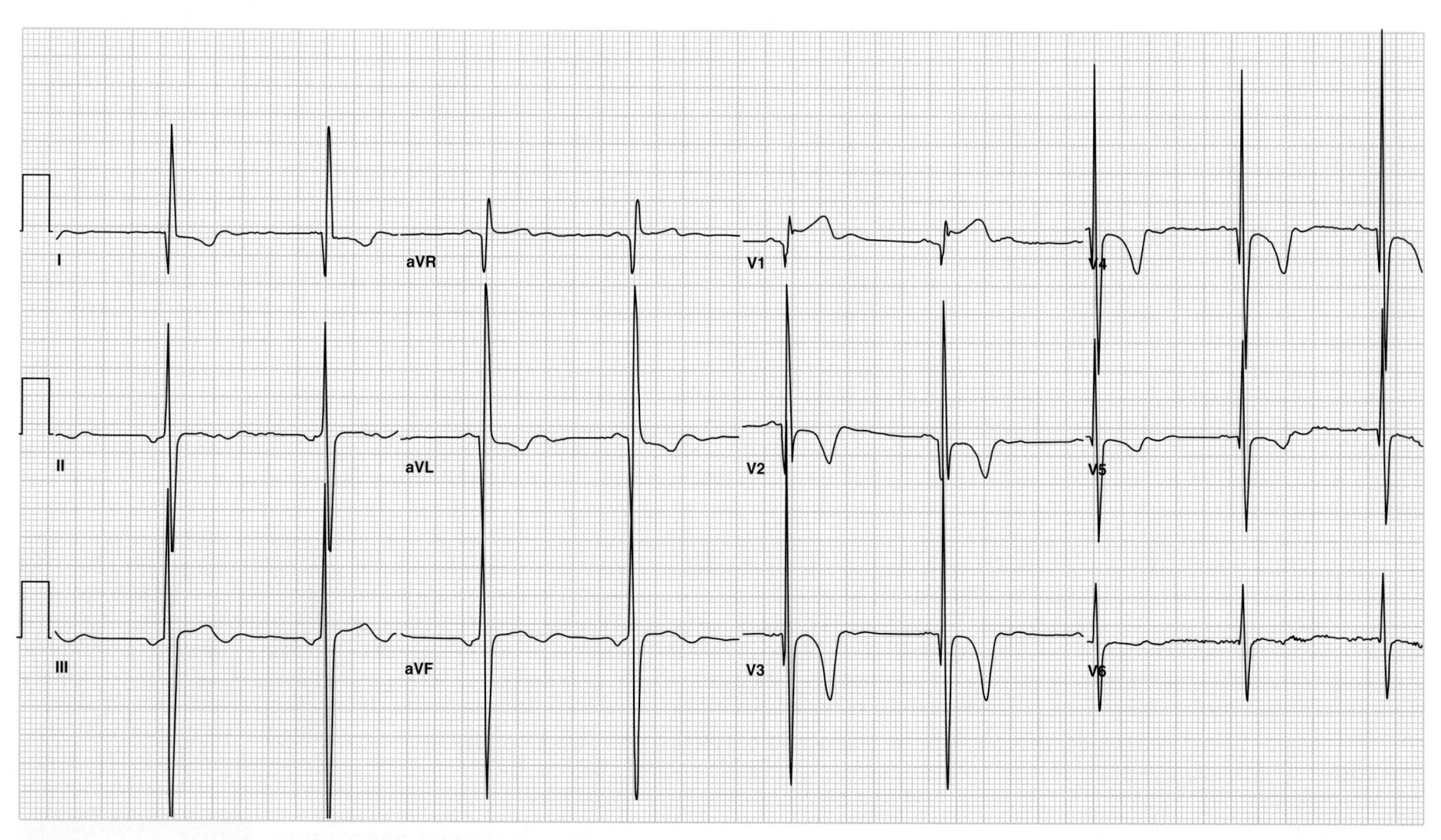

CHIEF COMPLAINT: Chest pain

HISTORY OF PRESENT ILLNESS	An advanced provider responds to a report of a 74-year-old male who experienced left-sided chest pain earlier in the day. He is now pain free but feels weak and is profusely diaphoretic. He denies fever, chills, or loss of consciousness.
PAST MEDICAL HISTORY	Stroke, angina
MEDICATIONS	Isosorbide, aspirin 81 mg
ALLERGIES	Iodine
VITAL SIGNS	BP: 140/70 mm Hg, P: 80 beats/min., R: 18 breaths/min., SpO$_2$: 99%
EXAM	Patient is a thin, elderly male. He is profusely diaphoretic. Heart sounds are normal. His lungs are clear bilaterally. His abdomen is nontender. No pedal edema. Distal pulses are strong bilaterally.

CLINICAL CHALLENGES AND QUESTIONS

1. What does this 12-lead ECG show?

2. How would you treat this patient?

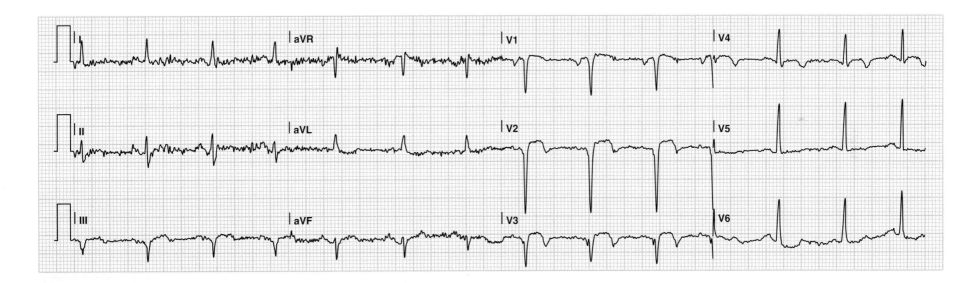

CASE 9   CHIEF COMPLAINT: Chest pain

HISTORY OF PRESENT ILLNESS	You are transporting a 53-year-old male patient from the local community hospital to a referral center for an emergent cardiac catheterization. The patient presented to the local hospital approximately 2 hours ago. He reported chest pain, nausea and diaphoresis at the time of arrival.
PAST MEDICAL HISTORY	Hypertension
MEDICATIONS	Lisinopril
VITAL SIGNS	BP: 150/100 mm Hg, P: 50-60 beats/min., R: 20 breaths/min., SpO$_2$: 98% on nasal cannula
EXAM	The patient is an anxious–appearing adult male. Lung sounds reveal crackles bilaterally. His abdomen is soft and nontender. He has no edema in his lower extremities.

CLINICAL CHALLENGES AND QUESTIONS

1. What does this 12-lead ECG show?
2. How would you treat this patient?

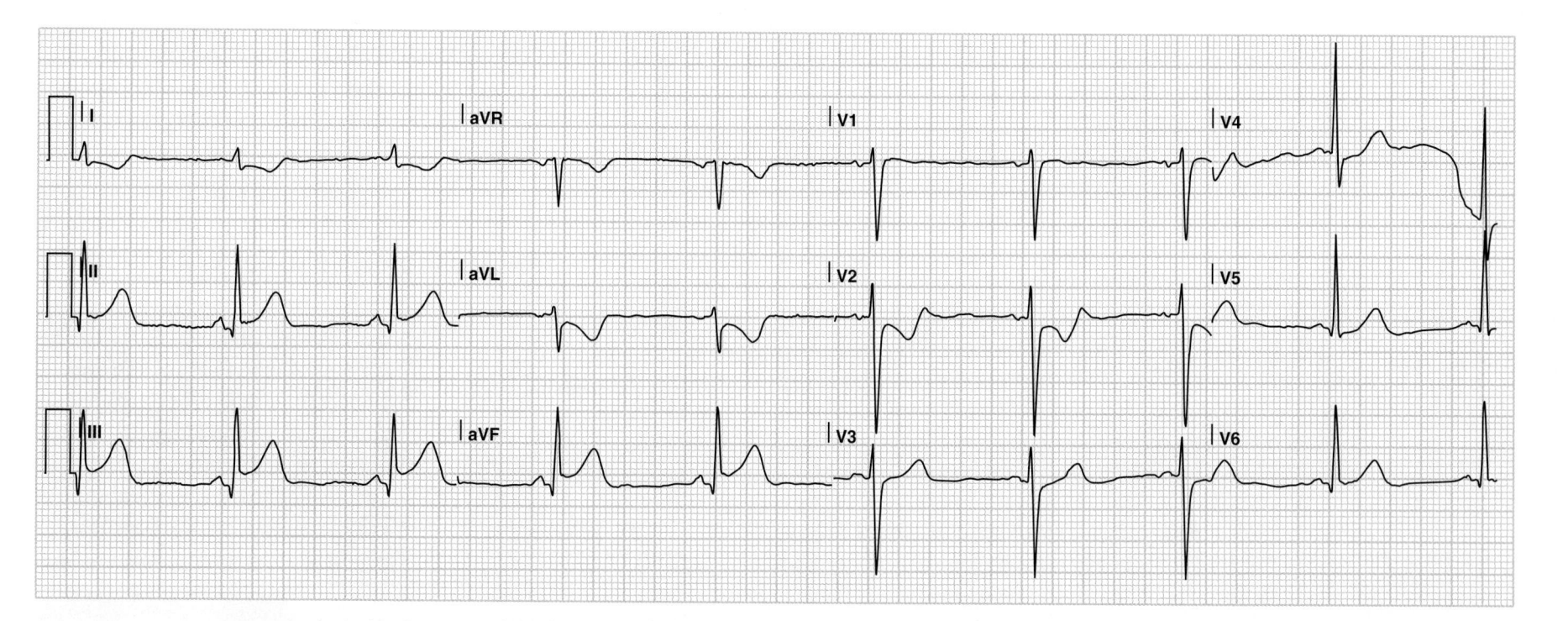

HISTORY OF PRESENT ILLNESS	Advanced providers arrive on the scene of a 10-year-old male experiencing shortness of breath. He was sitting in math class when his symptoms began. The patient also reports palpitations. There is no history of recent trauma or illness.
PAST MEDICAL HISTORY	None
MEDICATIONS	None
ALLERGIES	None
VITAL SIGNS	BP: 94/62 mm Hg, P: 210s, R: 24 breaths/min., SpO$_2$: 96%
EXAM	The patient does not seem to be in any distress, and is awake and alert. Heart sounds reveal significant tachycardia. Lung sounds are clear bilaterally. Radial pulses are weak and rapid. Skin is cool and clammy.

CLINICAL CHALLENGES AND QUESTIONS

1. What does this rhythm strip show?
2. How would you treat this patient?

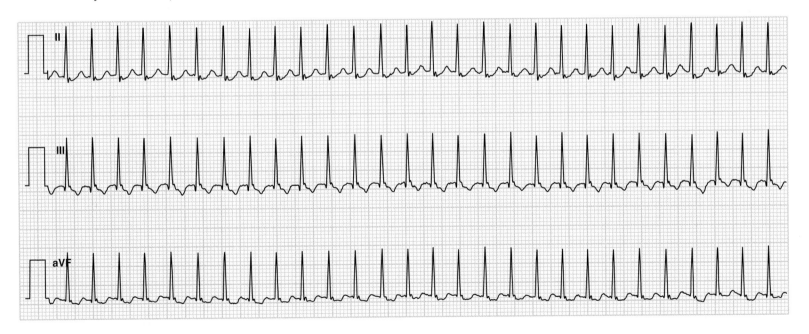

CASE 11   **CHIEF COMPLAINT:** Chest pain

HISTORY OF PRESENT ILLNESS	You respond to the scene of a 57-year-old man who reports "chest pressure." It started while he was shoveling snow. The pain does not radiate and is constant at a 4 on a 10-point pain scale. He reports associated nausea and shortness of breath. The patient has not experienced syncope, exertional dyspnea, or chills.
PAST MEDICAL HISTORY	Hypertension
MEDICATIONS	Aspirin, verapamil
ALLERGIES	None
VITAL SIGNS	BP: 158/84 mm Hg, P: 60 beats/min., R: 12 breaths/min., SpO$_2$: 96%
EXAM	The patient is an adult male in mild distress. He is awake, alert, and oriented. Heart sounds are normal. His lungs are clear and his abdomen is soft and nontender. Extremities are warm and well perfused; no cyanosis or edema is present. Radial pulses are strong and equal. His skin is warm and dry.

CLINICAL CHALLENGES AND QUESTIONS

1. What does this 12-lead ECG show?

2. How would you treat this patient?

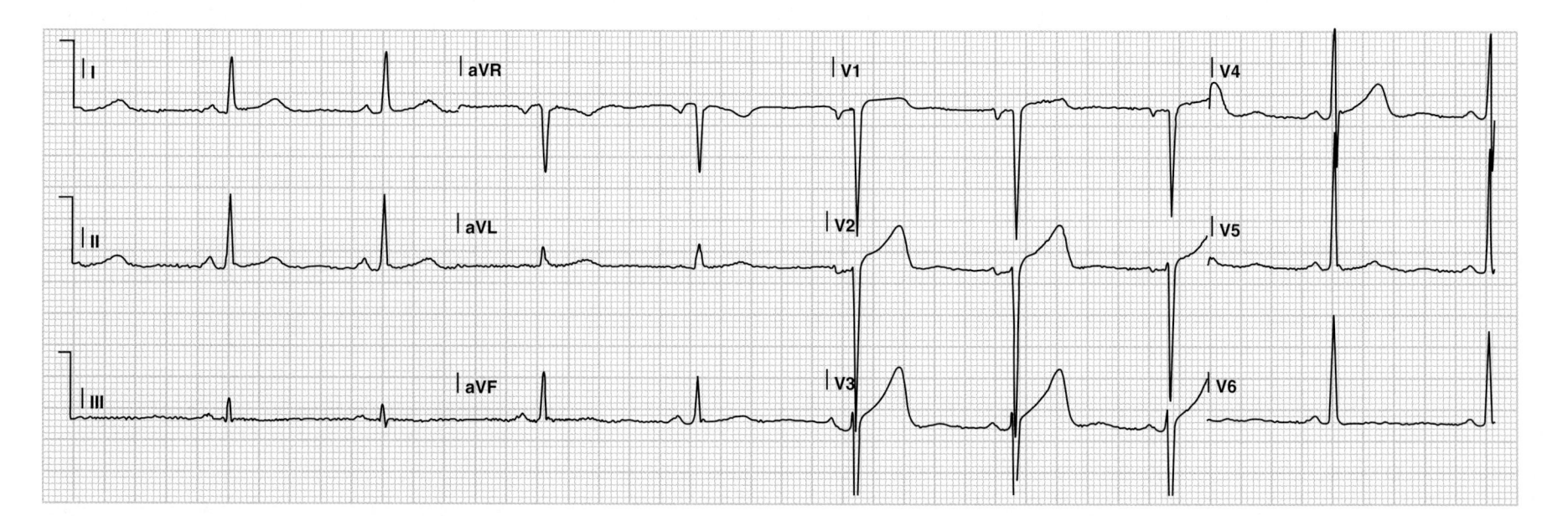

CHIEF COMPLAINT: Chest pain

HISTORY OF PRESENT ILLNESS	Advanced providers respond to a report of a 72-year-old male who has been experiencing chest pain for approximately 45 minutes. The patient reports that the pain came on suddenly while he was walking on the treadmill. He describes the pain as sharp and stabbing, and located in his right chest. He rates the pain a 9 on a 10-point scale.
PAST MEDICAL HISTORY	None
MEDICATIONS	None
ALLERGIES	Seasonal allergies
VITAL SIGNS	BP: 134/70 mm Hg, P: 70 beats/min., R: 18 breaths/min., SpO$_2$: 99%
EXAM	The patient is a well-appearing male in mild distress. Heart sounds are normal. Lung sounds are clear bilaterally. The abdomen is non-distended and soft. There is no lower extremity edema. Pulses are strong bilaterally. Skin is warm and well perfused.

CLINICAL CHALLENGES AND QUESTIONS

1. What does this 12-lead ECG show?

2. How would you treat this patient?

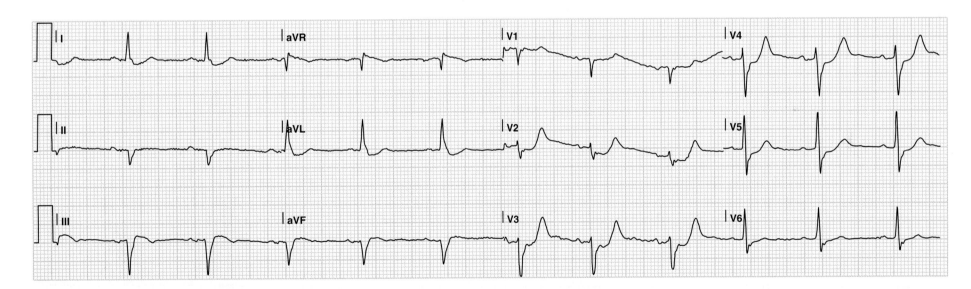

CASE 13   **CHIEF COMPLAINT:** Fever, change in mental status

HISTORY OF PRESENT ILLNESS	Advanced providers are transferring a 73-year-old male from a long-term care facility to an acute care hospital. The nursing home physician is concerned about the man's increasing oxygen requirements, episodic desaturations, and a recent fever. The providers find a nonverbal elderly male receiving oxygen by tracheal collar at an FiO_2 of 40%. Nursing home staff members report that the patient is less responsive than usual.
PAST MEDICAL HISTORY	Pneumonia, dementia, sepsis, myocardial infarction, pacemaker
MEDICATIONS	Aspirin, subcutaneous enoxaparin, colace, metoprolol, lorazepam as needed
ALLERGIES	None
VITAL SIGNS	BP: 90/52 mm Hg, P: 70–80 beats/min., R: 24 breaths/min., SpO_2: 92% on 40% oxygen by tracheal collar
EXAM	The patient is an elderly male in obvious respiratory distress. Heart sounds are normal. Coarse rhonchi are heard in all fields. The abdomen is slightly distended but without rebound or guarding. A gastric feeding tube and Foley catheter are in place. There are flexion contractures in the upper extremities. 1+ radial pulses are present bilaterally. The patient's skin is hot and dry. The urine in the reservoir appears cloudy and dark yellow.

CLINICAL CHALLENGES AND QUESTIONS

1. What does this 12-lead ECG show?

2. How would you treat this patient?

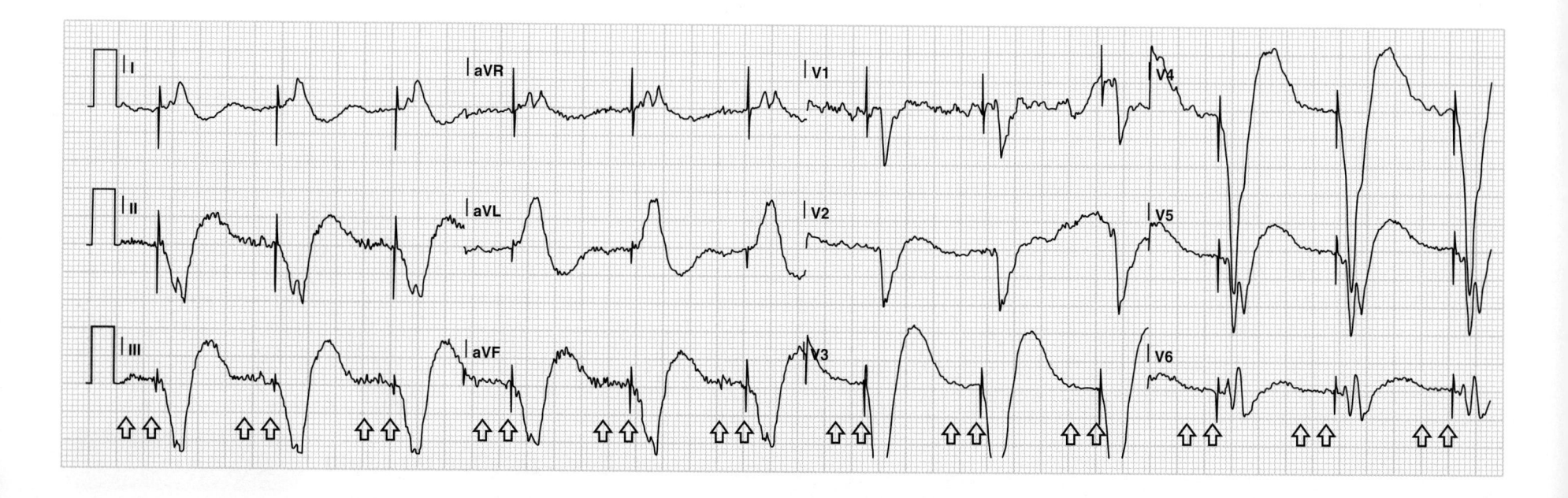

CHIEF COMPLAINT: Acute pericarditis

HISTORY OF PRESENT ILLNESS	A 55-year-old man is being evaluated for positional chest pain associated with a cough. The patient states that he has been unwell for the past 3 days. He reports intermittent and "achy" retrosternal chest discomfort. It is worse with movement and reproducible with chest wall palpation. The patient rates the pain a 5 on a 10-point scale, and states that he has been taking ibuprofen and aspirin with little relief. An ECG was obtained in the triage area and interpreted by the machine as "acute pericarditis." The patient has been placed in a treatment room and is awaiting evaluation by the attending ED physician. You review the ECG as you start an intravenous line and collect routine laboratory samples.
PAST MEDICAL HISTORY	Diabetes mellitus, hypertension, coronary artery disease, bronchitis
MEDICATIONS	Aspirin, ibuprofen, guaifenesin, metformin, sliding-scale insulin
ALLERGIES	None
VITAL SIGNS	BP: 136/80 mm Hg, P: 80 beats/min., R: 18 breaths/min., SpO$_2$: 96%
EXAM	Mildly ill, middle-aged man in no acute distress. The patient is awake and alert. Heart sounds are normal. Lungs are clear to auscultation. Abdomen is soft and not tender to palpation. Extremity exam reveals no cyanosis or clubbing. Strong radial pulses are present bilaterally. Skin is warm and dry.

CLINICAL CHALLENGES AND QUESTIONS

1. What does this 12-lead ECG show?

2. How would you treat this patient?

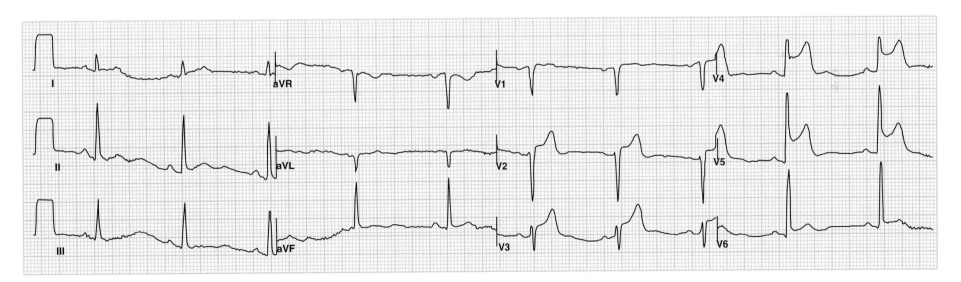

CASE 15   CHIEF COMPLAINT: Shortness of breath

HISTORY OF PRESENT ILLNESS	You are in the triage area, evaluating a 45-year-old man who has shortness of breath. You are orienting a new provider. The patient reports having shortness of breath for the past few days. His symptoms are worse at night and not associated with nausea. He has not been taking his antihypertensive medications and does not have access to a primary care physician. The patient denies chest pain, hemoptysis, vomiting, or syncope.
PAST MEDICAL HISTORY	Hypertension, uncontrolled diabetes
MEDICATIONS	Noncompliant with clonidine and diabetes medications
ALLERGIES	"Sulfur drugs" and intravenous dye
VITAL SIGNS	BP: 160/110 mm Hg; P: 88 beats/min., R: 16 breaths/min., SpO$_2$: 99%
EXAM	A well-developed, well-nourished male is sitting in the triage area. His skin is warm and dry. He is awake, alert, and oriented. The patient's heart sounds are normal and his lungs are clear. He does not have abdominal tenderness. No extremity edema is present. Strong radial pulses are present bilaterally.

(Continued)

CHIEF COMPLAINT: Shortness of breath

CLINICAL CHALLENGES AND QUESTIONS

1. What does this 12-lead ECG show?

2. How would you treat this patient?

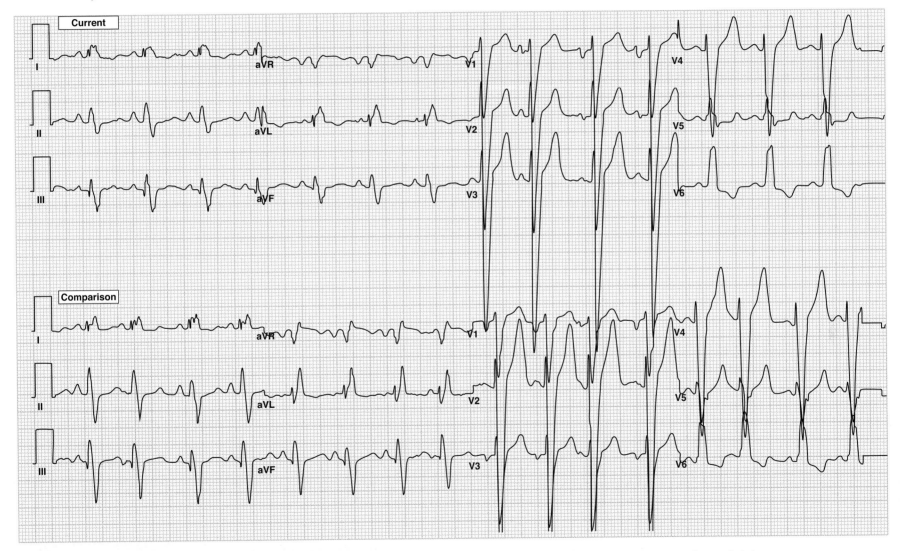

Your orientee retrieves an old ECG for comparison and asks if this patient should be brought back to the treatment area immediately.

CASE 16   CHIEF COMPLAINT: Syncope

HISTORY OF PRESENT ILLNESS	Advanced providers arrive on the scene of a 30-year-old male who experienced an episode of syncope. The patient is a professional cyclist and runner, and he has been training for a marathon. The weather has been very hot. The patient denies chest pain or shortness of breath. He reports increased thirst and states that he has not urinated in the past 8 hours.
PAST MEDICAL HISTORY	None
MEDICATIONS	None
ALLERGIES	None
VITAL SIGNS	BP: 118/62 mm Hg, P: 80s, R: 18 breaths/min., SpO$_2$: 99%
EXAM	The patient is aware and alert. Heart sounds are irregular. Lung sounds are clear to auscultation. The extremities are warm and well perfused. Radial pulses are equal and strong. The skin is hot and dry.

CLINICAL CHALLENGES AND QUESTIONS

1. What does the 3-lead ECG show?
2. How would you treat this patient?

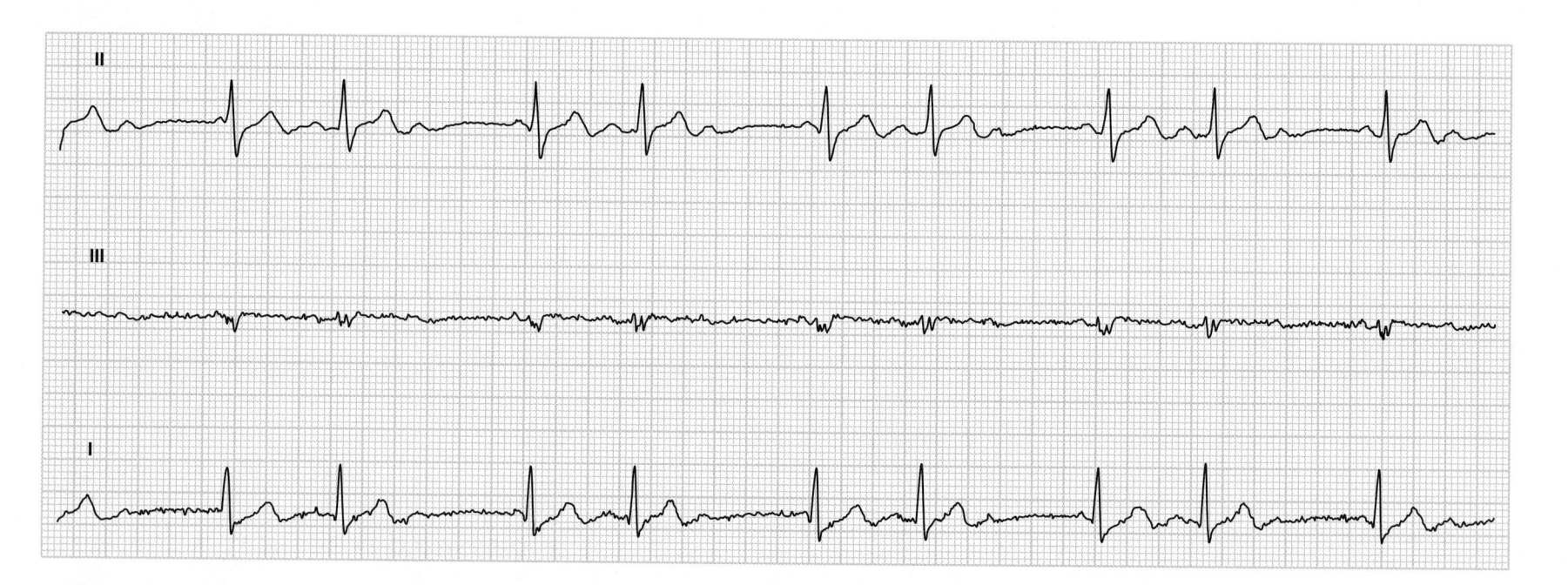

CHIEF COMPLAINT: Weakness, dyspnea

HISTORY OF PRESENT ILLNESS	Your patient is a 63-year-old female who reports weakness and shortness of breath. She states that her symptoms started several hours before her presentation at the ED.
PAST MEDICAL HISTORY	Unknown
MEDICATIONS	Unknown
ALLERGIES	Unknown
VITAL SIGNS	BP: 118/78 mm Hg, P: 70s, R: breaths/min., 16, SpO$_2$: 98%
EXAM	The patient appears anxious but is alert and oriented. Lung sounds are clear bilaterally. Extremity exam reveals no edema. Her abdomen is soft and nontender. Radial pulses are strong. Skin is warm and well perfused.

CLINICAL CHALLENGES AND QUESTIONS

1. What does this 12-lead ECG show?

2. How would you treat this patient?

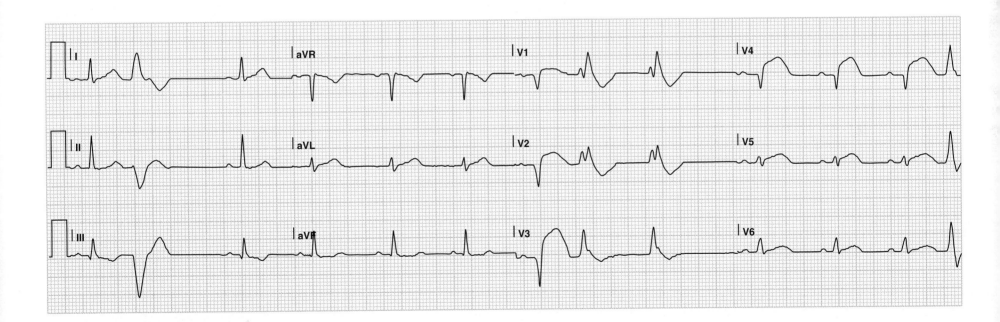

CASE 18

CHIEF COMPLAINT: Chest pain

HISTORY OF PRESENT ILLNESS	You are paged to a long-term care facility. A 60-year-old resident at the facility is experiencing chest pain. She was recently transferred from an acute care hospital for rehabilitation. The patient reports nausea, diaphoresis, midsternal chest discomfort, and shortness of breath. The pain began 30 minutes before your arrival and has not lessened with nitroglycerin or oxygen. While waiting for the ALS transport unit, you obtain a 12-lead ECG tracing.
PAST MEDICAL HISTORY	Cardiac disease, hypertension
MEDICINES	Aspirin, clopidogrel, metoprolol
ALLERGIES	"Sulfa drugs"
VITAL SIGNS	BP: 100/60 mm Hg; P: 72 beats/min.; R: 16 breaths/min., non-labored; SpO$_2$: 95%
EXAM	Elderly female who is anxious but oriented. Heart sounds are normal. Lung sounds are diminished bilaterally. Abdominal exam reveals no tenderness or guarding. Extremities are well perfused; 2+ peripheral pulses are present. Pitting edema (2+) is present and symmetric on lower legs.

CLINICAL CHALLENGES AND QUESTIONS

1. What does this 12-lead ECG show?

2. How would you treat this patient?

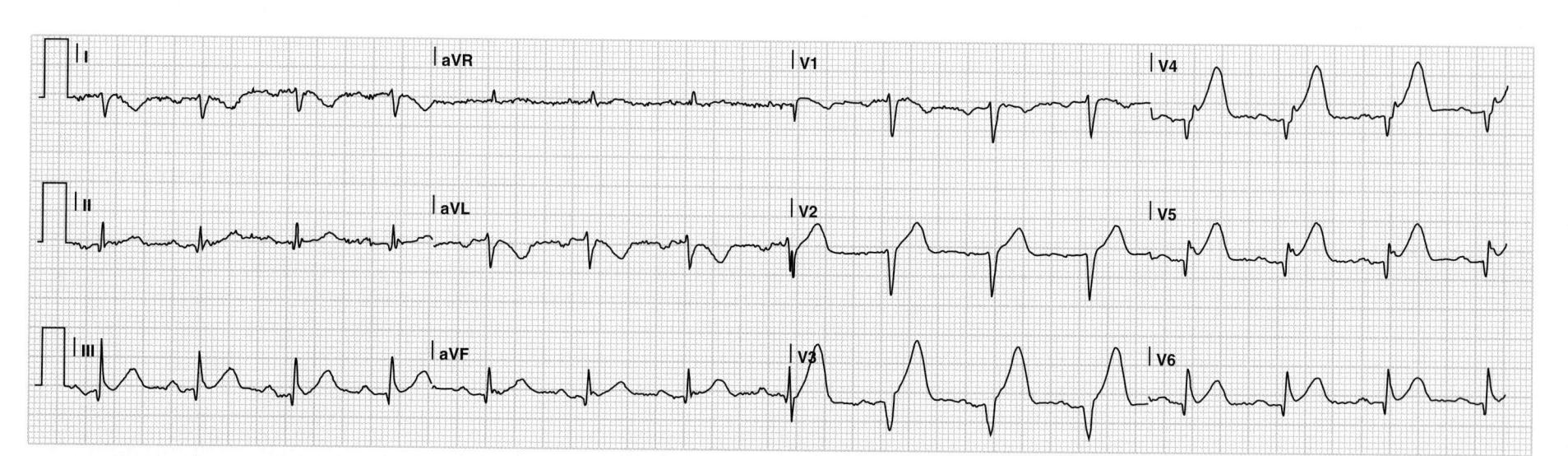

CHIEF COMPLAINT: Burning in chest

HISTORY OF PRESENT ILLNESS	You respond to a call regarding a 38-year-old man reporting a burning in his chest and throat. It started about an hour after he ate spicy chili. The pain radiates to his throat and is associated with dyspepsia; it remains constant at a 3 on a 10-point pain scale. He does not report diaphoresis and denies shortness of breath. The patient volunteers that he is in excellent physical health and has never experienced exercise intolerance or fatigue. A 12-lead ECG is obtained.
PAST MEDICAL HISTORY	Gastroesophageal reflux
MEDICATIONS	Omeprazole
ALLERGIES	None
VITAL SIGNS	BP: 138/76 mm Hg, P: 80 beats/min., R: 16 breaths/min., SpO$_2$, 97%
EXAM	The patient is a fit adult male who appears anxious. He is otherwise awake, alert, and oriented. Heart sounds are normal. Lung sounds are clear to auscultation. There is slight epigastric tenderness on palpation; the remainder of the abdominal exam is unremarkable. There is no extremity edema. Pulses are 2+ and strong. Skin is warm and dry.

CLINICAL CHALLENGES AND QUESTIONS

1. What does this 12-lead ECG show?

2. How would you treat this patient?

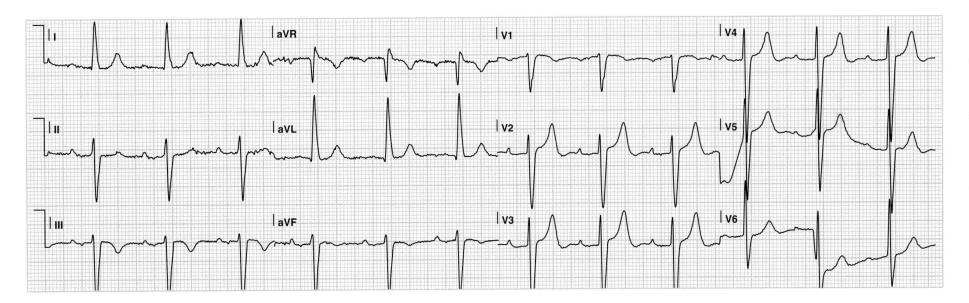

CASE 20 CHIEF COMPLAINT: Weakness

HISTORY OF PRESENT ILLNESS	Advanced providers respond to a call regarding a 68-year-old woman who reports weakness. It began several days ago, when she started taking a newly prescribed pain medicine. She denies nausea or shortness of breath.
PAST MEDICAL HISTORY	Hypertension, chronic lower back pain
MEDICATIONS	Daily aspirin, atenolol, acetaminophen with codeine
ALLERGIES	None
VITAL SIGNS	BP: 110/70 mm Hg, P: 60 beats/min, R: 16 breaths/min, SpO$_2$: 99%
EXAM	The patient is a pleasant, well-nourished elderly female in no obvious distress. She is awake, alert, and oriented. Heart sounds are normal, and lung sounds are clear. The patient's abdomen is soft, nontender, and nondistended. Her pupils are constricted. Extremities are without cyanosis or clubbing. Radial pulses are equal and strong. Skin is cool and dry.

CLINICAL CHALLENGES AND QUESTIONS

1. What does this 12-lead ECG show?

2. How would you treat this patient?

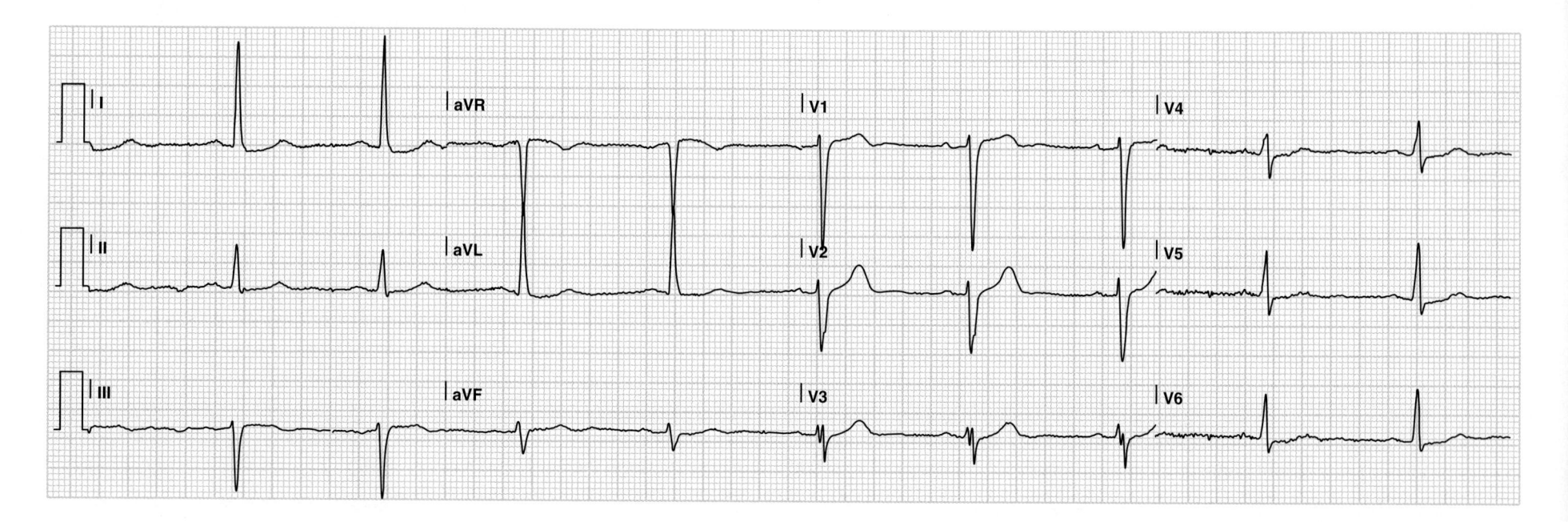

CHIEF COMPLAINT: Weakness, dyspnea

HISTORY OF PRESENT ILLNESS	An emergency department paramedic is triaging a 72-year-old woman with ongoing weakness. The patient has experienced fatigue and generalized shortness of breath for several days. She came to the emergency department today because of the worsening dyspnea and the development of a dry, persistent cough. The patient denies fever or chills. The patient states she has been more tired than usual and has experienced new dyspnea on exertion. She describes having some occasional "soreness" in her left shoulder. The pain is dull and constant, and she rates its intensity as a 3 on a 10-point scale.
PAST MEDICAL HISTORY	Hypertension, high cholesterol, urinary tract infections, diabetes, osteoarthritis, and "mild" chronic obstructive pulmonary disorder.
MEDICATIONS	Aspirin, atenolol, amlodipine, simvastatin
ALLERGIES	Codeine (hives), ketorolac
VITAL SIGNS	BP: 180/90 mm Hg, P: 92 beats/min., R: 22 breaths/min., SpO$_2$: 94%
EXAM	Patient is an elderly woman who appears ill. She is alert and oriented. Heart sounds are normal. Lungs are clear; chest wall is without retraction. Abdomen is soft and nontender. Extremities are without cyanosis or clubbing. 1+ pitting edema is present in the lower extremities. Skin is cool.

CLINICAL CHALLENGES AND QUESTIONS

1. What does this 12-lead ECG show?

2. How would you treat this patient?

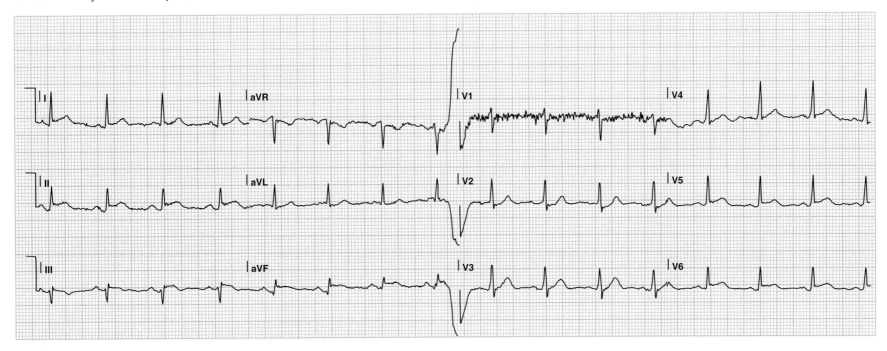

CASE 22

CHIEF COMPLAINT: Chest pain, weakness

HISTORY OF PRESENT ILLNESS	Advanced providers respond to a call regarding an 81-year-old man who reports weakness. He experienced an episode of chest pain while walking earlier in the day, but now the pain has completely resolved. The patient describes no associated nausea, vomiting, or diaphoresis.
PAST MEDICAL HISTORY	Unknown
MEDICATIONS	Unknown
ALLERGIES	None
VITAL SIGNS	BP: 140/70 mm Hg, P: 50 beats/min., R: 18 breaths/min., SpO$_2$: 99%
EXAM	Elderly male in no obvious distress. He is awake, alert, and oriented. Heart sounds are present. Lung sounds are clear to auscultation bilaterally. The abdomen is soft, nontender, and nondistended. Extremities are warm and well perfused; there is trace edema. Strong radial pulses with good capillary refill are present. Skin is warm and dry.

CLINICAL CHALLENGES AND QUESTIONS

1. What does this 12-lead ECG show?

2. How would you treat this patient?

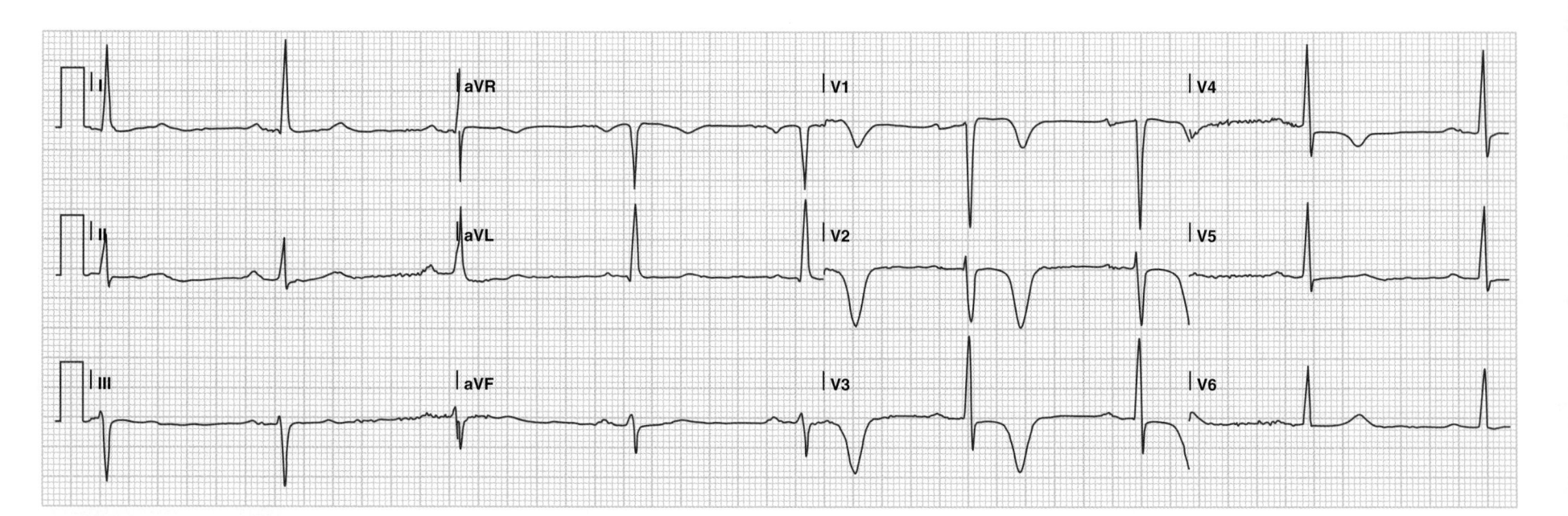

CHIEF COMPLAINT: Chest pain

HISTORY OF PRESENT ILLNESS	Advanced providers respond to a report of a 48-year-old man who has experienced retrosternal chest pain for 30 minutes. He recently finished running a marathon. Although his heart rate returned to baseline, he experienced persistent chest pain, diaphoresis, and nausea. The chest pain prompted him to seek help at the nearest aid station. He states that the pain radiates to his left arm and neck. He denies any recent fevers, chills, or loss of consciousness.
PAST MEDICAL HISTORY	None, previously healthy
MEDICATIONS	Herbal supplements
ALLERGIES	Seasonal allergies
VITAL SIGNS	BP: 140/70 mm Hg, P: 72 beats/min., R: 18 breaths/min., SpO$_2$: 99%
EXAM	The patient is a thin, athletic male who is awake, alert, and oriented. He is in mild distress. Heart sounds are normal. Lung sounds are clear. Abdomen is soft to palpation. Extremities are without cyanosis, clubbing, or edema. Pulses are 2+ bilaterally. Skin is diaphoretic and warm.

CLINICAL CHALLENGES AND QUESTIONS

1. What does this 12-lead ECG show?

2. How would you treat this patient?

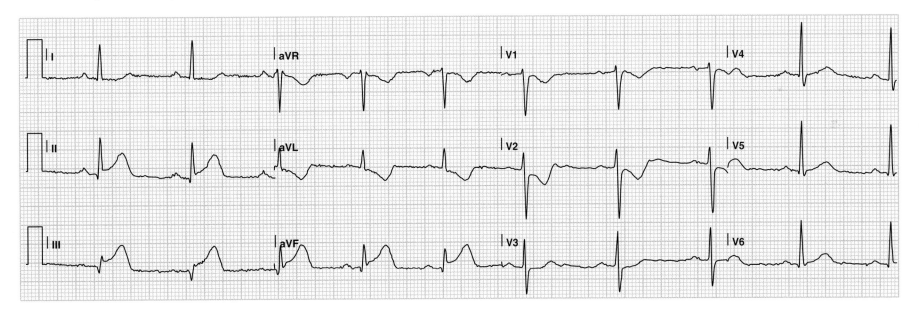

CASE 24   CHIEF COMPLAINT: Syncope

HISTORY OF PRESENT ILLNESS	A 60-year-old man called 9-1-1 after experiencing a syncopal episode. The event was not witnessed. The patient states that he suddenly felt weak and dizzy and then awoke on the floor of his bedroom. He reports some mild nausea. He has had a dry cough for the past 2 days. He denies chest pain, fever, or vomiting.
PAST MEDICAL HISTORY	Hypertension, diabetes
MEDICATIONS	Metformin, lisinopril, daily aspirin
ALLERGIC	Penicillin
VITAL SIGNS	BP: 110/70 mm Hg; P: 60 beats/min.; R: 16 breaths/min., non-labored; SpO$_2$: 96%
EXAM	Anxious, well-developed, and well-nourished male in no acute distress. He is alert, oriented, and cooperative. Heart sounds are normal. Lung sounds reveal bibasilar crackles. Abdomen is soft and nontender. Extremities have mild bilateral and symmetric pitting edema. Radial pulses are present and 1+ bilaterally. Skin is cool.

CLINICAL CHALLENGES AND QUESTIONS

1. What does this 12-lead ECG show?

2. How would you treat this patient?

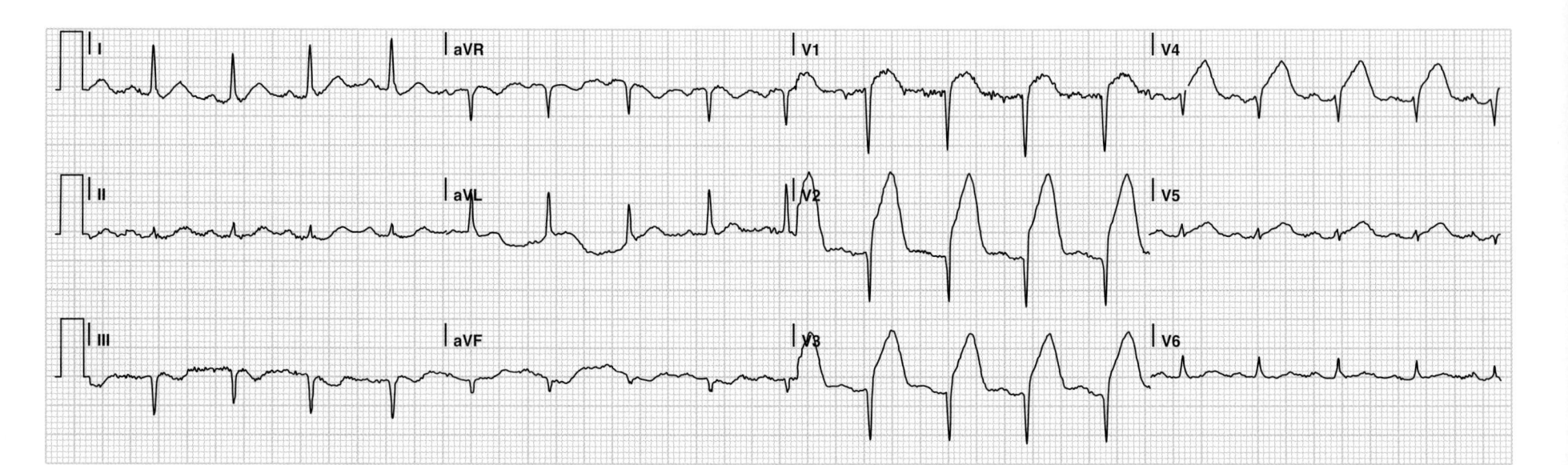

CHIEF COMPLAINT: Unresponsiveness

HISTORY OF PAST ILLNESS	You and a student provider are paged to assist an engine company on scene. The patient is a homeless 60-year-old man. Three hours earlier, he started to experience chest pain and shortness of breath. He rated the pain as a 9 on a 10-point scale. It radiated superiorly "up the center" of his chest. The patient reported associated nausea and "stomach pains." He was recently released from a local ED after being "ruled out" for myocardial infarction. Paramedics from the engine company established an intravenous line and administered sublingual nitroglycerin (NTG) according to protocol. When you arrive at the scene, the patient is unresponsive and supine.
PAST MEDICAL HISTORY	Chronic chest pain, alcohol abuse, diabetes mellitus
MEDICATIONS	Patient is noncompliant with medications but is supposed to take aspirin, lisinopril, hydrochlorothiazide, insulin, and metoprolol.
ALLERGIES	No known allergies
VITAL SIGNS	(After NTG administration) BP: 77 mm Hg (by palpation), P: 100 beats/min. and irregular, R: 17 breaths/min., SpO$_2$: 88%
EXAM	A disheveled male patient is supine on the ground; he moans in response to painful stimuli. Heart sounds are irregular and lungs are clear bilaterally. No lower extremity cyanosis or edema. Radial pulses are absent bilaterally. There is a strong and irregular femoral pulse. Skin is cool to the touch.

CLINICAL CHALLENGES AND QUESTIONS

1. What does this 12-lead ECG show?

2. How would you treat this patient?

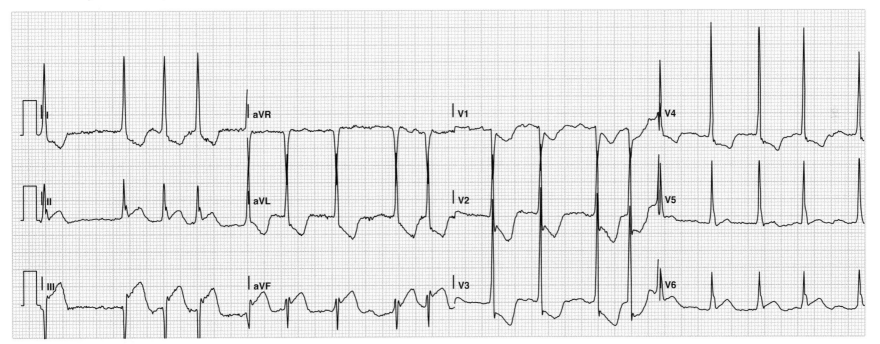

CASE 26   **CHIEF COMPLAINT:** Weakness, dyspnea

HISTORY OF PRESENT ILLNESS	The patient is an 87-year-old male who reports fatigue and shortness of breath for several hours. The patient also reports an episode of retrosternal chest pressure lasting for approximately 5 minutes. The patient is also nauseated. He denies vomiting or loss of consciousness.
PAST MEDICAL HISTORY	Hypertension, high cholesterol, diabetes
MEDICATIONS	Aspirin, atenolol, simvastatin, insulin
ALLERGIES	Penicillin
VITAL SIGNS	BP: 80/60 mm Hg, P: 106 beats/min., R: 18 breaths/min., SpO$_2$: 94%
EXAM	The patient appears ill. Lung sounds reveal bibasilar crackles. Extremities are cool and distal pulses are weak bilaterally.

CLINICAL CHALLENGES AND QUESTIONS

1. What does this 12-lead ECG show?

2. How would you treat this patient?

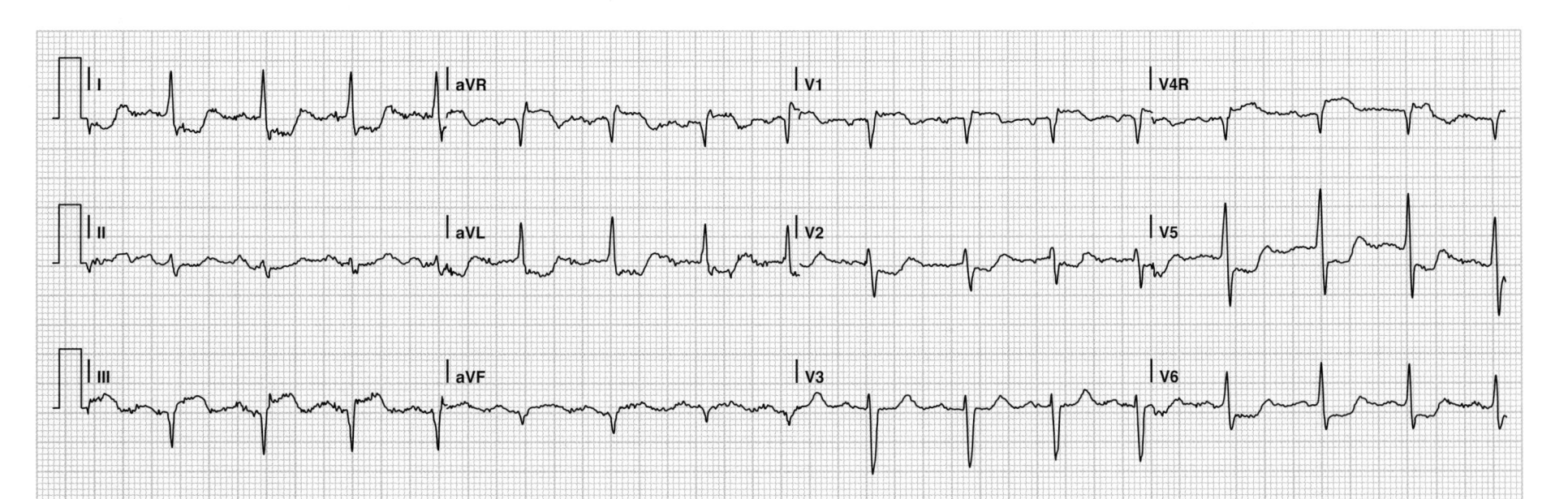

CHIEF COMPLAINT: Myocardial infarction

HISTORY OF PRESENT ILLNESS	You are transporting a 58-year-old male patient from the local community hospital for an emergent cardiac catheterization. The patient presented to the local hospital approximately 1 hour ago. He experienced chest pain, nausea and diaphoresis. His pain has been increasing and has required upward titration of a nitroglycerin (NTG) infusion. He still reports crushing, left-sided chest discomfort, which he describes as 10 on a 10-point scale.
PAST MEDICAL HISTORY	Hypertension, hyperlipidemia
MEDICATIONS	NTG infusion, 20 mcg/min/IV; heparin, 1200 units/hour/IV; aspirin; metoprolol; lisinopril; atorvastatin
ALLERGIES	None
VITAL SIGNS	BP: 150/100 mm Hg, P: 100 beats/min., R: 22 breaths/ min., SpO$_2$: 94% on nasal cannula
EXAM	The patient is an awake and alert elderly male. Lung sounds reveal crackles bilaterally. The abdomen is soft and nontender to palpation. There is no lower extremity edema. Pulses are strong and equal.

CLINICAL CHALLENGES AND QUESTIONS

1. What does this 12-lead ECG show?

2. How would you treat this patient?

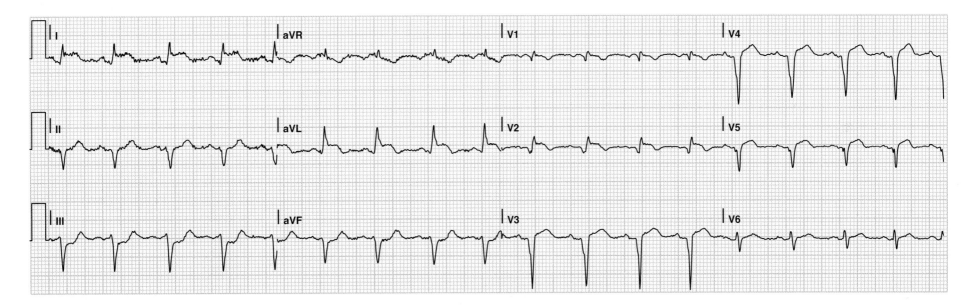

CASE 28   **CHIEF COMPLAINT:** Weakness, dyspnea

HISTORY OF PRESENT ILLNESS	You are triaging an 86-year-old female who reports several "fainting spells." She came to the emergency department today due to fatigue and mild shortness of breath. She states that she fainted after doing chores around the house. She denies chest pain, nausea, or vomiting.
PAST MEDICAL HISTORY	Urinary tract infections, osteoarthritis
MEDICATIONS	Ibuprofen
ALLERGIES	None
VITAL SIGNS	BP: 112/68mm Hg, P: 80 beats/min., R: 18 breaths/min., SpO$_2$: 98%
EXAM	The patient is a morbidly obese, elderly female. Lung sounds are clear bilaterally. The abdomen is soft and distended. Strong distal pulses are noted bilaterally.

CLINICAL CHALLENGES AND QUESTIONS

1. What does this 12-lead ECG show?

2. How would you treat this patient?

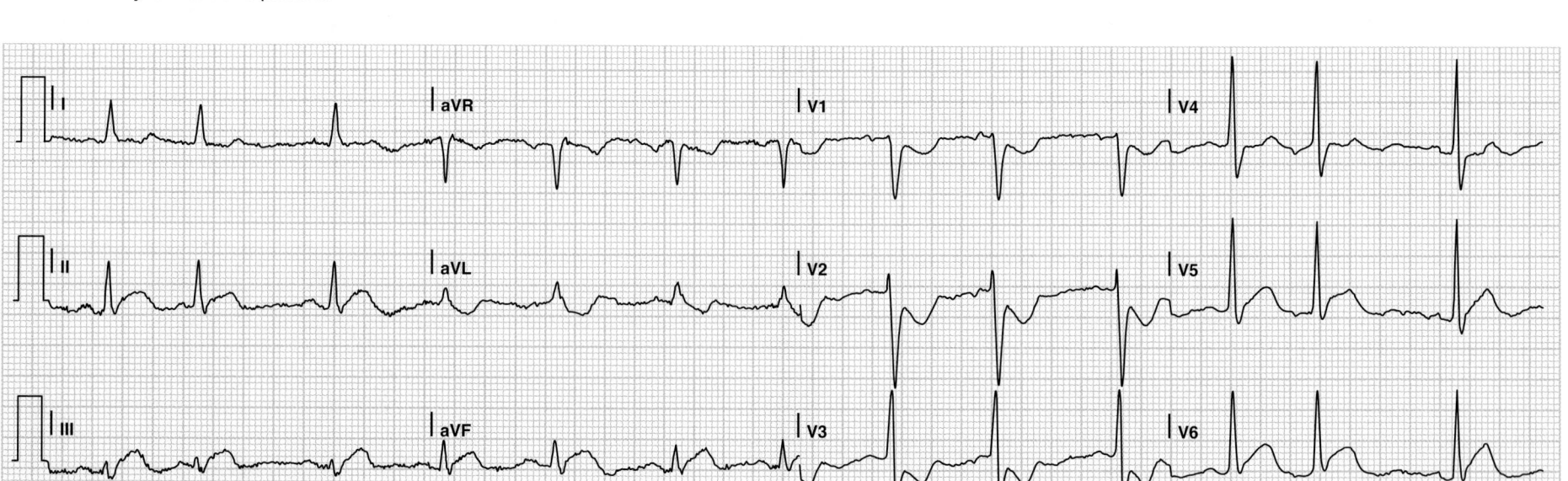

CHIEF COMPLAINT: Shortness of breath

HISTORY OF PRESENT ILLNESS	Advanced providers arrive on the scene of an 81-year-old male who became short of breath while watching television.
PAST MEDICAL HISTORY	Chronic obstructive pulmonary disease
MEDICATIONS	Albuterol, ipratropium, fluticasone
ALLERGIES	None
VITAL SIGNS	BP: 128/82 mm Hg, P: 130 beats/min., R: 28 breaths/min., SpO$_2$: 94%
EXAM	The patient is a pleasant, well-nourished male. Heart sounds are normal. Occasional bilateral wheezing is heard on auscultation. No pedal edema is noted in the lower extremities. Radial pulses are strong and equal at the radial arteries.

CLINICAL CHALLENGES AND QUESTIONS

1. What does this 12-lead ECG show?

2. How would you treat this patient?

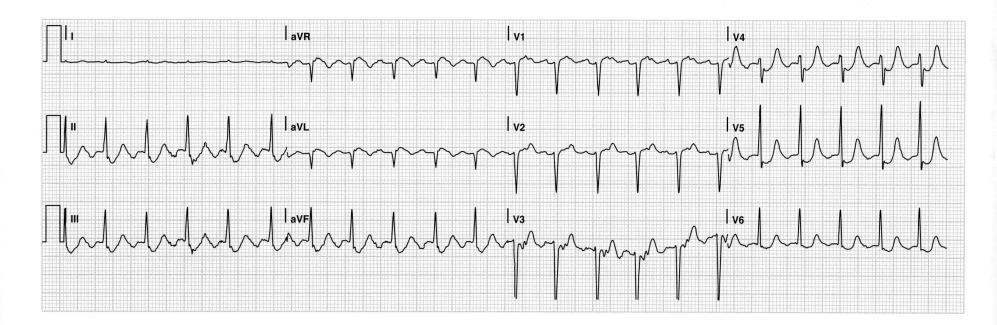

CASE 30

CHIEF COMPLAINT: Syncope

HISTORY OF PRESENT ILLNESS	The patient is a 57-year-old male who reports an acute onset of crushing, substernal chest pressure. He rates the pressure as a 10 on a 10-point scale. He also reports feeling nauseous.
PAST MEDICAL HISTORY	Hypertension, diabetes
MEDICATIONS	Metformin, atenolol, daily aspirin
ALLERGIES	None
VITAL SIGNS	BP: 132/64 mm Hg, P: 70 beats/min., R: 18 breaths/min., SpO$_2$: 96%
EXAM	Anxious, well-developed 57-year-old male. Lung sounds are clear bilaterally. The abdomen is soft. There is no edema in the lower extremities. Skin is clammy and cool.

CLINICAL CHALLENGES AND QUESTIONS

1. What does this 12-lead ECG show?

2. How would you treat this patient?

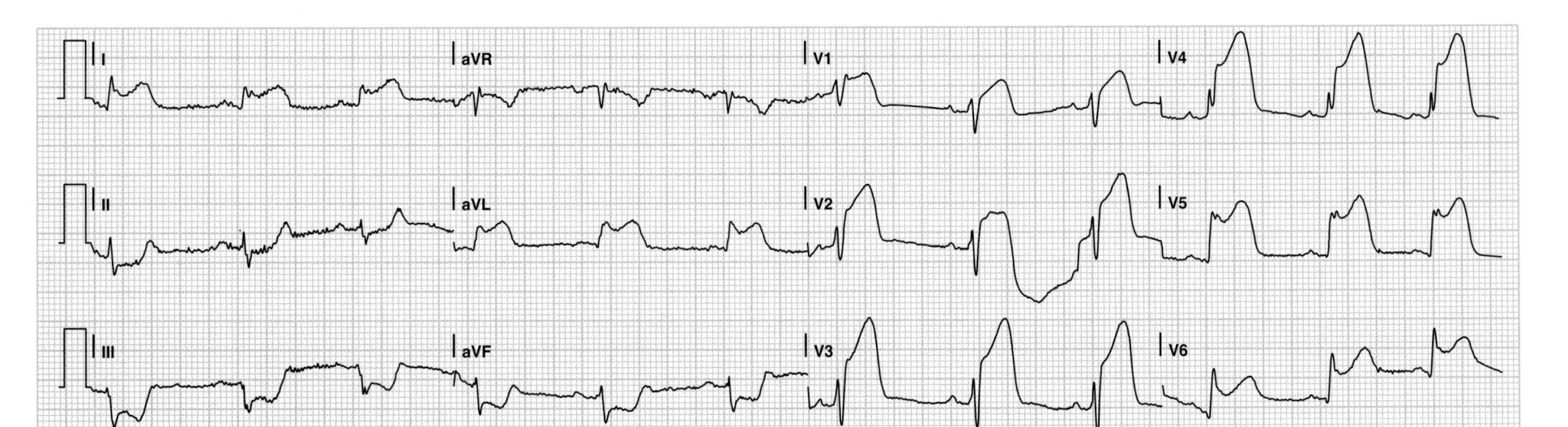

CHIEF COMPLAINT: Syncope

HISTORY OF PRESENT ILLNESS	Advanced providers respond to a call regarding a 45-year-old man who passed out while giving blood. Just before the event, the patient said he felt dizzy. The patient denies chest pain, shortness of breath, or dizziness.
PAST MEDICAL HISTORY	Hypertension
MEDICATIONS	Atenolol, lisinopril
ALLERGIES	Penicillin
VITAL SIGNS	BP: 160/90 mm Hg, R: 70 beats/min., R: 16 breaths/min., SpO$_2$: 99%
EXAM	The patient is an athletic male who is in no obvious distress. Heart sounds are normal. Lungs are clear to auscultation. The abdomen is soft, nontender, and nondistended. Extremities are warm and without edema. Pulses are symmetric and strong. Skin is cool and clammy.

CLINICAL CHALLENGES AND QUESTIONS

1. What does this 12-lead ECG show?

2. How would you treat this patient?

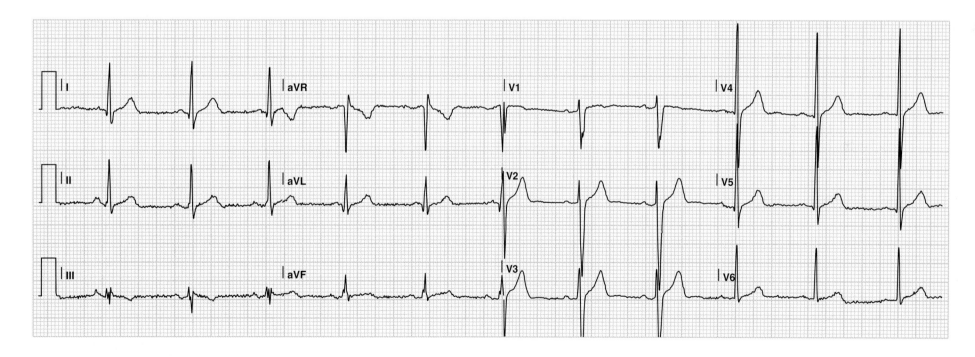

CASE 32   CHIEF COMPLAINT: Shortness of breath

HISTORY OF PRESENT ILLNESS	You respond to a call regarding a 67-year-old woman who reports shortness of breath. The condition started suddenly, while she was at rest, and is accompanied by diaphoresis. She reports associated nausea.
PAST MEDICAL HISTORY	Hypertension, hypercholesterolemia, diabetes mellitus
MEDICATIONS	Daily aspirin, amlodipine, metoprolol, atorvastatin, insulin
ALLERGIES	None
VITAL SIGNS	BP: 162/86mm Hg, P: 90 beats/min., R: 26 breaths/min., SpO$_2$: 97%
EXAM	The patient is an elderly female in respiratory distress. She is anxious but awake, alert, and oriented. Heart sounds are normal; lung sounds are clear to auscultation. The abdomen is soft and nontender to palpation. Extremity exam reveals trace edema bilaterally. Radial pulses are strong and symmetric. Skin is diaphoretic.

CLINICAL CHALLENGES AND QUESTIONS

1. What does this 12-lead ECG show?
2. How would you treat this patient?

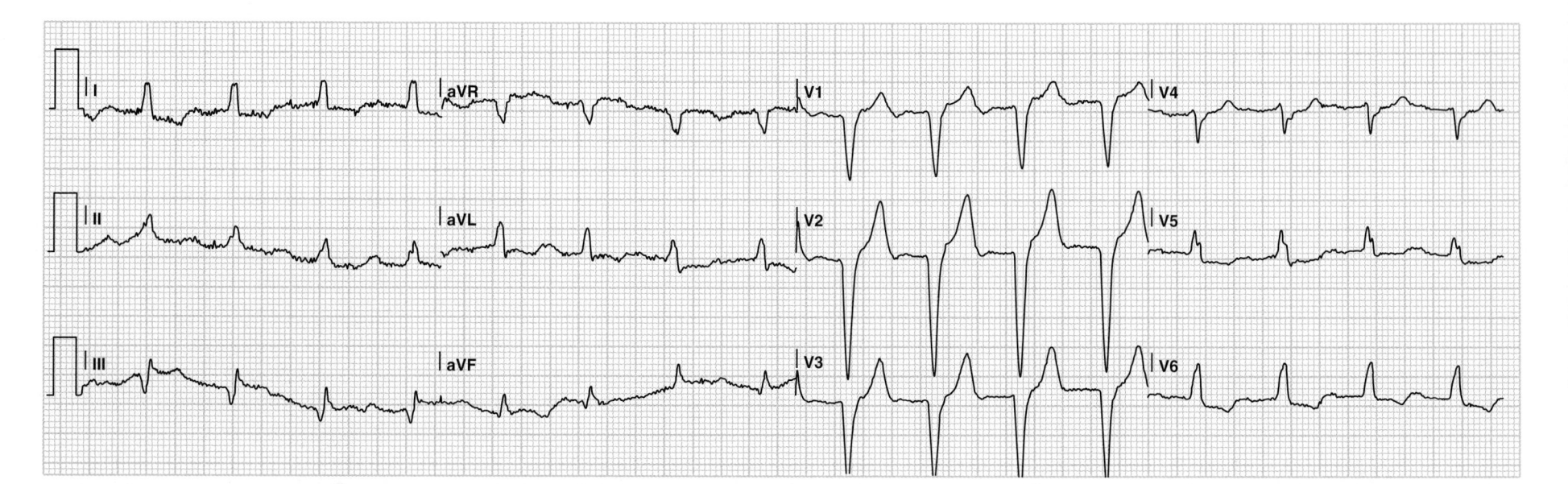

CHIEF COMPLAINT: Syncope

HISTORY OF PRESENT ILLNESS	You respond to a report of a 72-year-old man with syncope. The patient described feeling weak and slightly short of breath, and then waking up on the floor. The duration of his loss of consciousness is unknown. The patient currently feels left-sided chest pressure, with an intensity of 6 on a 10-point scale, and is still short of breath. He has had dyspnea on exertion and malaise for the past 2 weeks.
PAST MEDICAL HISTORY	Diabetes, hypertension
ALLERGIES	None
MEDICATIONS	Metformin, glipizide, sliding-scale insulin, aspirin, metoprolol
VITAL SIGNS	BP: 154/90 mm Hg, P: 62 beats/min., R: 18 breaths/min., SpO$_2$: 99%, fingerstick glucose reading: 126 mg/dL
EXAM	Well-developed, well-nourished elderly male who is awake and alert. The patient appears to be in mild distress. Heart sounds are normal. Lung sounds are clear with symmetric chest rise and fall. Abdomen is nontender and without masses or pulsations. Extremities show 1+ symmetric pitting edema without cyanosis or clubbing. Pulses are strong and equal bilaterally.

CLINICAL CHALLENGES AND QUESTIONS

1. What does this 12-lead ECG show?

2. How would you treat this patient?

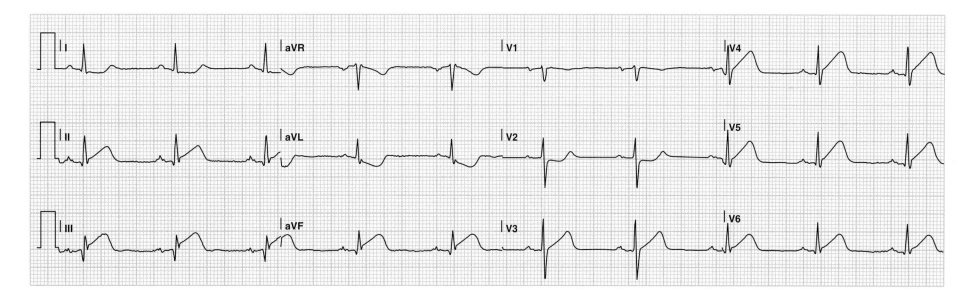

CASE 34   **CHIEF COMPLAINT:** Vomiting

HISTORY OF PRESENT ILLNESS	Advanced providers respond to a report of a 50-year-old man at a local stadium's first aid station. The patient went to the first aid station after vomiting three or four times. He had been drinking at the game and asked aid station personnel for some antacids. He now has epigastric burning, nausea, and vomiting. He admits that he is sweating but remarks that "it has been fairly warm outside." He denies syncope, chest pain, back pain, or fever. His symptoms started approximately 1 hour ago.
PAST MEDICAL HISTORY	Hypertension, anxiety, gastritis
MEDICATIONS	Omeprazole, calcium carbonate, ranitidine as needed
ALLERGIES	None
VITAL SIGNS	BP: 160/90 mm Hg, P: 90 beats/min., R: 20 breaths/min., SpO$_2$: 99%
EXAM	Obese 50-year-old male, slightly diaphoretic. Patient is alert and oriented. Heart sounds are regular. Lung sounds are clear to auscultation bilaterally. Abdomen is soft, and the patient has mild tenderness to deep palpation at the epigastrium. Extremities are without edema or cyanosis. Strong radial pulses are present bilaterally. Skin is warm and wet.

CLINICAL CHALLENGES AND QUESTIONS

1. What does this 12-lead ECG show?

2. How would you treat this patient?

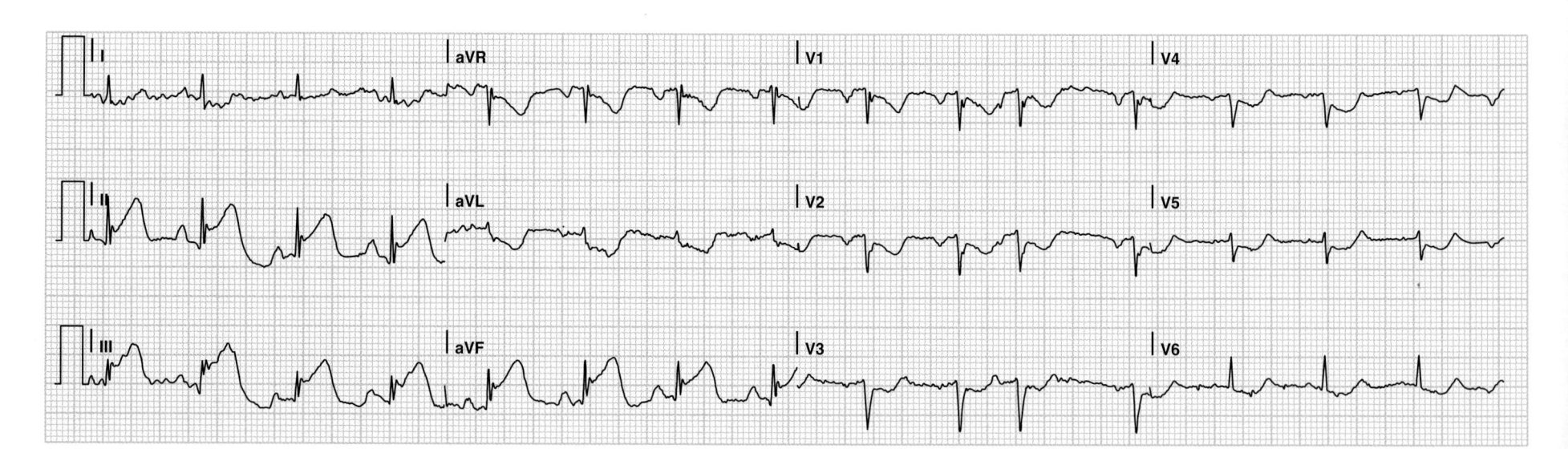

CHIEF COMPLAINT: Unconsciousness

HISTORY OF PRESENT ILLNESS	You arrive on the scene where a 30-year-old man is unconscious. The patient's girlfriend informs you that she called 9-1-1 because "he won't wake up." The patient recently recovered from a mild case of "flu" and has been adjusting his dose of insulin because of elevated blood glucose levels. Further history is unobtainable given the patient's level of consciousness. The blood glucose measurement reads "high" on the glucometer.
PAST MEDICAL HISTORY	Insulin-dependent diabetes
MEDICATIONS	Insulin
ALLERGIES	None
VITAL SIGNS	BP: 90/70 mm Hg, P: 90–100 beats/min., R: 42 breaths/min., SpO$_2$: 97%
EXAM	The patient is a well-developed, muscular adult male who is unconscious. He withdraws from painful stimuli. Heart sounds are normal but irregular. Lungs are clear to auscultation bilaterally. The abdomen is soft and nondistended. Extremities are warm to touch and without edema. Strong radial pulses are present in the upper extremities. Skin is dry.

CLINICAL CHALLENGES AND QUESTIONS

1. What does this 12-lead ECG show?
2. How would you treat this patient?

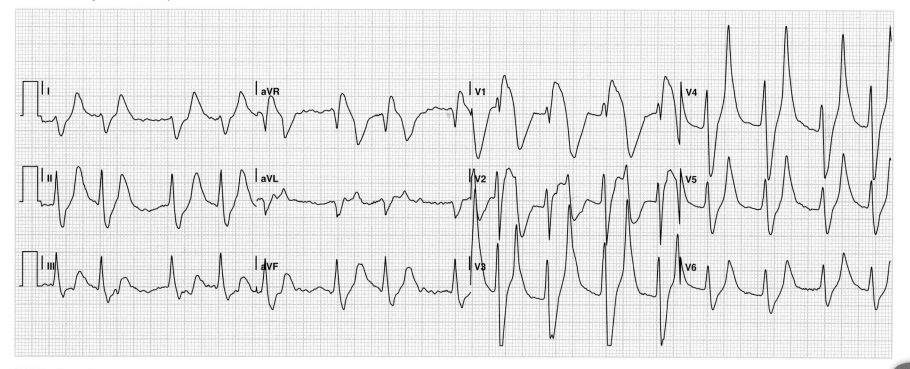

CASE 36   CHIEF COMPLAINT: STEMI

HISTORY OF PRESENT ILLNESS	You are transporting a 72-year-old man from a community hospital to a tertiary care facility for cardiac catheterization and balloon pump insertion. You initiated a dopamine drip before departure. The patient remains hypotensive despite intravenous saline boluses. A nitroglycerin (NTG) infusion was discontinued because of hypotension, and the patient is currently receiving heparin. You administer a third of a liter of normal saline and obtain a right-sided 12-lead ECG. Hypotension persists after the fluid bolus.
PAST MEDICAL HISTORY	Hypertension, coronary artery disease
MEDICATIONS	Intravenous NTG, 10 mcg/min (discontinued); intravenous heparin, 1000 units/hr; intravenous dopamine, 10 mcg/kg/min; aspirin; clopidogrel
ALLERGIES	Penicillin
VITAL SIGNS	BP: 70 by palpitation, P: 56 beats/min., R: 12 breaths/min.
EXAM	Patient appears ill and pale. He is conscious and answers questions appropriately. Heart sounds are normal. Lung sounds include bibasilar crackles. Extremities are cool and there is no edema. Radial pulses are weak and symmetric bilaterally. The skin is diaphoretic.

CLINICAL CHALLENGES AND QUESTIONS

1. What does this 12-lead ECG show?

2. How would you treat this patient?

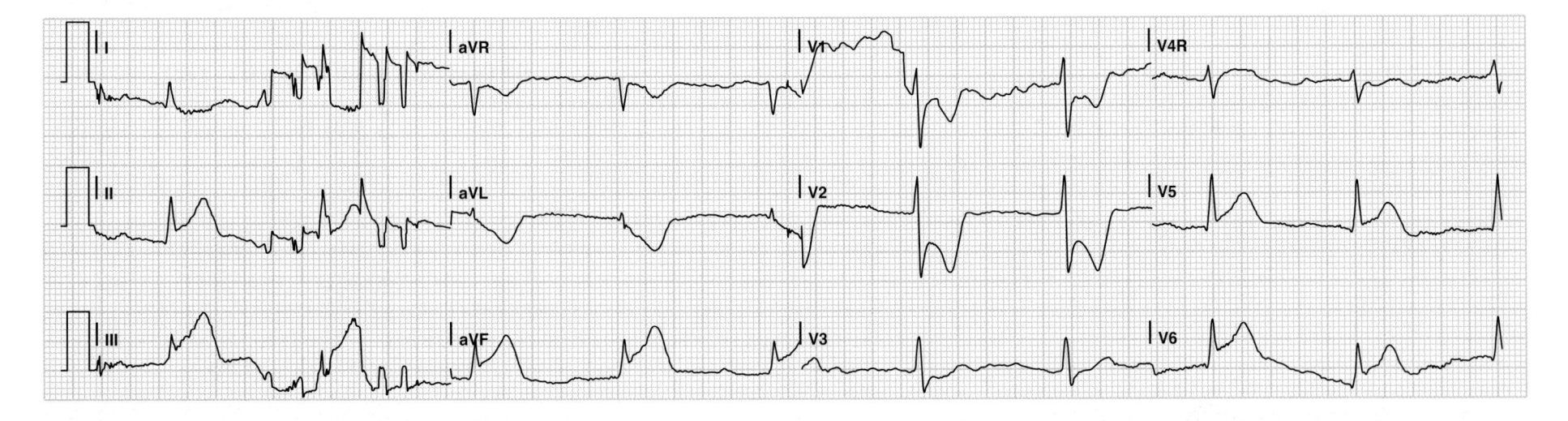

Note: V$_4$ is placed on the right chest (V$_4$R).

HISTORY OF PRESENT ILLNESS	Advanced providers respond to a report of an 80-year-old man in respiratory distress at a local long-term care facility. The nursing staff reports that the patient had been well until 2 days ago, when he experienced coughing, restlessness, and shortness of breath. He had been treated effectively with an albuterol inhaler and an increased dose of furosemide. Today, the patient is much more uncomfortable and cannot be calmed down. He is confused and cannot offer additional history.
PAST MEDICAL HISTORY	Full code, congestive heart failure, myocardial infarction, hypertension, diabetes mellitus, coronary artery disease
MEDICATIONS	No list available
ALLERGIES	Unknown
VITAL SIGNS	BP: 200/110 mm Hg, P: 101 beats/min., R: 24 breaths/min., SpO_2: 88%
EXAM	Patient is an elderly male who appears ill and is in obvious respiratory distress. The patient is confused but cooperative. Heart sounds are normal. Lung exam reveals coarse crackles in all fields. Intercostal and abdominal accessory muscle use is present. The abdomen is soft and without any palpable masses. 2+ pitting edema are present in the lower extremities. Skin is warm and dry.

CLINICAL CHALLENGES AND QUESTIONS

1. What does this 12-lead ECG show?

2. How would you treat this patient?

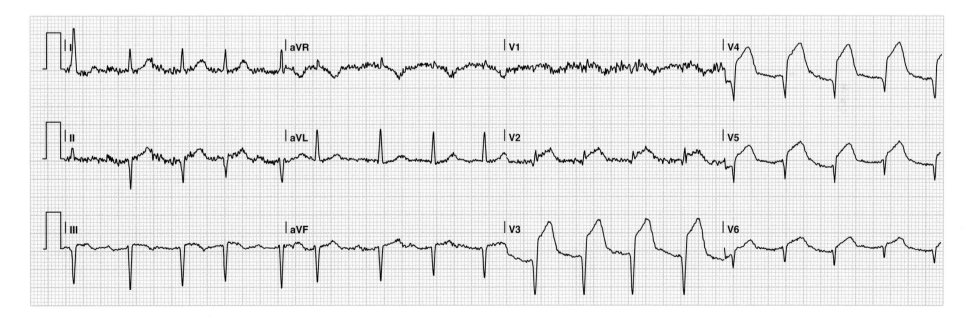

CASE 38

CHIEF COMPLAINT: Postoperative pain

HISTORY OF PRESENT ILLNESS	You are transferring a 72-year-old woman from a hospital to a rehabilitation facility about 1 hour away. The patient is on a morphine pump for postoperative pain management. She is without acute complaint and is resting comfortably. A routine ECG is obtained before the extended interfacility transport.
PAST MEDICAL HISTORY	Osteoporosis, fractured hip, complete right hip replacement
MEDICATIONS	Enoxaparin, morphine
ALLERGIES	None
VITAL SIGNS	BP: 128/64 mm Hg; P: 60 beats/min.; R: 12 breaths/min.; SpO$_2$: 99% on oxygen, 2 liters/min
EXAM	The patient is an elderly female who appears to be resting comfortably on the transport stretcher. She is awake, alert, and oriented. Heart sounds are normal. Lung sounds are clear to auscultation bilaterally. The abdomen is soft, nontender, and nondistended. There are 2+ nonpitting edema bilaterally. Pedal pulses are 1+. Skin is warm and dry.

CLINICAL CHALLENGES AND QUESTIONS

1. What does this 12-lead ECG show?

2. How would you treat this patient?

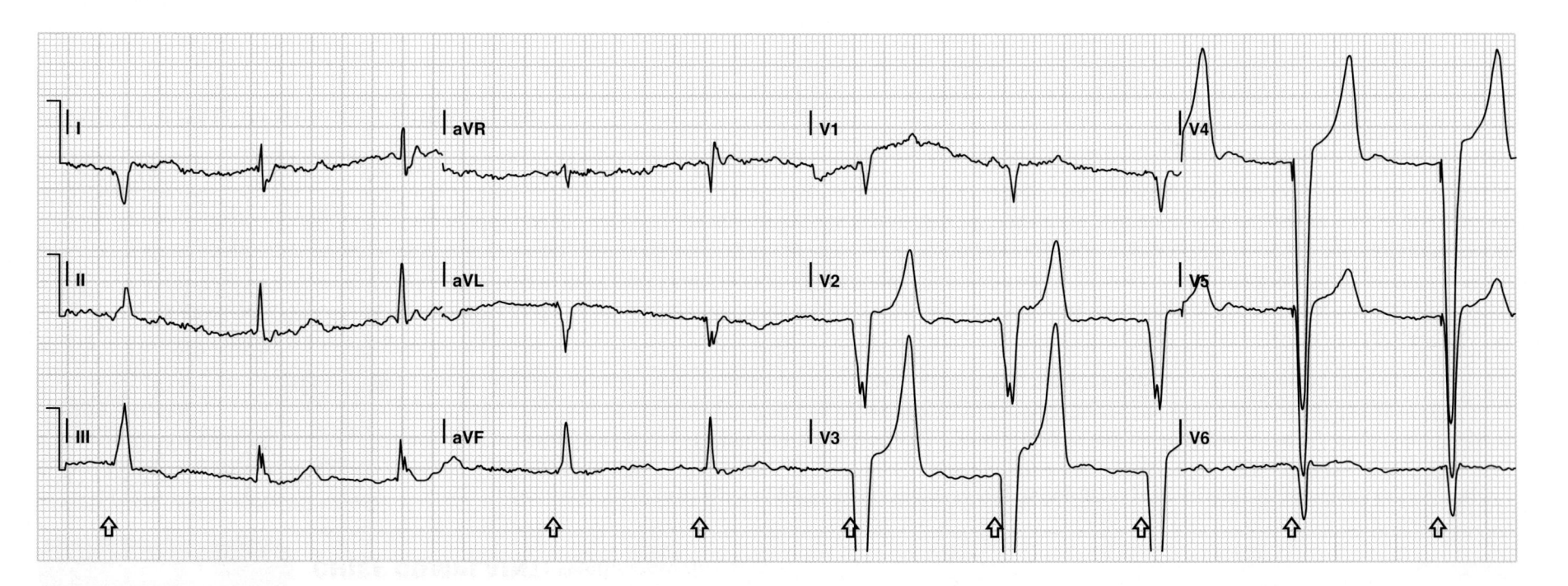

CHIEF COMPLAINT: Weakness

HISTORY OF PRESENT ILLNESS	You are triaging a 75-year-old female who presents for weakness and fatigue, which she has had for several days. The patient thinks she is recovering from a viral illness. She states that she has been coughing. The cough has been worse at night and occasionally prevents her from sleeping. She reports mild shortness of breath today but denies nausea, vomiting, or sweating.
PAST MEDICAL HISTORY	Arthritis
MEDICATIONS	Naproxen
ALLERGIES	None
VITAL SIGNS	BP: 110/64 mm Hg, P: 90 beats/min., R: 18 breaths/min., SpO$_2$: 95%
EXAM	Patient is an obese 75-year-old female. She is awake, alert, and oriented. Lung exam reveals crackles at the bases. Strong radial pulses and good capillary refill are present.

CLINICAL CHALLENGES AND QUESTIONS

1. What does this 12-lead ECG show?

2. How would you treat this patient?

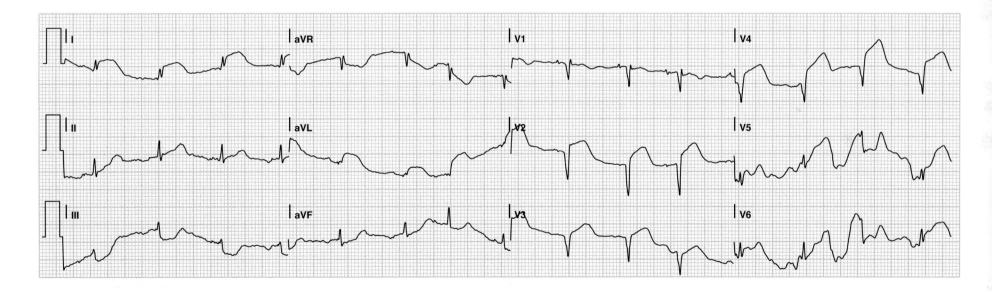

CASE 40   **CHIEF COMPLAINT:** Unresponsiveness

HISTORY OF PRESENT ILLNESS	You respond to a nursing home, where a 92-year-old female has been found unresponsive on the floor. She was at the facility for long-term cardiac rehabilitation. According to the staff, the patient was found unconscious and apneic at shift change. She has a history of falling and loss of consciousness. Cardiopulmonary resuscitation was performed for 10 minutes. One shock from an automatic external defibrillator was administered. The patient's pulse was restored 5 minutes before your arrival. She had been suffering from "cold-type" symptoms for the last 2 days. The patient remains unresponsive. No "do not resuscitate" or advance directive is on file.
PAST MEDICAL HISTORY	Unobtainable
MEDICATIONS	Unobtainable
ALLERGIES	Unobtainable
VITAL SIGNS	BP: 70 mm Hg (by palpation); P: faint carotid pulse is palpable; R: 20 breaths/min., assisted with bag-valve-mask ventilation
EXAM	Unconscious, unresponsive elderly woman. Pupils are 3 mm and sluggish bilaterally, and periorbital ecchymosis is present above the right eye. Heart sounds are diminished. Lung sounds are coarse but equal bilaterally with bag-valve-mask ventilation. Abdomen is soft and nontender. Extremities are without cyanosis or edema. Radial pulses are not palpable. Skin is cool.

CLINICAL CHALLENGES AND QUESTIONS

1. What does this 12-lead ECG show?

2. How would you treat this patient?

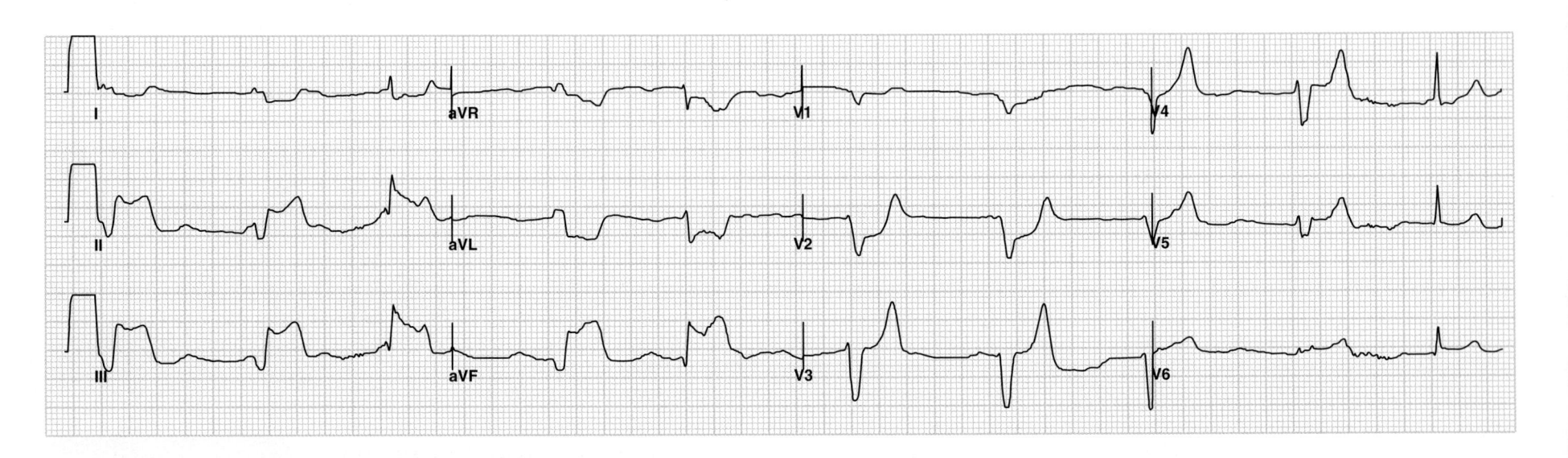

CHIEF COMPLAINT: Chest pain

HISTORY OF PRESENT ILLNESS	Advanced providers respond to a report of a 52-year-old man experiencing mid-sternal chest pain. The pain is a 10 on a 10-point scale and radiates to his left arm. The patient reports diaphoresis but no nausea, vomiting, or loss of consciousness. The pain began during minimal exertion. Pain has been ongoing and constant for approximately 1 hour. The patient denies any previous symptoms or poor health until the onset of the pain.
PAST MEDICAL HISTORY	None
MEDICATIONS	Occasional use of ibuprofen
ALLERGIES	None
VITAL SIGNS	BP: 132/70 mm Hg, P: 62 beats/min., R: 16 breaths/min., SpO$_2$: 99%
EXAM	Patient is well developed and well nourished. He seems to be in mild distress but is awake, alert, and oriented. Heart sounds are normal. Lung sounds are clear. Abdomen is soft and nontender. Extremities are without cyanosis or edema. Strong pulses are present bilaterally. Skin is warm and dry.

CLINICAL CHALLENGES AND QUESTIONS

1. What does this 12-lead ECG show?
2. How would you treat this patient?

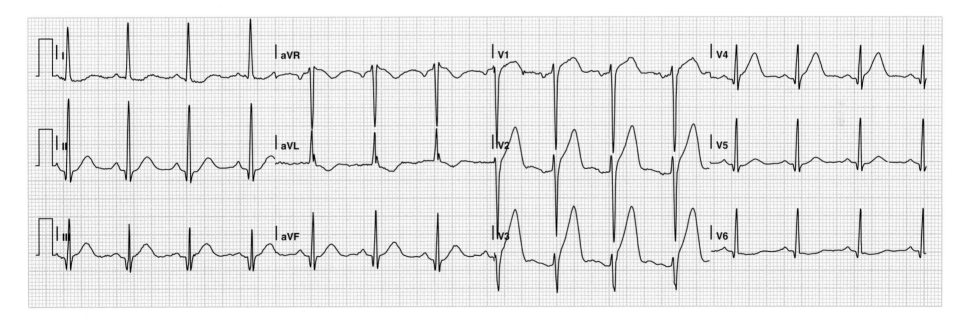

CASE 42   CHIEF COMPLAINT: Syncope

HISTORY OF PRESENT ILLNESS	You and your partner respond to a call from a 34-year-old male who experienced an episode of syncope while shopping. He has no complaints and states, "I am fine. Sorry for bothering you guys." The patient denies nausea, vomiting, diaphoresis, or chest pain.
PAST MEDICAL HISTORY	None
MEDICATIONS	None
ALLERGIES	None
VITAL SIGNS	BP: 118/62 mm Hg, P: 80 beats/min., R: 18 breaths/min., SpO$_2$: 99%
EXAM	Well-developed, muscular man in no obvious distress. The patient is alert and oriented. Heart sounds are normal. Lungs are clear. Abdomen is soft and nontender to palpation. Extremities are without edema. The radial pulses are equal and strong. Skin is warm and dry.

CLINICAL CHALLENGES AND QUESTIONS

1. What does this 12-lead ECG show?

2. How would you treat this patient?

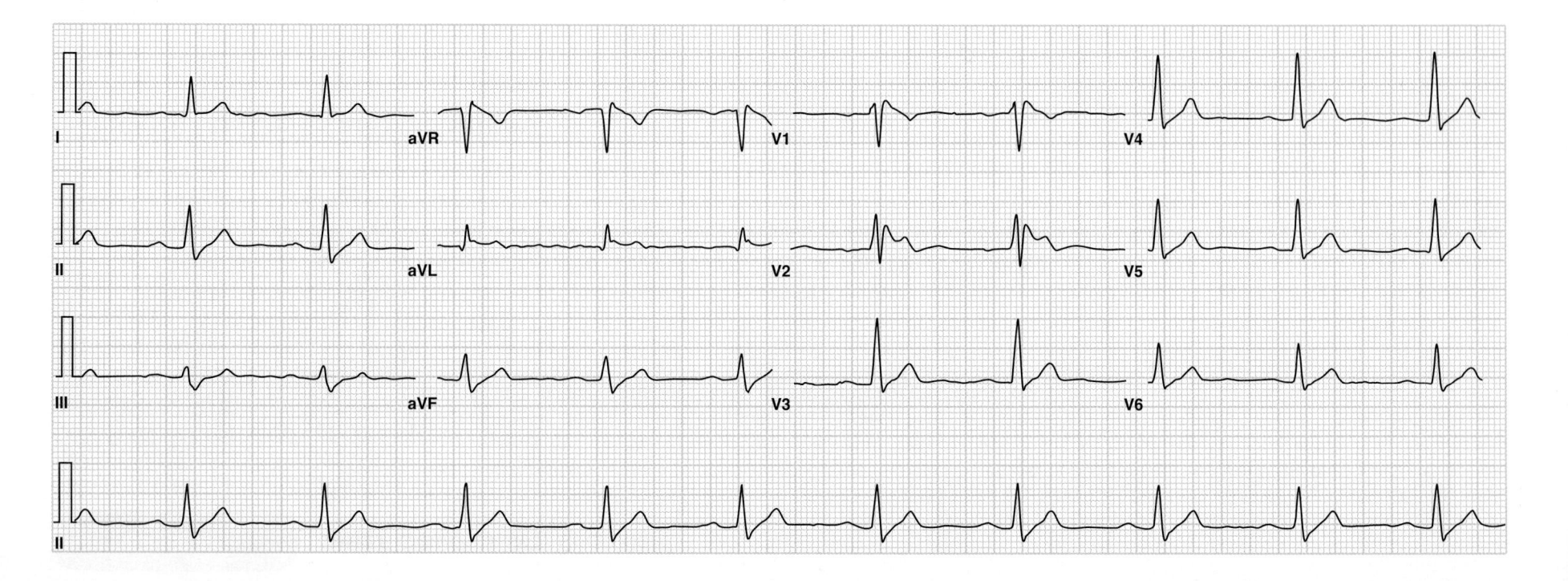

HISTORY OF PRESENT ILLNESS	The patient is a 57-year-old male who experienced a syncopal episode. He recalls feeling dizzy and weak after returning home from his daily walk. The patient lost consciousness and awoke to find himself on the kitchen floor. He reports a "weird feeling" in his chest.
PAST MEDICAL HISTORY	Hypertension, diabetes
MEDICATIONS	Metformin, lisinopril, daily aspirin
ALLERGIES	None
VITAL SIGNS	BP: 110/70 mm Hg; P: 100 beats/min.; R: 18 breaths/min., nonlabored; SpO$_2$: 96%
EXAM	The patient is alert and oriented. Heart sounds are normal. Lung sounds are clear bilaterally. The patient's abdomen is distended. Extremities are cool. Radial pulses are strong bilaterally.

CLINICAL CHALLENGES AND QUESTIONS

1. What does this 12-lead ECG show?

2. How would you treat this patient?

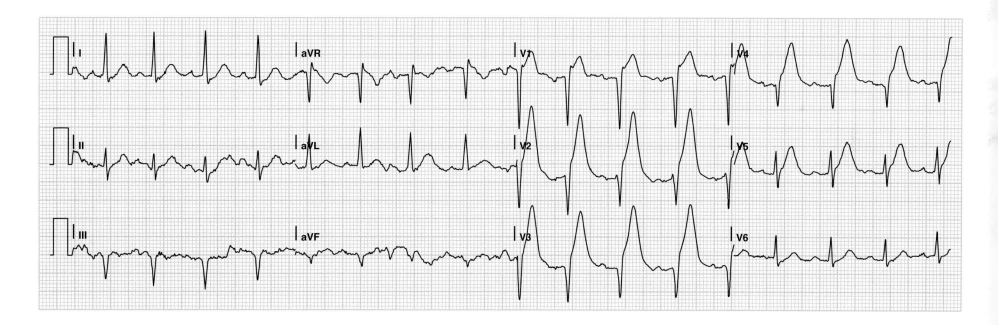

CASE 44   **CHIEF COMPLAINT:** Altered mental status

HISTORY OF PRESENT ILLNESS	Advanced providers arrive on scene of a 14-year-old male reporting extreme fatigue.
PAST MEDICAL HISTORY	No significant history of medical illness. No history of recent falls, head injury, or drug or alcohol use. The patient was bitten by a tick 1 month ago.
MEDICATIONS	None
ALLERGIES	None
VITAL SIGNS	BP: 108/56 mm Hg, P: 30s, R: 18 breaths/min., SpO$_2$: 99%, blood glucose: 94 mg/dL
EXAM	The patient is prone on the couch. He responds to loud verbal stimuli and answers questions appropriately. Heart sounds are bradycardic but otherwise normal. Lung sounds are clear to auscultation. The abdomen is soft and nontender. There are no ecchymoses or contusions on the skin. No pedal edema is present. Pulses are strong and regular at the radial arteries.

CLINICAL CHALLENGES AND QUESTIONS

1. What does this rhythm strip show?

2. How would you treat this patient?

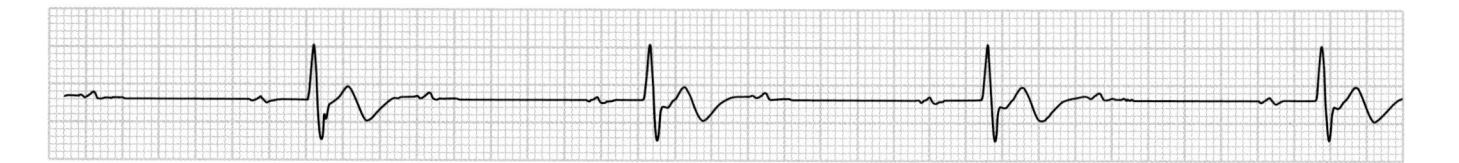

CHIEF COMPLAINT: Weakness

HISTORY OF PRESENT ILLNESS	You respond to the home of an 84-year-old female who is experiencing fatigue and weakness. The patient states that her symptoms have been ongoing for a few days. She has had mild nausea but has not vomited. The patient reports a lack of appetite and grew concerned when she became tired while performing routine activities. She does not have chest pain or shortness of breath, and she denies recent illness, fever, or chills.
PAST MEDICAL HISTORY	Diabetes mellitus, hypercholesterolemia, hypertension, arthritis
MEDICATIONS	Aspirin, propranolol, metformin, ibuprofen, acetaminophen, lisinopril
ALLERGIES	None
VITAL SIGNS	BP: 120/70 mm Hg, P: 82 beats/min., R: 18 breaths/min., SpO$_2$: 95%
EXAM	An elderly female is seated in her living room chair. She is awake and alert. Heart sounds are present. Lung sounds reveal crackles at both bases. Abdomen is flat, nondistended, and soft. Extremity exam reveals trace pedal edema. Pulses at the radial site are strong bilaterally. Skin is slightly dry.

CLINICAL CHALLENGES AND QUESTIONS

1. What does this 12-lead ECG show?

2. How would you treat this patient?

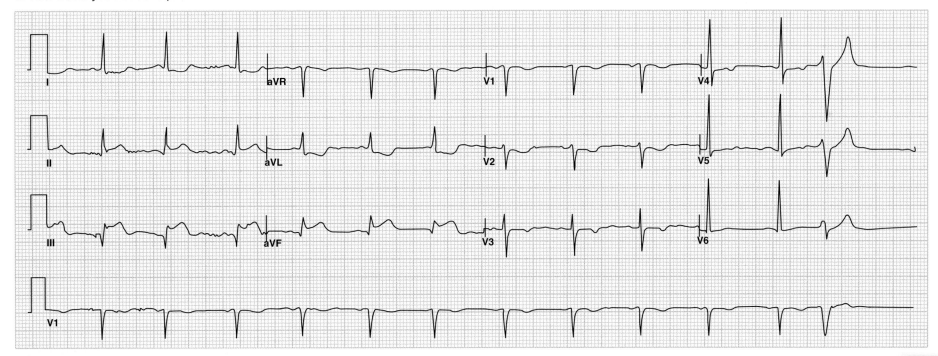

CASE 46

CHIEF COMPLAINT: Disorientation

HISTORY OF PRESENT ILLNESS	Advanced providers respond to a hemodialysis center for an adult male in the waiting area who is disoriented. The patient has a history of renal failure and receives dialysis three times per week. Because of a severe snow storm, he missed two dialysis sessions the previous week.
PAST MEDICAL HISTORY	Renal failure, hypertension
MEDICATIONS	Lisinopril, atenolol, aspirin
ALLERGIES	None
VITAL SIGNS	BP: 148/92 mm Hg, P: 152 beats/min., R: 22 breaths/min., SpO$_2$: 97%
EXAM	The patient is an adult male who is slouched over in a chair. He responds to questions but is disoriented. Heart sounds are normal. His lung sounds are clear but diminished, and his abdomen is firm and nontender. Extremities are warm and well perfused, and pitting edema is present from mid-thigh to the feet. The patient has strong and equal radial pulses.

CLINICAL CHALLENGES AND QUESTIONS

1. What does this 12-lead ECG show?

2. How would you treat this patient?

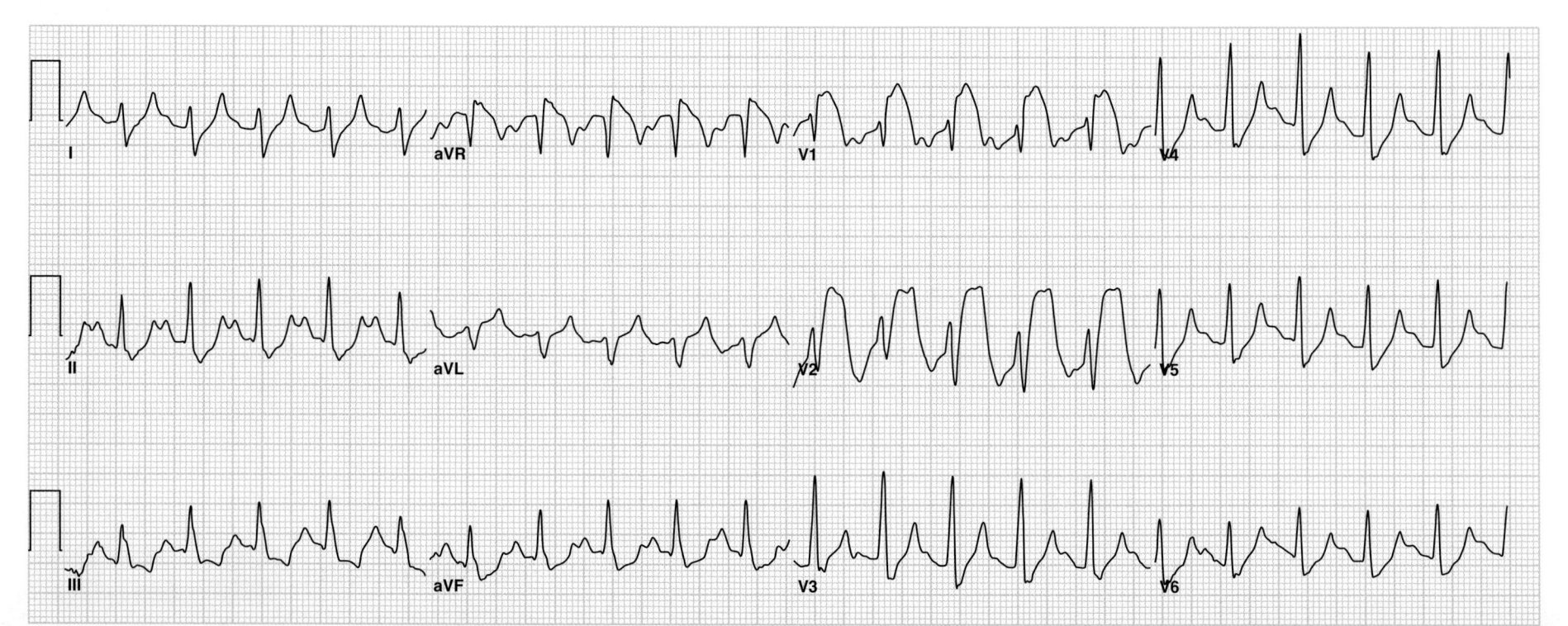

CHIEF COMPLAINT: Stomach burning

HISTORY OF PRESENT ILLNESS	You are dispatched to assist a 39-year-old male who reports "burning in his stomach." It started after exercise, does not radiate, and is constant at a 5 on a 10-point pain scale. He feels nauseated and is short of breath.
PAST MEDICAL HISTORY	Hypertension
MEDICATIONS	Daily aspirin, hydrochlorothiazide
ALLERGIES	None
VITAL SIGNS	BP: 160/70 mm Hg, P: 80 beats/min., R: 16 breaths/min., SpO$_2$: 99%
EXAM	Well-developed, well-nourished male in mild distress. The patient is alert and oriented. Cardiac examination reveals normal heart sounds. Lungs are clear to auscultation. Extremities are warm and well perfused; no edema is noted. Radial pulses are strong and equal bilaterally. Skin is warm and dry.

CLINICAL CHALLENGES AND QUESTIONS

1. What does this 12-lead ECG show?

2. How would you treat this patient?

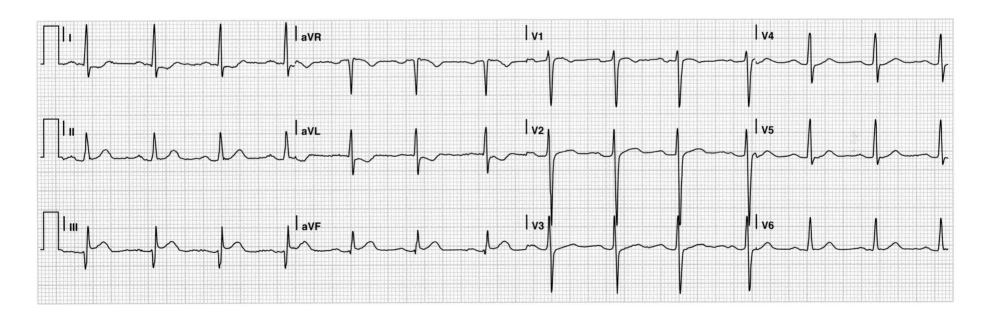

CASE 48   CHIEF COMPLAINT: Sharp chest pain

HISTORY OF PRESENT ILLNESS	You respond to a call regarding a 19-year-old male reporting sharp, stabbing chest pain. It started earlier in the day and does not radiate. The patient rates it as an 8 on a 10-point pain scale but says it decreases to a 3 when he leans forward. He reports having a low-grade fever for the past 3 days.
PAST MEDICAL HISTORY	None
MEDICATIONS	None
ALLERGIES	None
VITAL SIGNS	BP: 100/70 mm Hg, P: 70–80 beats/min., R: 22 breaths/min., SpO$_2$: 97%, T: 100.7°F
EXAM	The patient is an adult male in moderate distress. Heart sounds are normal, and lung sounds are clear. Abdomen is soft, nontender, and nondistended. The patient's extremities are warm and without edema. Radial pulses are 2+ bilaterally. Skin is warm and slightly diaphoretic.

CLINICAL CHALLENGES AND QUESTIONS

1. What does this 12-lead ECG show?
2. How would you treat this patient?

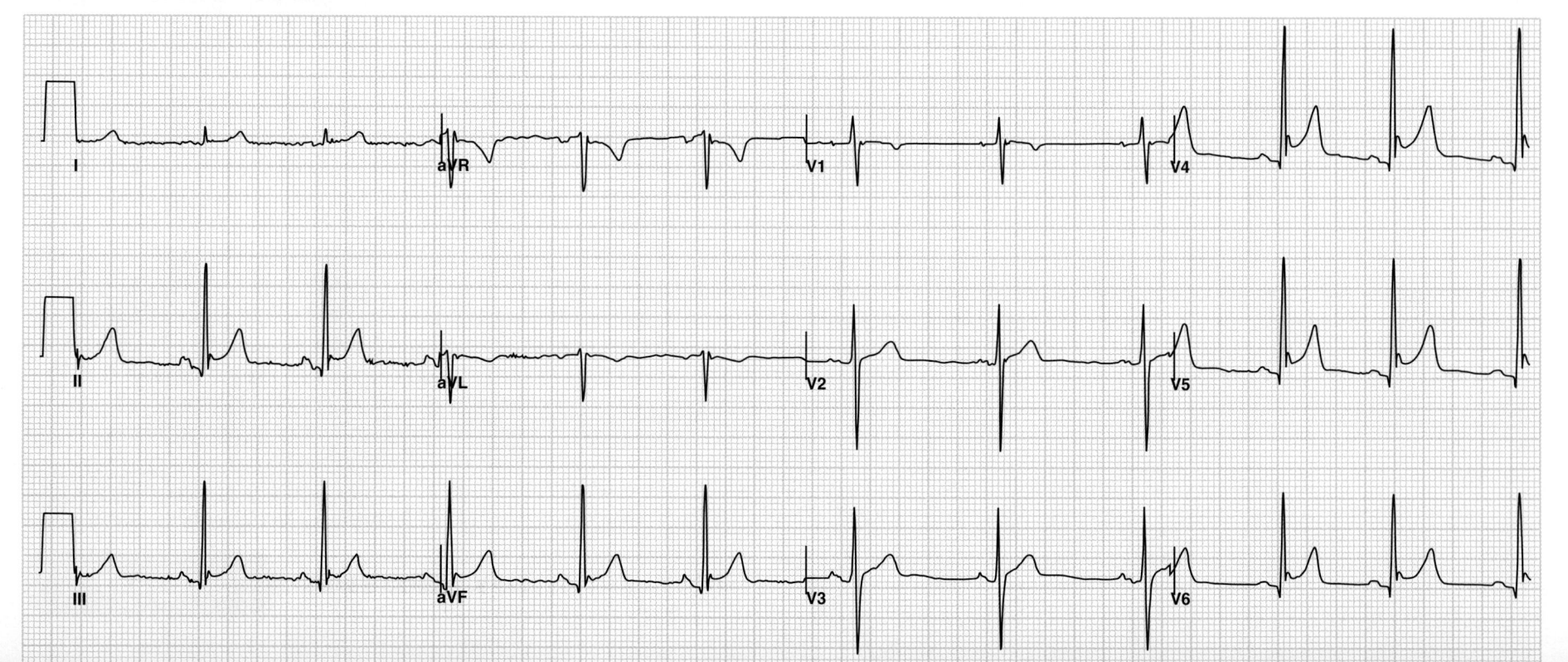

CHIEF COMPLAINT: Unconsciousness

HISTORY OF PRESENT ILLNESS	Advanced providers are dispatched to a local health care provider's office. The patient initially reported weakness and an ECG was obtained by the primary care provider. The patient, a 78-year-old male, lost consciousness before the arrival of emergency medical services personnel.
PAST MEDICAL HISTORY	Hypertension, congestive heart failure, diabetes, dementia, atrial fibrillation
MEDICATIONS	Metoprolol, furosemide, hydrochlorothiazide, amiodarone
ALLERGIES	None
VITAL SIGNS	BP: 0 mm Hg, P: 0 beats/min., R: 0 breaths/min., SpO$_2$: not obtainable
EXAM	The patient has no pulse and is apneic. Heart and lung sounds are absent. Extremities are cool.

CLINICAL CHALLENGES AND QUESTIONS

1. What does this rhythm strip show?

2. How would you treat this patient?

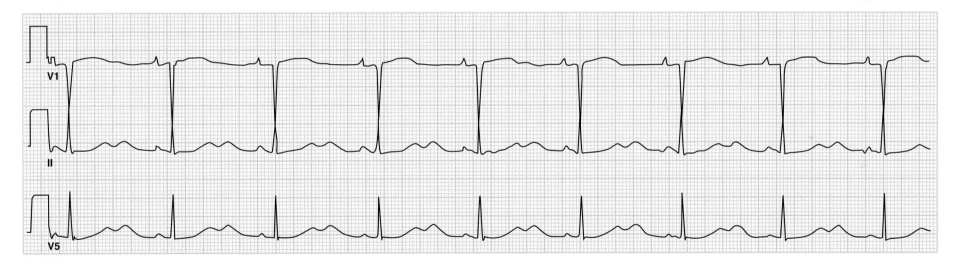

(Continued)

CASE 49   **CHIEF COMPLAINT:** Unconsciousness

Several seconds after displaying the initial rhythm, the patient's rhythm converts to this:

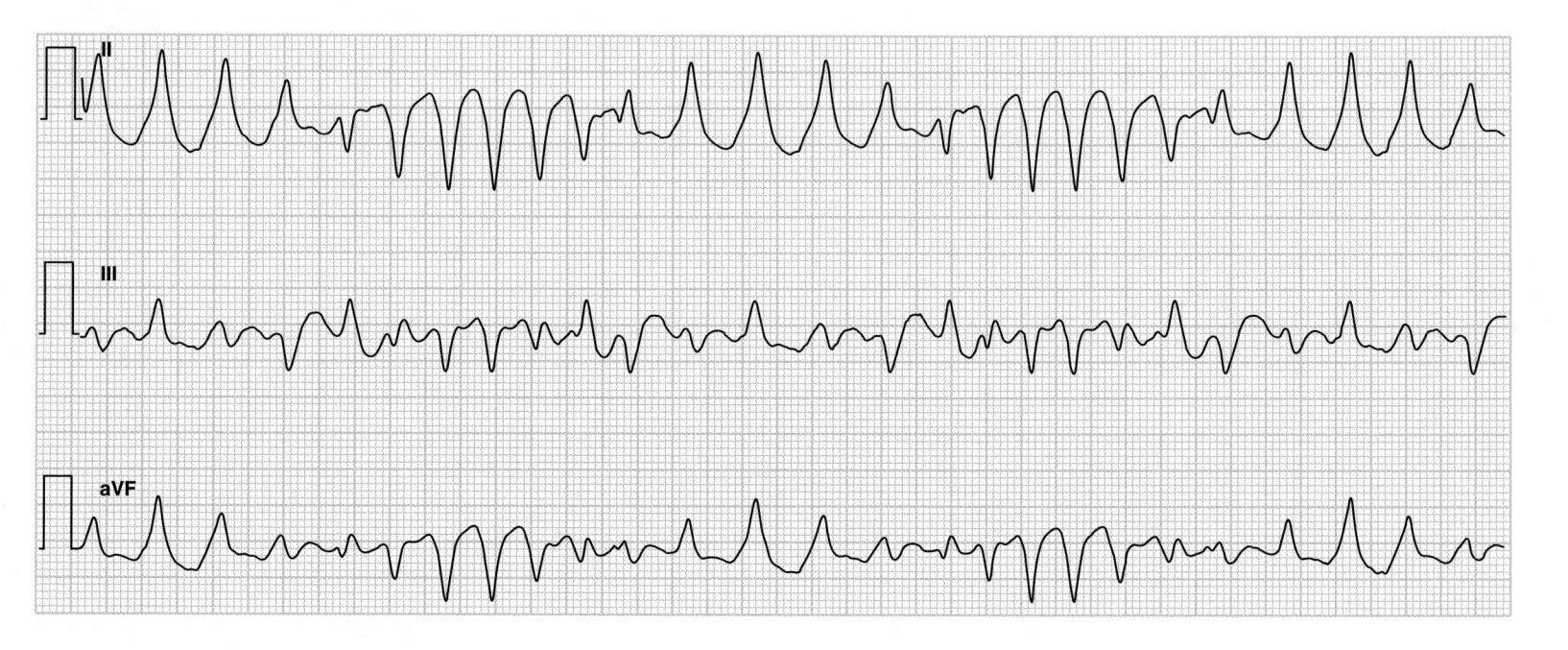

CHIEF COMPLAINT: Weakness

HISTORY OF PRESENT ILLNESS	You are triaging a 70-year-old female who presents with weakness and fatigue that has lasted for several days. The patient thinks she is recovering from a mild cold. She states that she has been coughing. The cough has been worse at night and occasionally prevents her from getting to sleep. She reports mild shortness of breath today but denies nausea, vomiting, sweating, or loss of consciousness.
PAST MEDICAL HISTORY	Diabetes mellitus, hypertension, arthritis
MEDICATIONS	Glipizide, atenolol, amlodipine
ALLERGIES	Sulfa drugs
VITAL SIGNS	BP: 150/90 mm Hg, P: 90 beats/min., R: 18 breaths/min., SpO$_2$: 95%
EXAM	Patient is awake, alert, and oriented. The lung examination reveals crackles at the bases. There is mild bilateral pitting edema. 2+ radial pulses are present. Capillary refill is good.

CLINICAL CHALLENGES AND QUESTIONS

1. What does this 12-lead ECG show?

2. How would you treat this patient?

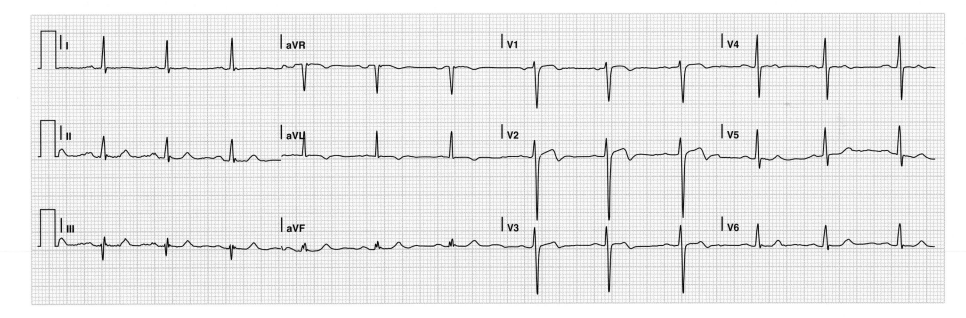

CASE 51   **CHIEF COMPLAINT:** Chest pain

HISTORY OF PRESENT ILLNESS	You respond to a call from a 46-year-old male experiencing chest pain and having trouble breathing. He was walking his dog when he became acutely short of breath and developed chest pain. The pain is constant and retrosternal, and does not radiate. The patient denies associated loss of consciousness, nausea, or vomiting.
PAST MEDICAL HISTORY	None
MEDICATIONS	None
ALLERGIES	None
VITAL SIGNS	BP: 100/60 mm Hg, P: 100 beats/min., R: 22 breaths/min., SpO$_2$: 96%
EXAM	Adult male, tachypneic, anxious. He is otherwise alert and cooperative. Heart sounds are normal; lungs sounds are slightly diminished bilaterally. The abdomen is soft and nontender. Extremities are warm and well perfused. Strong radial pulses are present. Skin is dry.

CLINICAL CHALLENGES AND QUESTIONS

1. What does this 12-lead ECG show?

2. How would you treat this patient?

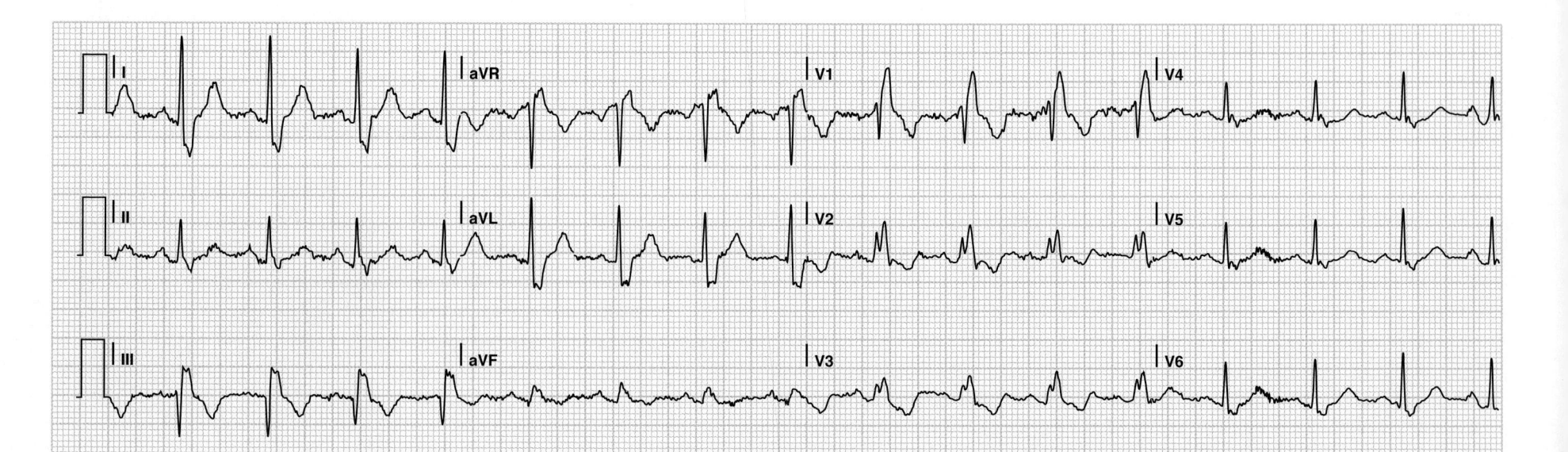

CHIEF COMPLAINT: Syncope

HISTORY OF PRESENT ILLNESS	You are an EMS instructor at the local public safety training facility. A 50-year-old police officer collapses during routine morning exercise drills. You grab the advanced life support gear and respond to the outdoor basketball courts. On arrival, police officers are attending a man who is lying on the ground. Witnesses state that he was "out of it" for about 30 seconds. He appears anxious and pale, and states that he has midsternal chest pressure, which he rates as a 6 on a 10-point pain scale. He reports nausea and recalls a sensation of weakness before the event.
PAST MEDICAL HISTORY	None
MEDICATIONS	None
ALLERGIES	None
VITAL SIGNS	BP: 80 mm Hg (by palpation), P: 150 beats/min., R: 16 breaths/min., SpO$_2$: 88%
EXAM	A well-developed male is supine. He is awake, alert, oriented, and visibly anxious. Heart sounds are not muffled, and you auscultate what sounds like a gallop. Lung examination reveals bibasilar crackles with some poor inspiratory effort. The abdomen is soft and nontender. The patient has faint radial pulses. The skin is cool and diaphoretic.

CLINICAL CHALLENGES AND QUESTIONS

1. What does this 12-lead ECG show?

2. How would you treat this patient?

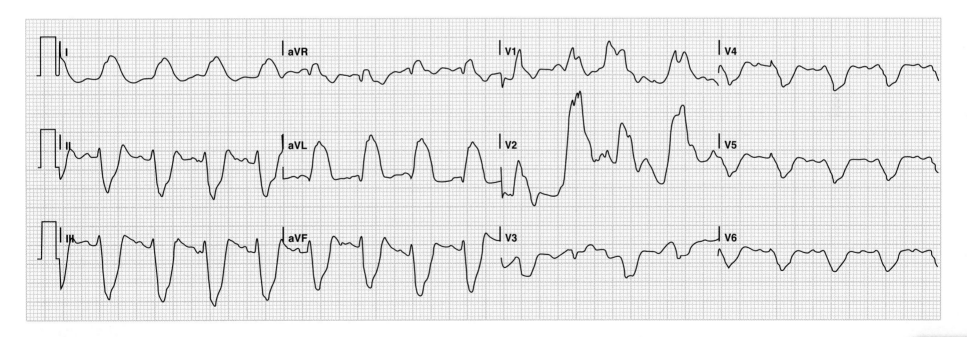

CASE 53

CHIEF COMPLAINT: Chest pain, fever, cough

HISTORY OF PRESENT ILLNESS	Your patient is a 38-year-old male who reports sharp chest pain, fever, and cough. The chest pain started earlier in the day, prompting the 9-1-1 call. The fever and cough started several days ago. The pain worsens when the patient coughs. He rates it as a 6 on a 10-point pain scale.
PAST MEDICAL HISTORY	Bronchitis, pneumonia, hypertension
MEDICATIONS	Atenolol
ALLERGIES	None
VITAL SIGNS	T: 101°F, BP: 140/70 mm Hg, P: 60 beats/min., R: 24 breaths/min., SpO$_2$: 94%
EXAM	The patient is an adult male in mild respiratory distress. He is awake, alert, and oriented. Heart sounds are normal. Lung sounds are coarse with scattered wheezing in all fields. Air movement is good. There is mild tenderness to palpation of the epigastrium. Abdomen is otherwise soft, nontender, and nondistended. Extremities are warm and well perfused. Radial pulses are strong and equal. Skin is dry.

CLINICAL CHALLENGES AND QUESTIONS

1. What does this 12-lead ECG show?

2. How would you treat this patient?

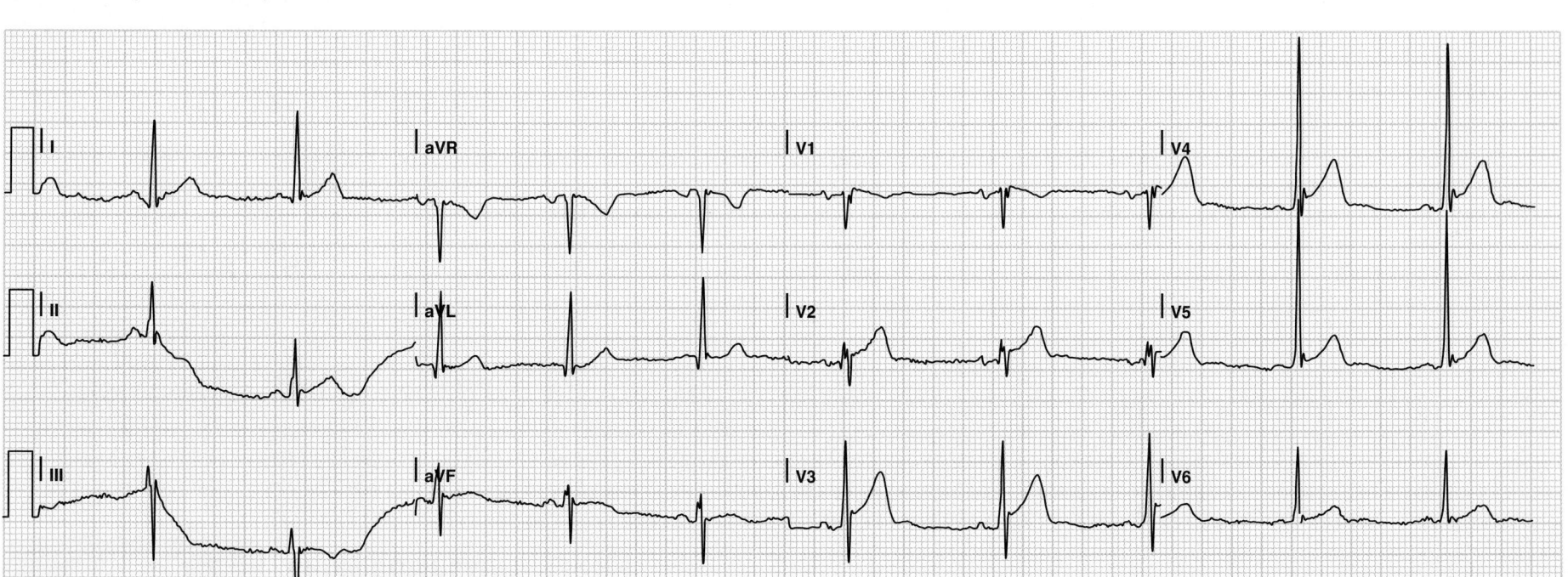

HISTORY OF PRESENT ILLNESS	Advanced providers respond to an outpatient surgical center, where a 21-year-old male has experienced a syncopal episode. The patient was undergoing a laser vision correction procedure when he lost consciousness for several minutes. The patient is alert on the arrival of paramedics and denies chest pain, shortness of breath, or dizziness.
PAST MEDICAL HISTORY	Myopia
MEDICATIONS	None
ALLERGIES	None
VITAL SIGNS	BP: 110/70 mm Hg, P: 80 beats/min., R: 16 breaths/min., SpO$_2$: 99%
EXAM	The patient is a healthy-looking male in no obvious distress. He is alert and oriented. Heart sounds are normal without any obvious murmur. The lungs are clear, and the abdomen is soft and nontender. Extremities are without edema. The skin is warm and slightly diaphoretic.

CLINICAL CHALLENGES AND QUESTIONS

1. What does this 12-lead ECG show?
2. How would you treat this patient?

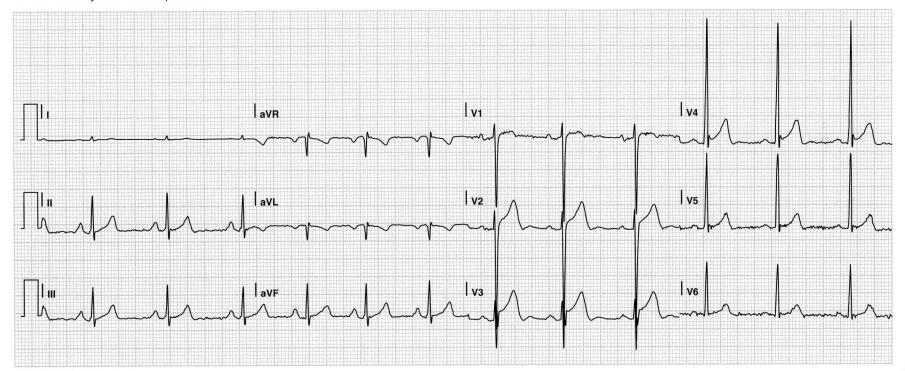

CASE 55   CHIEF COMPLAINT: Chest pain

HISTORY OF PRESENT ILLNESS	You arrive on the scene of a 74-year-old female who reports having chest pain for 30 minutes. The pain is constant and localized to the right anterior chest. The pain is worse with palpation. The patient denies shortness of breath, nausea, or vomiting.
PAST MEDICAL HISTORY	Parkinson disease
MEDICATIONS	Carbidopa/levodopa
ALLERGIES	None
VITAL SIGNS	BP: 146/84 mm Hg, P: 120s, R: 16 breaths/min., SpO$_2$: 97%
EXAM	The patient is awake, alert, and oriented. Heart sounds are normal. Lungs sounds are clear to auscultation. The abdomen is soft. Skin is warm and dry.

CLINICAL CHALLENGES AND QUESTIONS

1. What does this 12-lead ECG show?

2. How would you treat this patient?

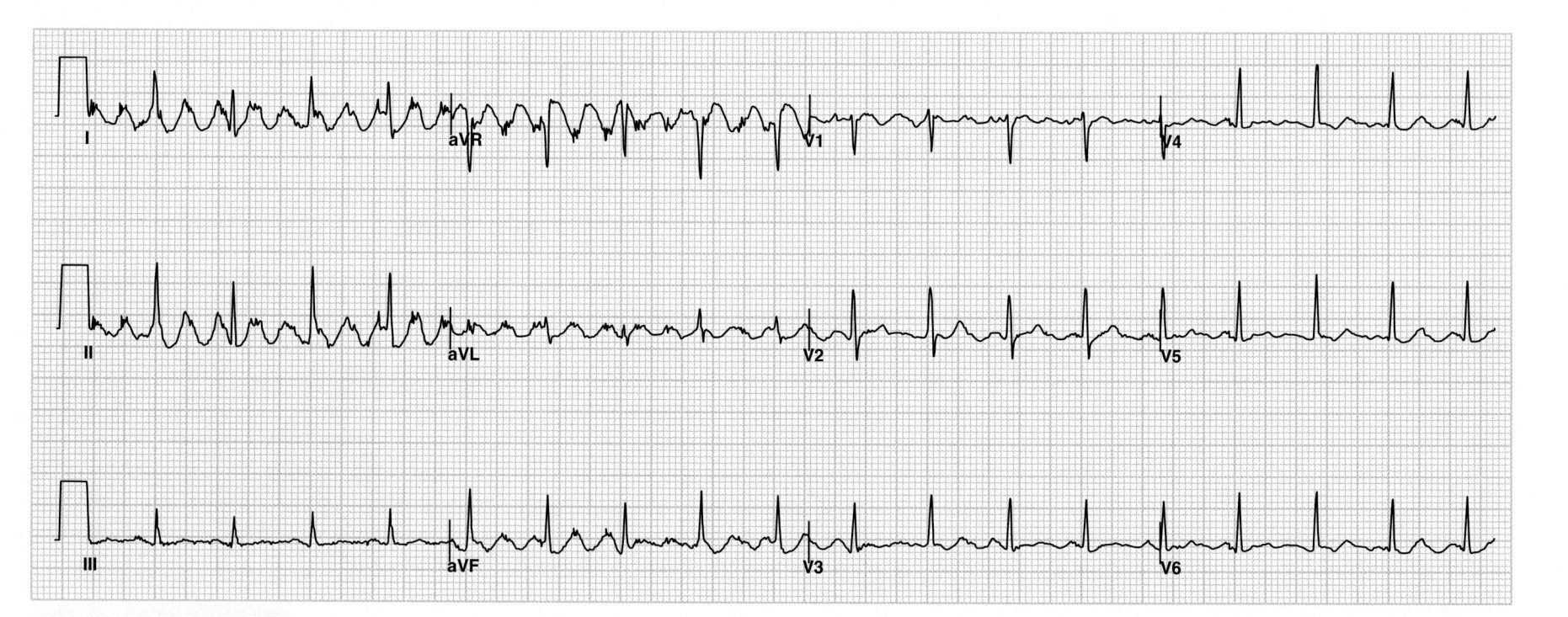

CHIEF COMPLAINT: Chest pain

HISTORY OF PRESENT ILLNESS	You are transporting a 70-year-old male from the local community hospital to a regional cardiac referral center for emergent cardiac catheterization. The patient presented to the local hospital approximately 30 minutes ago. He had chest pain, nausea, and diaphoresis. His pain has been increasing, requiring upward titration of a nitroglycerin infusion. He still reports crushing, left-sided chest pain, which he describes as a 10 on a 10-point scale.
PAST MEDICAL HISTORY	Diabetes mellitus, hypertension, hyperlipidemia
MEDICATIONS	Intravenous nitroglycerin infusion, 20 µg/min; intravenous heparin, 1,200 units/hr; aspirin; metoprolol; lisinopril; atorvastatin daily
VITAL SIGNS	BP: 150/100 mm Hg, P: 100 beats/min., R: 22 breaths/min., SpO$_2$: 94% on nasal cannula
EXAM	The patient is an anxious elderly male in moderate distress. Heart sounds are normal; crackles are present in all lung fields, with mild chest wall retraction. Abdomen is soft to palpation. No lower extremity edema. Radial pulses are 2+ bilaterally. Skin is diaphoretic.

CLINICAL CHALLENGES AND QUESTIONS

1. What does this 12-lead ECG show?

2. How would you treat this patient?

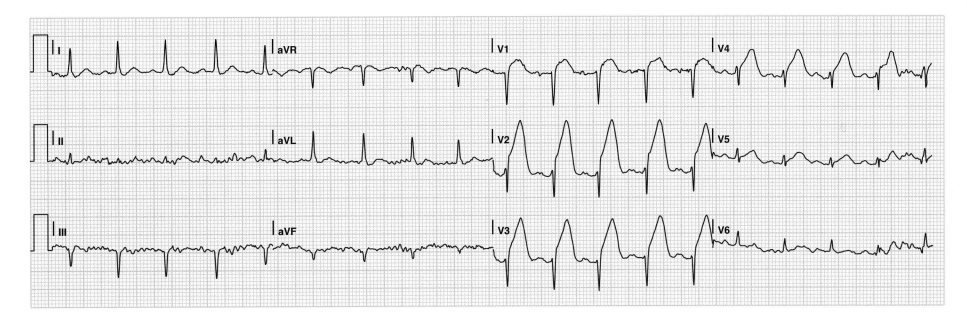

CASE 57

CHIEF COMPLAINT: Shortness of breath

HISTORY OF PRESENT ILLNESS	Advanced providers respond to a call regarding a 76-year-old male who began having difficulty catching his breath while watching a football game. He did not experience chest pain but did break out in a sweat around the same time the shortness of breath started.
PAST MEDICAL HISTORY	Unknown
MEDICATIONS	Unknown
ALLERGIES	None
VITAL SIGNS	BP: 124/70 mm Hg, P: 150–200 beats/min., R: 24 breaths/min., SpO$_2$: 97%
EXAM	Elderly male in moderate respiratory distress. Heart sounds are normal. Lungs are clear in all fields. The abdomen is soft, nontender, and nondistended. Extremities are warm and well perfused. No edema. Radial pulses are equal and symmetric, and distal pulses are strong. The skin is cool and clammy.

CLINICAL CHALLENGES AND QUESTIONS

1. What do you notice right away in the 3-lead ECG below? What do you think about the rate? What is the underlying rhythm?
2. What are your immediate treatment options?

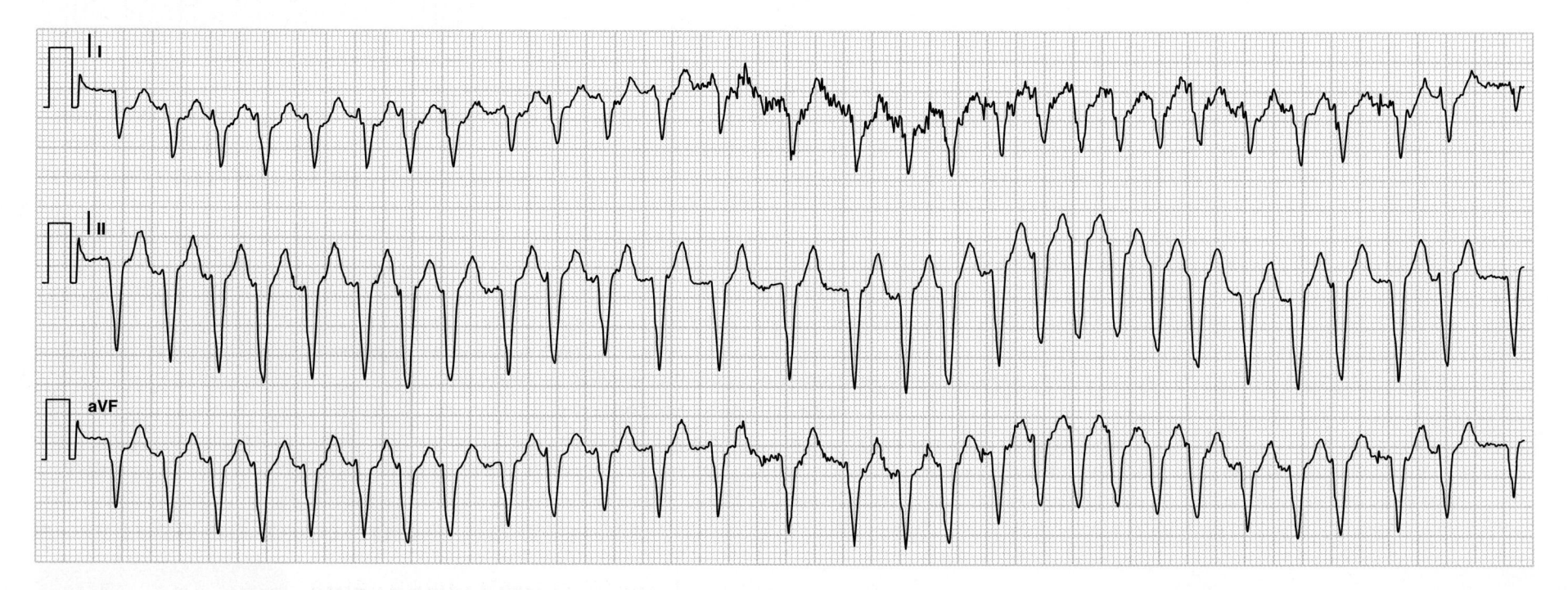

(Continued)

CHIEF COMPLAINT: Shortness of breath

CLINICAL CHALLENGES AND QUESTIONS

A 12-lead ECG (shown below) from the same patient was obtained several minutes later. He remains symptomatic and stable. What is the goal of your treatment?

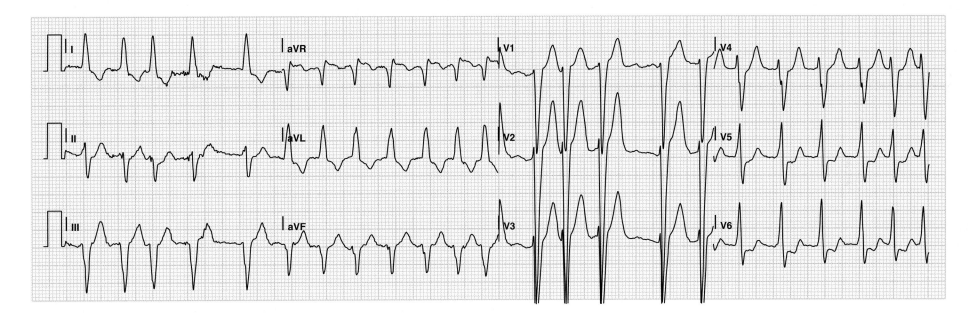

CASE 58

CHIEF COMPLAINT: Chest pain

HISTORY OF PRESENT ILLNESS	Advanced providers respond to a residence for a report of a 49-year-old male with chest pain. The patient states that the pain began 3 hours ago. It is retrosternal and radiates inferiorly to the epigastrium. He rates the pain as a constant 5 on a 10-point scale. The pain is associated with nausea, vomiting, and weakness.
PAST MEDICAL HISTORY	None
MEDICATIONS	None
ALLERGIES	None
VITAL SIGNS	BP: 180/100 mm Hg, P: 92 beats/min., R: 16 breaths/min., SpO₂: 96%
EXAM	Patient is awake and oriented. He is cooperative and in no acute distress. Heart sounds are normal. Lungs are clear. Abdominal examination is unremarkable. Extremities are without edema. Radial pulses are 2+ bilaterally. Skin is cool and dry.

CLINICAL CHALLENGES AND QUESTIONS

1. What does this 12-lead ECG show?

2. How would you treat this patient?

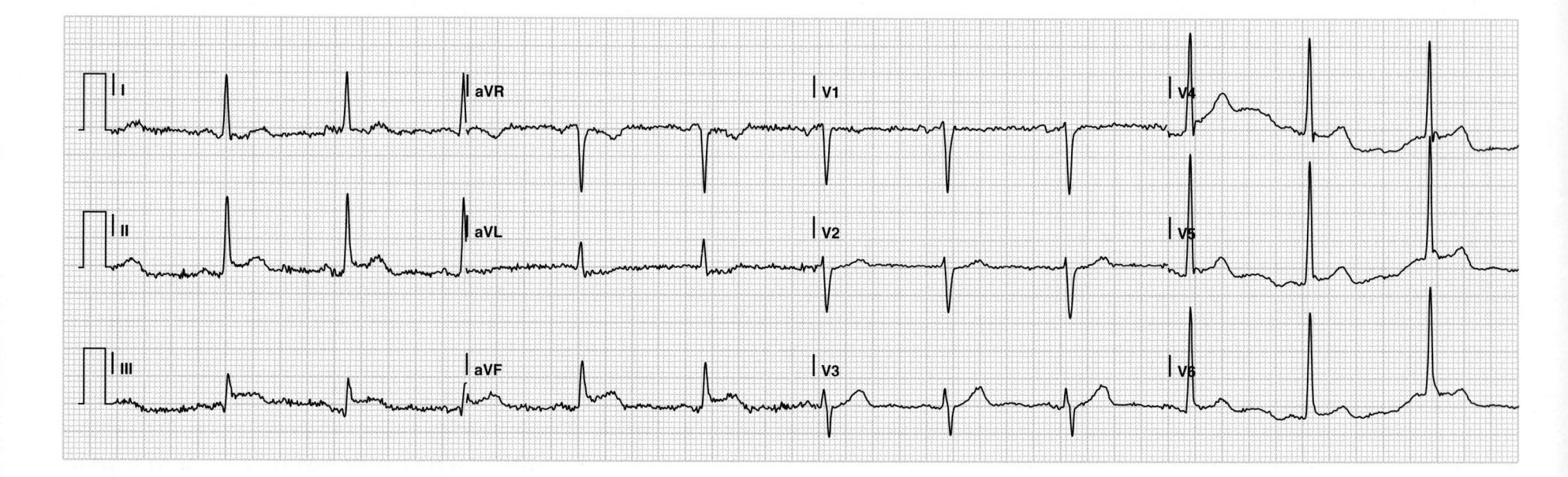

CHIEF COMPLAINT: Chest pain

HISTORY OF PRESENT ILLNESS	Your medevac crew is transporting a 71-year-old female to a cardiac catheterization facility. At the sending facility, the patient was judged to be "high risk" because of her history of stent placement and coronary artery disease, and an ECG was performed. The patient is on a nitroglycerin drip and received 324 mg of aspirin before your arrival. During transport, the patient becomes hypotensive and diaphoretic. You repeat the 12-lead ECG.
PAST MEDICAL HISTORY	Coronary artery disease, high cholesterol, hypertension, peripheral vascular disease
MEDICATIONS	Nitroglycerin intravenous drip, 10 μg/min; ASA; fentanyl, 50 μg every 30 min for pain; metoprolol; furosemide; nifedipine
ALLERGIES	None
VITAL SIGNS	BP: 96/50 mm Hg, P: 110 beats/min., R: 20 breaths/min., SpO$_2$: 96%
EXAM	Well-developed, well-nourished female in mild distress. Cardiac and lung examination cannot be performed because of helicopter noise. Extremities are cool; 1+ distal pulses bilaterally. No edema. Skin is cool to touch.

CLINICAL CHALLENGES AND QUESTIONS

1. What does this 12-lead ECG show?

2. How would you treat this patient?

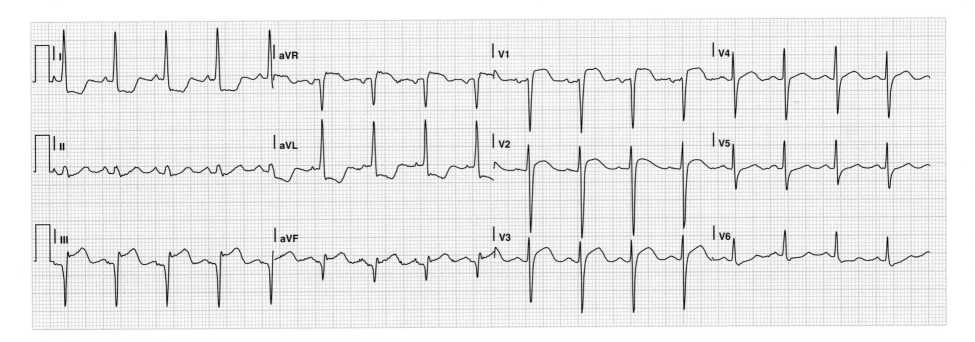

CASE 60

CHIEF COMPLAINT: Interfacility transport

HISTORY OF PRESENT ILLNESS	Advanced providers are transferring a 24-year-old trauma victim to a rehabilitation facility. Three weeks earlier, he was stabbed in the chest multiple times, causing a puncture wound to the right ventricle and interventricular septum. The patient currently has no acute complaint; he denies chest pain, shortness of breath, nausea, vomiting, or diaphoresis. A routine ECG is acquired before transfer.
PAST MEDICAL HISTORY	Thoracotomy, ventricular pacemaker, respiratory failure
MEDICATIONS	Enoxaparin, multivitamins, albuterol inhaler, morphine sulfate, oxycodone, Colace
ALLERGIES	None
VITAL SIGNS	BP: 108/54 mm Hg; P: 80 beats/min.; R: 12 breaths/min.; SpO$_2$: 96% on oxygen, 2 L/min.
EXAM	The patient is sleeping but easily arousable. He is oriented to person, place, and time. Heart sounds are normal; lung sounds are diminished at the bases. Abdominal exam reveals a large midline surgical scar but is otherwise soft and nontender to palpation. Trace nonpitting pedal edema is present bilaterally. Radial pulses are strong and equal. Skin is warm and dry.

CLINICAL CHALLENGES AND QUESTIONS

1. What does this 12-lead ECG show?

2. How would you treat this patient?

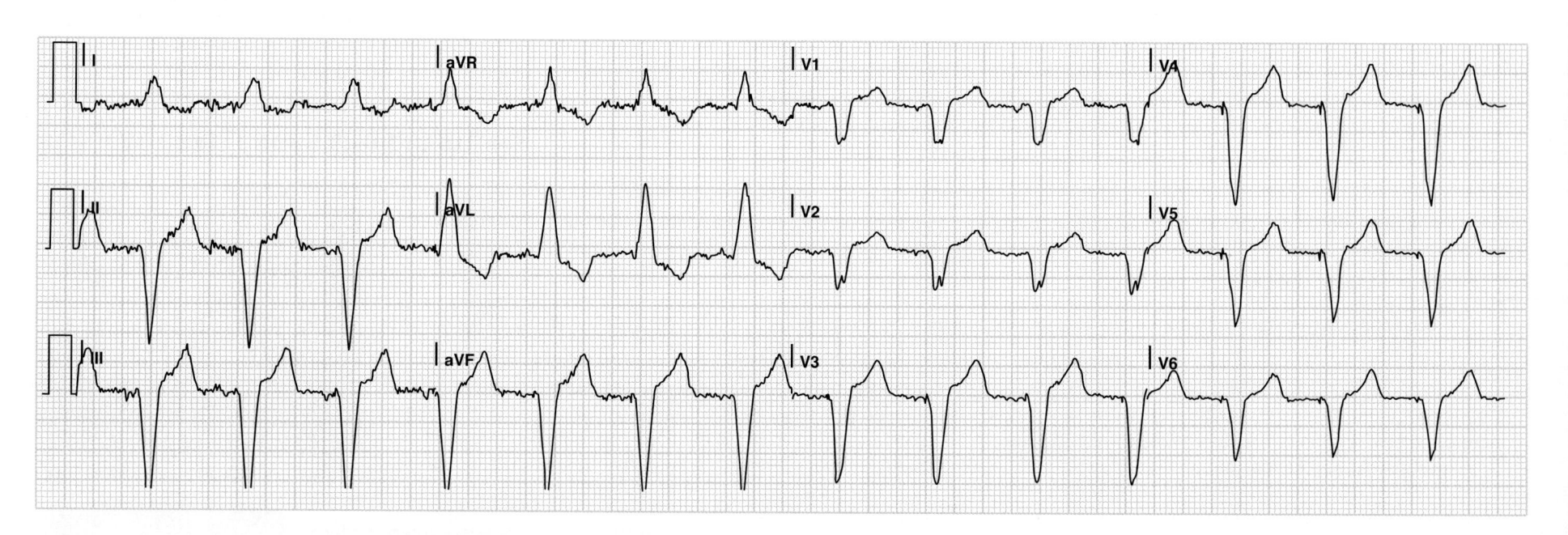

CHIEF COMPLAINT: Chest pain

HISTORY OF PRESENT ILLNESS	You arrive on the scene, where a 35-year-old male reports retrosternal chest pain. The pain began 3 days ago, after "cold" symptoms resolved. His pain gets worse when he leans forward or coughs. The patient reports a mild fever but has not experienced nausea, vomiting, or hemoptysis. Otherwise, he appears well.
PAST MEDICAL HISTORY	None
MEDICATIONS	Ibuprofen
ALLERGIES	None
VITAL SIGNS	BP: 132/70 mm Hg, P: 110 beats/min., R: 20 breaths/min., SpO$_2$: 96%
EXAM	Patient appears anxious, but is awake, alert, aware, and cooperative. Heart sounds are tachycardic. Lungs are clear to auscultation. Abdomen is soft and nontender. Extremities are warm and well perfused. Skin is warm and dry.

CLINICAL CHALLENGES AND QUESTIONS

1. What does this 12-lead ECG show?

2. How would you treat this patient?

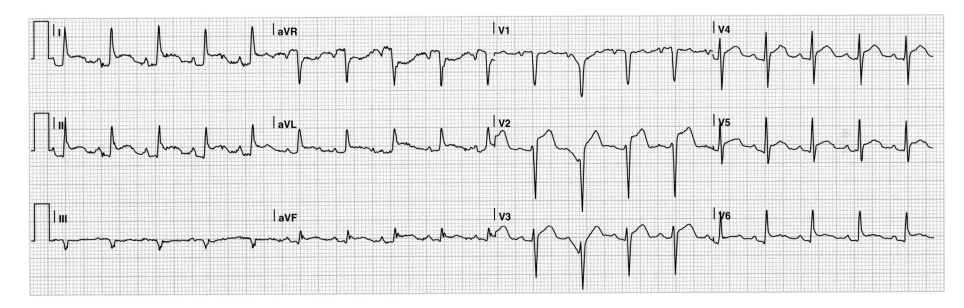

CASE 62   CHIEF COMPLAINT: Weakness

HISTORY OF PRESENT ILLNESS	You are triaging a 70-year-old female who has come to the ED after experiencing weakness and fatigue for several days. She thinks she is recovering from a mild cold. She states that she has been coughing. The cough has been worse at night and occasionally prevents her from sleeping. She reports mild shortness of breath today but denies nausea, vomiting, sweating, or loss of consciousness.
PAST MEDICAL HISTORY	Diabetes mellitus, hypertension, arthritis
MEDICATIONS	Glipizide, atenolol, amlodipine
ALLERGIES	Sulfa drugs
VITAL SIGNS	BP: 150/90, P: 90 beats/min., R: 18 breaths/min., SpO$_2$: 95%
EXAM	The patient is an obese female who is awake, alert, and oriented. She is mildly distressed. Heart sounds are normal. Lung exam reveals basilar crackles. Abdomen is soft and nontender, without rigidity or guarding. Mild pitting edema is present bilaterally. 2+ radial pulses are present, and capillary refill time is brisk. Skin is warm and dry.

CLINICAL CHALLENGES AND QUESTIONS

1. What does this 12-lead ECG show?

2. How would you treat this patient?

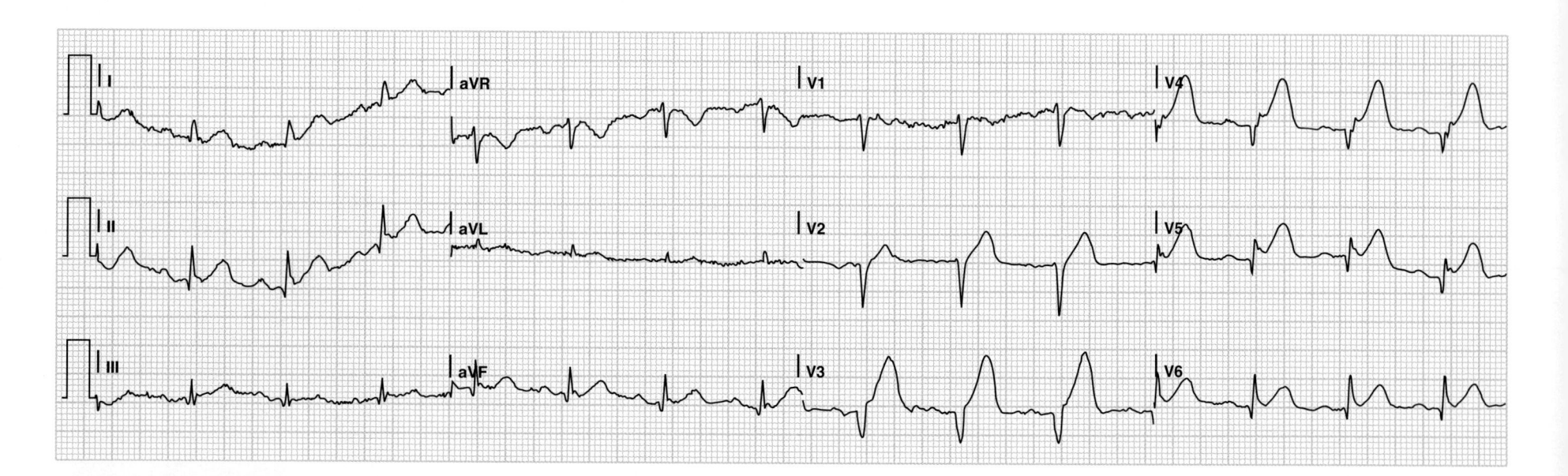

CHIEF COMPLAINT: Chest pain

HISTORY OF PRESENT ILLNESS	Advanced providers respond to a call regarding a 16-year-old male who reports stabbing chest pain. The pain started while he was playing basketball, and it does not radiate. He describes it as a constant 5 on a 10-point pain scale. He denies shortness of breath. The pain worsens when he moves his right arm and with deep breathing, but it is relieved by rest.
PAST MEDICAL HISTORY	None
MEDICATIONS	None
ALLERGIES	None
VITAL SIGNS	BP: 140/70 mm Hg, P: 70–80 beats/min., R: 18 breaths/min., SpO$_2$: 99%
EXAM	The patient is a well-developed, muscular adolescent male in moderate distress. Heart sounds are normal, and lungs are clear. The abdomen is soft and nontender. Extremities are warm and well perfused. Radial pulses are strong. Skin is warm.

CLINICAL CHALLENGES AND QUESTIONS

1. What does this 12-lead ECG show?

2. How would you treat this patient?

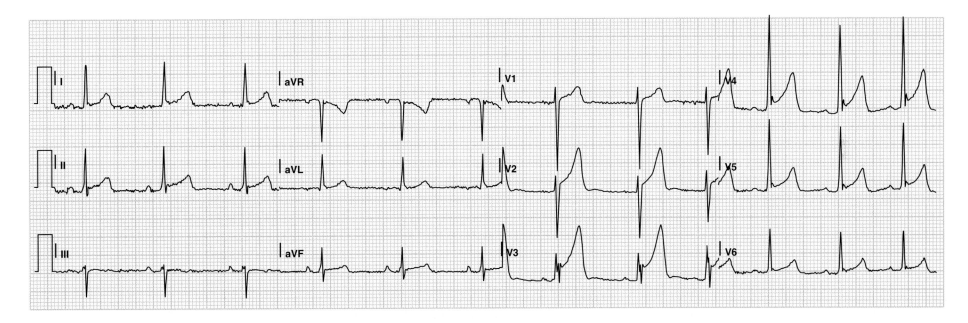

CASE 64   CHIEF COMPLAINT: Respiratory distress

HISTORY OF PRESENT ILLNESS	You respond to the report of a 65-year-old male in respiratory distress at a local grocery store. He reports feeling weak and mildly short of breath over the past few days, and he experienced mild chest pain and nausea earlier in the day.
PAST MEDICAL HISTORY	Hypertension, diabetes mellitus, coronary artery disease, hyperlipidemia
MEDICATIONS	Unknown
ALLERGIES	Unknown
VITAL SIGNS	BP: 134/76 mm Hg, P: 60 beats/min., R: 22 breaths/min., SpO$_2$: 98%
EXAM	The patient is a fit 65-year-old male who appears restless. His pupils are equal and reactive. Lung sounds are normal. His abdominal is soft to palpation. No pedal edema is present. Radial pulses are strong and equal.

CLINICAL CHALLENGES AND QUESTIONS

1. What does this 12-lead ECG show?

2. How would you treat this patient?

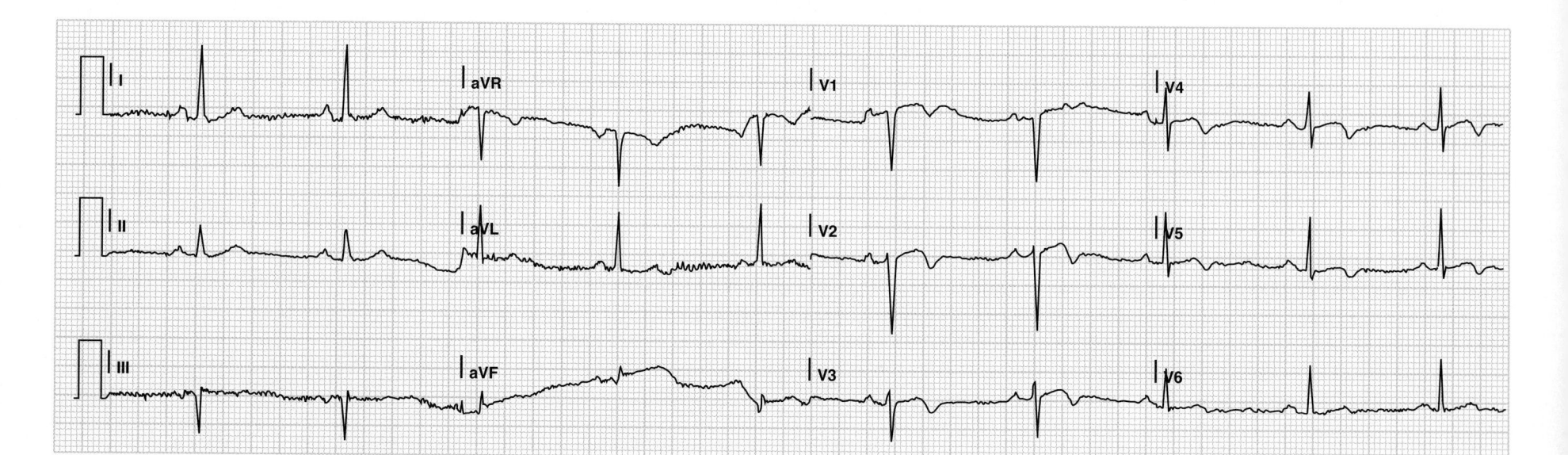

CHIEF COMPLAINT: Respiratory distress

HISTORY OF PRESENT ILLNESS	Advanced providers arrive on the scene of an 81-year-old female who reports feeling short of breath and extremely fatigued. The patient denies chest pain.
PAST MEDICAL HISTORY	Heart failure, hypertension
MEDICATIONS	Furosemide, potassium chloride, aspirin, metoprolol
ALLERGIES	None
VITAL SIGNS	BP: 110/54 mm Hg, P: 30s, R: 14 breaths/min., SpO$_2$: 95%
EXAM	The patient is restless and anxious. Heart sounds reveal a systolic murmur. Lung sounds reveal crackles in the bases bilaterally on auscultation. The abdomen is soft. There is 1+ pitting edema bilaterally. Radial pulses are present.

CLINICAL CHALLENGES AND QUESTIONS

1. What does this 12-lead ECG show?

2. How would you treat this patient?

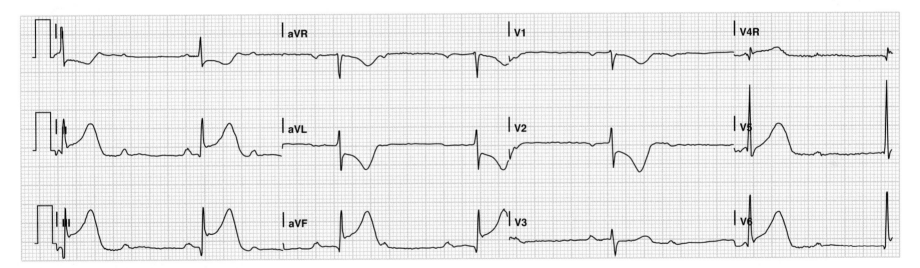

CASE 66

CHIEF COMPLAINT: Weakness

HISTORY OF PRESENT ILLNESS	You arrive at the home of a 73-year-old male who experienced a sudden onset of weakness. He denies loss of consciousness, shortness of breath, or chest pain. The patient denies any recent sickness or injury.
PAST MEDICAL HISTORY	Diabetes, hypercholesterolemia, left bundle branch block
MEDICATIONS	Daily aspirin, insulin, atorvastatin
ALLERGIES	None
VITAL SIGNS	BP: 140/70 mm Hg, P: 60 beats/min., R: 14 breaths/min., SpO$_2$: 97%
EXAM	The patient is an elderly male in no obvious distress. He is slow to respond to questions. Heart sounds are normal. Lung sounds are clear. Abdomen is soft, nontender, and nondistended. Extremities reveal trace edema. Radial pulses are equal and strong. The skin is cool and clammy.

CLINICAL CHALLENGES AND QUESTIONS

1. What does this 12-lead ECG show?

2. How would you treat this patient?

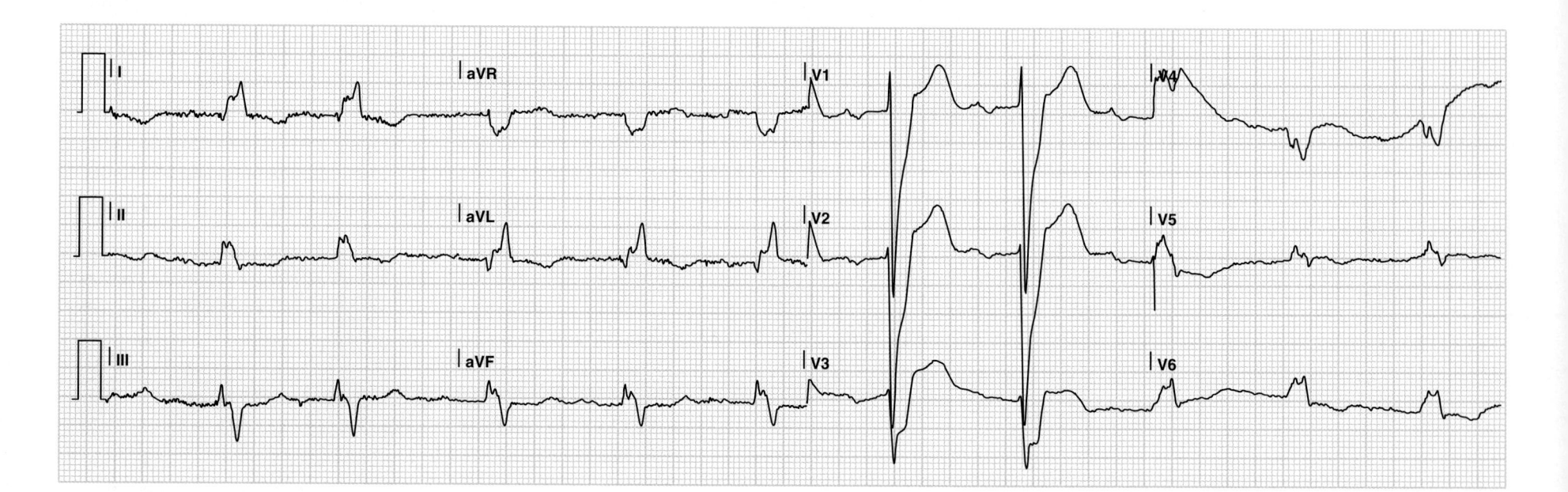

CHIEF COMPLAINT: Chest pain

HISTORY OF PRESENT ILLNESS	Advanced providers arrive on the scene, where a 68-year-old man has been coughing up blood and having chest pain for the past 20 minutes. He states that he cannot breathe.
PAST MEDICAL HISTORY	Total left hip replacement 4 days ago
MEDICATIONS	Takes numerous prescribed medications; cannot recall their names
ALLERGIES	None
VITAL SIGNS	BP: 110/54 mm Hg, P: 110 beats/min., R: 28 breaths/min., SpO$_2$: 94%
EXAM	Elderly male, tachycardic, tachypneic, anxious. Patient has a cough that occasionally produces blood-tinged mucus. Lung sounds are clear, but a pleural friction rub is heard. The abdomen is soft and nontender. The skin is cool and clammy.

CLINICAL CHALLENGES AND QUESTIONS

1. What does this 12-lead ECG show?

2. How would you treat this patient?

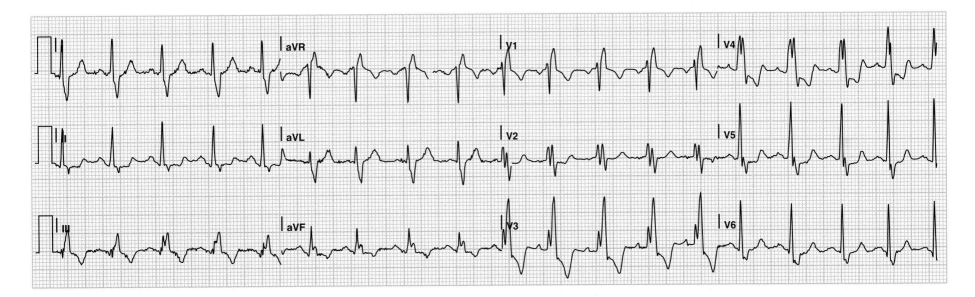

CASE 68

CHIEF COMPLAINT: Weakness

HISTORY OF PRESENT ILLNESS	You respond to the home of a 60-year-old patient with weakness. On arrival, you find an obese male seated in a recliner. He reports feeling weak for the past several days. He also has been lightheaded and states that he "almost passed out" today. The patient has experienced some recent diarrhea and subjective fever. He denies any chest pain or dyspnea on exertion. The patient reports persistent nausea but denies any vomiting.
PAST MEDICAL HISTORY	Diabetes mellitus, hypertension
MEDICATIONS	Metformin, metoclopromide, lisinopril
ALLERGIES	Aspirin (stomach upset)
VITAL SIGNS	BP: 110/70 mm Hg, P: 140 beats/min., R: 16 breaths/min., SpO$_2$: 96%
EXAM	Obese 60-year-old male in no acute distress. He is alert and oriented. Heart sounds are normal. Lungs are clear to auscultation bilaterally. Abdomen is soft and nontender. Extremities are well perfused; 2+ edema is present bilaterally. Radial pulses are strong and equal bilaterally. Skin is somewhat dry and exhibits poor turgor.

CLINICAL CHALLENGES AND QUESTIONS

1. What does this 12-lead ECG show?

2. How would you treat this patient?

Your partner asks if he should apply the defibrillator pads and shock this rhythm. He states that the patient is symptomatic and may be relatively hypotensive. The patient confirms that his blood pressure usually runs between 150 and 160 mm Hg. You attach defibrillator pads in case the patient's condition deteriorates.

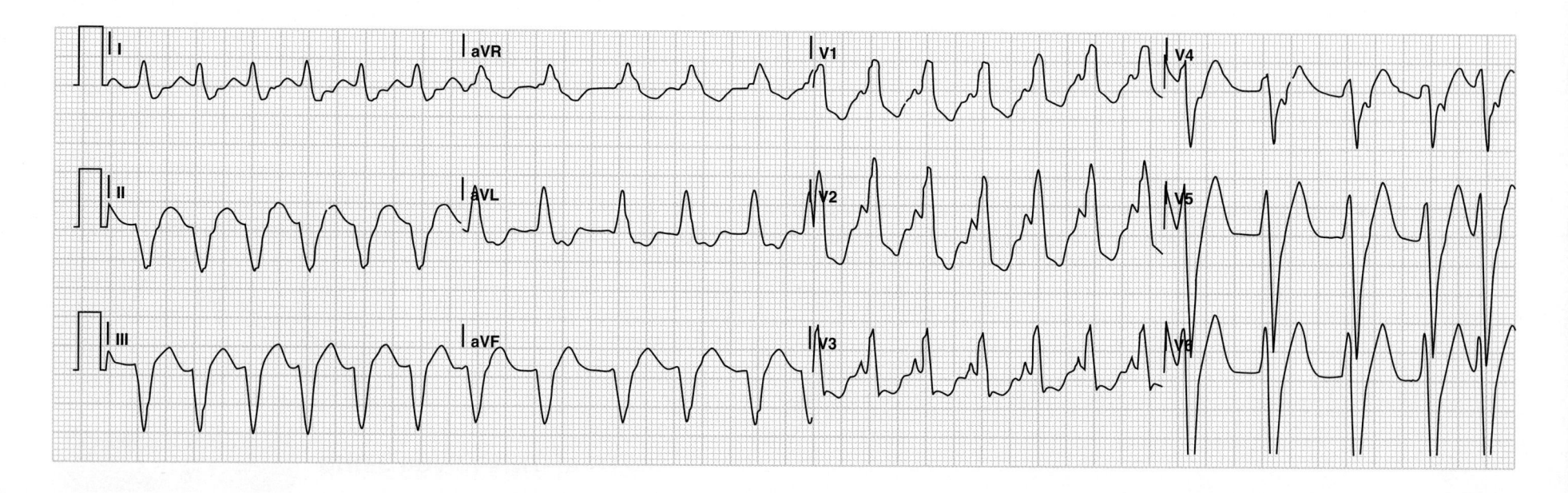

CASE 69   CHIEF COMPLAINT: Syncope

HISTORY OF PRESENT ILLNESS	Advanced providers arrive on scene of a 90-year-old male who experienced multiple episodes of syncope while trying to stand.
PAST MEDICAL HISTORY	None
MEDICINES	None
ALLERGIES	None
VITAL SIGNS	BP: 84/52 mm Hg, P: 30s, R: 14 breaths/min., SpO$_2$: 92%
EXAM	The patient answers questions appropriately but is very slow to respond. His skin is pale and clammy. Lung sounds are clear to auscultation. The abdomen is soft. No pedal edema is noted. Blood sugar is 88 mg/dL. Pupils are 4 mm and reactive to light.

CLINICAL CHALLENGES AND QUESTIONS

1. What does this rhythm strip show?
2. How would you treat this patient?

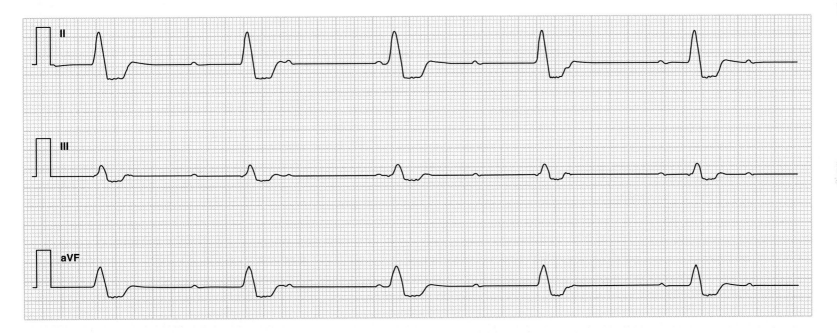

CASE 70   **CHIEF COMPLAINT:** Respiratory distress

HISTORY OF PRESENT ILLNESS	Advanced providers respond to the report of a 74-year-old female in respiratory distress at a local long-term care facility. The nursing staff reports the patient had been well until 2 days before when she experienced coughing, restlessness, and shortness of breath. She had been treated effectively with an albuterol inhaler and an increased dose of furosemide. Today, the patient is much more uncomfortable and cannot be calmed down. The patient is confused at baseline and does not offer additional history.
PAST MEDICAL HISTORY	Full code, congestive heart failure, myocardial infarction, hypertension
MEDICATIONS	No list available
ALLERGIES	Unknown
VITAL SIGNS	BP: 200/110 mm Hg, P: 60 beats/min., R: 24 breaths/min., SpO$_2$: 88%
EXAM	Elderly 74-year-old female in obvious respiratory distress. The patient appears anxious. Heart exam is remarkable for the presence of an S$_3$. Lung sounds reveal coarse crackles bilaterally. Significant pitting pedal edema is noted. Radial pulses are bounding and equal.

CLINICAL CHALLENGES AND QUESTIONS

1. What does this 12-lead ECG show?

2. How would you treat this patient?

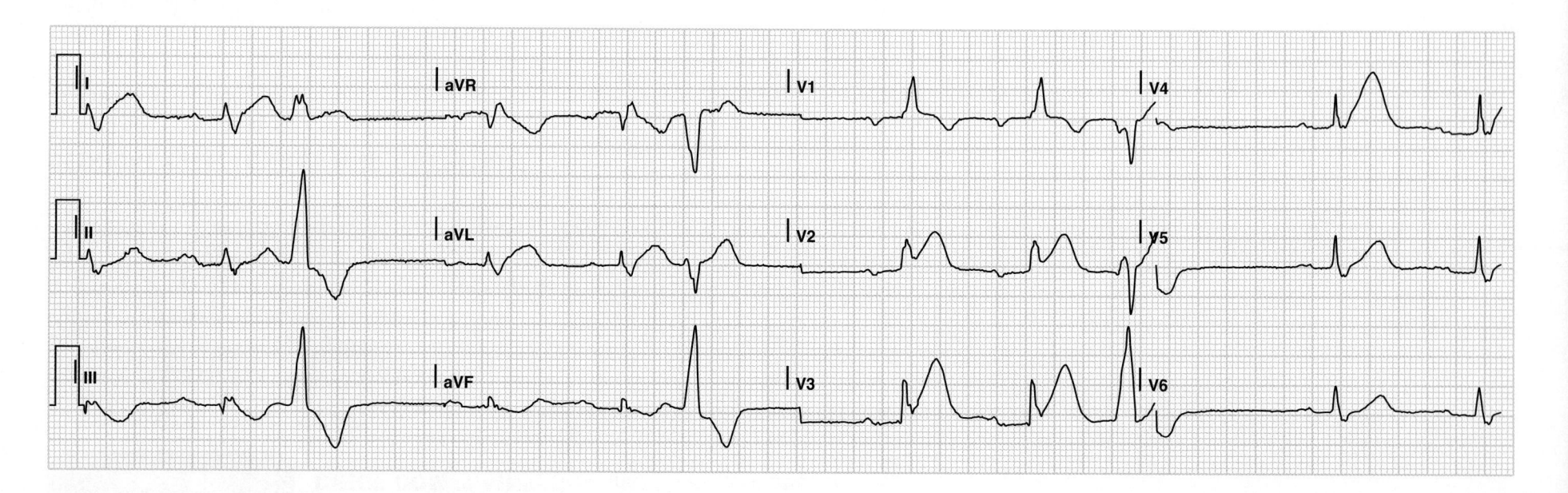

CHIEF COMPLAINT: Abdominal pain, vomiting, diarrhea

HISTORY OF PRESENT ILLNESS	You arrive at the home of a 72-year-old male with stomach pain. He reports associated nausea, vomiting, and diarrhea. He has had three episodes of nonbilious, nonbloody emesis. Lower abdominal cramping has been followed by episodes of diarrhea. His symptoms started several hours after eating lunch at the local diner and are worsened by eating. The patient denies chest pain, shortness of breath, or syncope.
PAST MEDICAL HISTORY	Myocardial infarction, pacemaker
MEDICATIONS	Daily aspirin
ALLERGIES	None
VITAL SIGNS	BP: 140/68 mm Hg, P: 70 beats/min., R: 14 breaths/min., SpO$_2$: 98%
EXAM	The patient is an elderly male who is actively vomiting. He is awake, alert, and oriented. Heart sounds are normal. The lungs are clear, and the patient is afebrile. His abdomen is soft, mildly distended, and tender in all quadrants. Extremities are without edema and are warm and well perfused. Radial pulses are 1+ and equal bilaterally. Skin is warm and dry.

CLINICAL CHALLENGES AND QUESTIONS

1. What does this 12-lead ECG show?
2. How would you treat this patient?

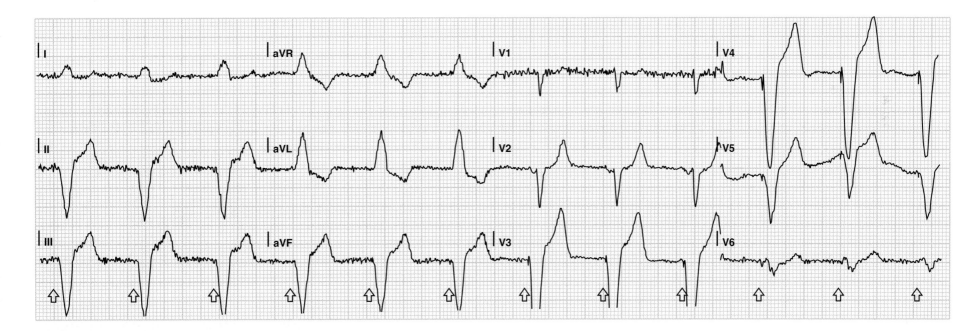

CASE 72   **CHIEF COMPLAINT:** Unresponsiveness

HISTORY OF PRESENT ILLNESS	You are transporting a 70-year-old female who has a history of cardiomyopathy and stent placement. The patient requires further management at a tertiary care facility. When the patient is transferred to you, she is receiving a dopamine drip at 10 mg/kg/min. The patient is awake, alert, and oriented. Once onboard, the patient reports a sudden onset of palpitations and shortness of breath. She feels faint and states that her head is "pounding." Her heart monitor alarm sounds.
PAST MEDICAL HISTORY	Coronary artery disease, hypertension, cardiac stents, myocardial infarction, stroke
MEDICATIONS	Clopidogrel, aspirin, lisinopril, simvastatin, tramadol
ALLERGIES	None
VITAL SIGNS	BP: 72 mm Hg (by palpation); P: 170 beats/min.; R: 16 breaths/min., regular; SpO$_2$: does not register
EXAM	Patient's eyes open to verbal stimuli. Heart sounds are muffled and tachycardic. Lung sounds are symmetric and clear. Abdomen is soft and nontender. Extremity exam reveals no edema. Weak distal radial pulses are palpable. Capillary refill is prolonged.

CLINICAL CHALLENGES AND QUESTIONS

1. What does this 12-lead ECG show?

2. How would you treat this patient?

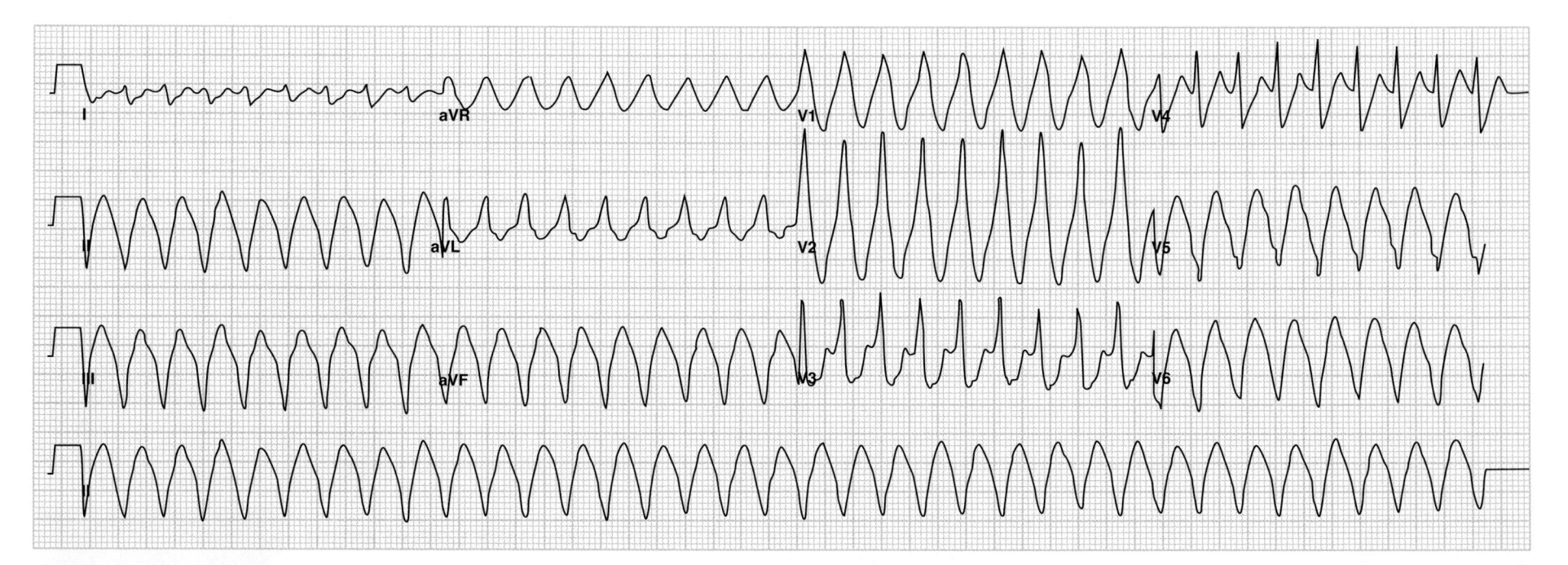

CHIEF COMPLAINT: Shortness of breath

HISTORY OF PRESENT ILLNESS	You respond to a call from a 55-year-old male with chest pain. The patient reports that he has felt tired and nauseated over the past few days. His pain is intermittent, worse with activity, and relieved by rest. There is occasional radiation of the pain to the epigastric region. When your unit arrives at the scene, the patient states that his chest pain has just "vanished." He feels slightly better and denies vomiting, fever, or cough.
PAST MEDICAL HISTORY	Hypertension, diabetes mellitus, cocaine use
MEDICATIONS	Noncompliant with prescribed antihypertensives
ALLERGIES	None
VITAL SIGNS	BP: 126/80 mm Hg; P: 100 beats/min., irregular; R: 16 breaths/min.; SpO_2: 95%
EXAM	A well-developed, well-nourished male is seated in the living room. He is alert, oriented, and cooperative. Heart sounds are irregular, with an apparent systolic murmur best heard at the apex. Lung sounds are slightly diminished at the bases. Abdomen is distended but nontender. Extremities are warm and well perfused. Pulses are also irregular at the radial site bilaterally. Skin is dry.

CLINICAL CHALLENGES AND QUESTIONS

1. What does this 12-lead ECG show?

2. How would you treat this patient?

3. Your paramedic student wonders why the patient has an irregular pulse in the **absence** of atrial fibrillation. When counted for a full minute, the patient's pulse varies between 40 and 80 beats/min. What might explain the variation in heart rate?

(Continued)

CASE 73   **CHIEF COMPLAINT:** Shortness of breath

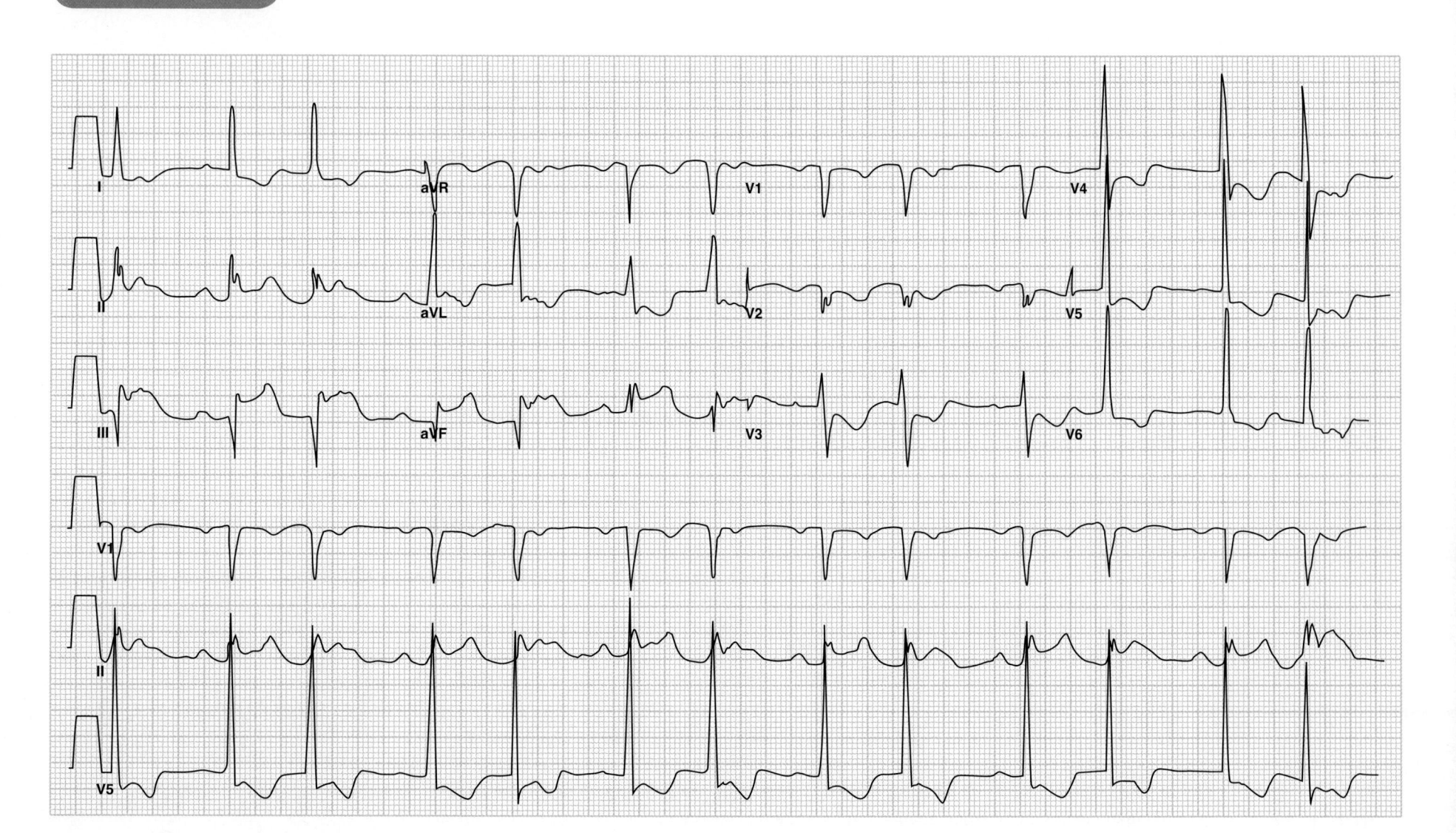

CHIEF COMPLAINT: Palpitations

HISTORY OF PRESENT ILLNESS	Advanced providers arrive on the scene of a 67-year-old female experiencing palpitations and unexplained sweating.
PAST MEDICAL HISTORY	Myocardial infarction, hypertension
MEDICATIONS	Does not remember but takes "a lot of them"
ALLERGIES	None
VITAL SIGNS	BP: 84/52 mm Hg, P: 80s, R: 24 breaths/min., SpO$_2$: 97%
EXAM	The patient is an ill-appearing female. She is awake, alert, and oriented. Lung sounds are clear. The abdomen is soft and nontender. Extremities are without edema. Radial pulses are weak and irregular. Skin is wet and cool.

CLINICAL CHALLENGES AND QUESTIONS

1. What does this 12-lead ECG show?
2. How would you treat this patient?

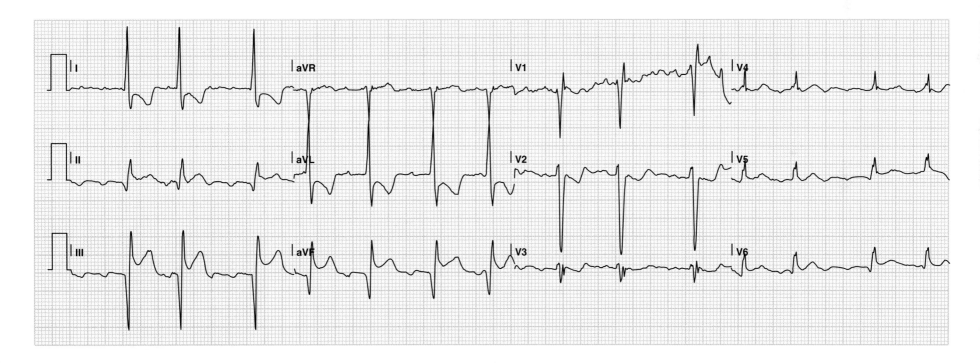

CASE 75   CHIEF COMPLAINT: Syncope

HISTORY OF PRESENT ILLNESS	Advanced providers arrive on the scene of a 48-year-old teacher who passed out while lecturing.
PAST MEDICAL HISTORY	None
MEDICATIONS	None
ALLERGIES	None
VITAL SIGNS	BP: 104/62 mm Hg, P: 160s, R: 18 breaths/min., SpO$_2$: 99%
EXAM	The patient appears to be calm and in no obvious distress. Heart sounds are irregular. Lung sounds are clear to auscultation. The abdomen is soft and nontender. Extremities are warm and well perfused. Strong distal pulses are present bilaterally. Skin is warm and dry.

CLINICAL CHALLENGES AND QUESTIONS

1. What does this rhythm strip show?

2. How would you treat this patient?

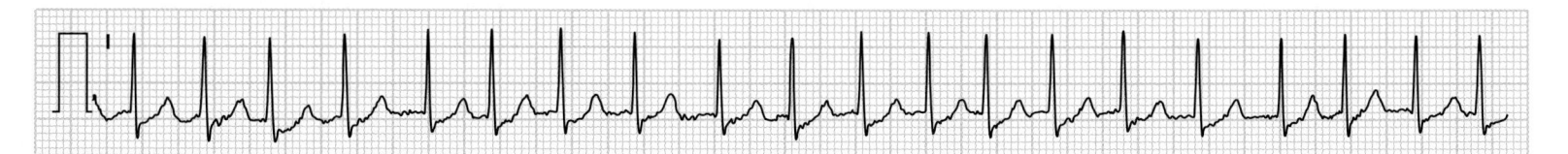

CHIEF COMPLAINT: Chest pain

HISTORY OF PRESENT ILLNESS	You are triaging a 52-year-old male with chest pain. He states that it began approximately 1 hour before his arrival at the emergency department. The pain is retrosternal, rates a 10 on a 10-point scale, and is associated with left upper extremity paresthesia. The patient states that the onset correlated with mild exercise and the pain is relieved when he rests. He has no shortness of breath. The patient denies diaphoresis, loss of consciousness, or nausea. A 12-lead ECG is obtained.
PAST MEDICAL HISTORY	Mild hypertension, obesity
MEDICATIONS	None
ALLERGIES	None.
VITAL SIGNS	BP: 126/90 mm Hg; P: 82 beats/min.; R: 14 breaths/min., nonlabored
EXAM	A well-developed, well-appearing man is sitting in the emergency department triage area. He appears to be in no acute distress and is awake, alert, and oriented. Heart sounds are normal. Lungs are clear to auscultation bilaterally. Abdomen is soft, nontender, and nondistended. Extremities are well perfused and without edema. The patient has 2+ radial pulses. Skin is warm and dry.

CLINICAL CHALLENGES AND QUESTIONS

1. What does this 12-lead ECG show?

2. The patient exhibits relatively stable vital signs. The emergency department is crowded and no treatment beds are available. What immediate interventions might you consider? Does this patient warrant triage to the immediate care area?

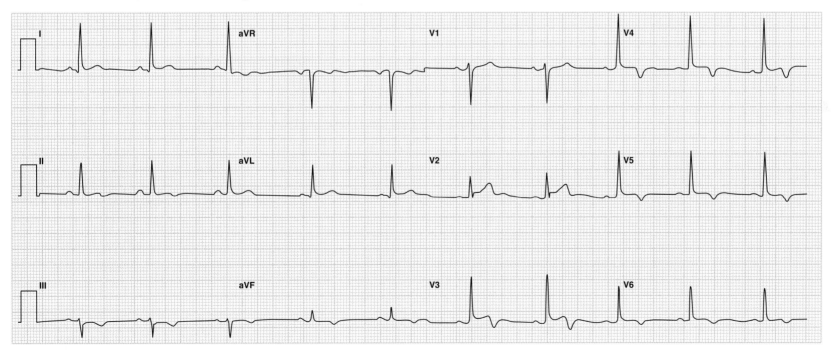

CASE 77

CHIEF COMPLAINT: Unresponsiveness

HISTORY OF PRESENT ILLNESS	You respond to a report of a "man down." The patient is a 23-year-old male found in an alley. He has obvious blunt force trauma to the head. The patient has sonorous respirations and only withdraws from pain. Additional history and information are unobtainable.
PAST MEDICAL HISTORY	Unknown
MEDICATIONS	Unknown
ALLERGIES	Unknown
VITAL SIGNS	BP: 170/100 mm Hg; P: 60 beats/min.; R: 8 breaths/min, sonorous; SpO_2: 88%
EXAM	A well-developed man is lying on the ground. He grimaces and withdraws in response to painful stimuli. Pupils are 4 mm bilaterally and sluggish; there is a prominent left parietal hematoma. Heart sounds are regular. Lungs are clear to auscultation bilaterally. Abdomen is soft and nondistended. Extremities are without obvious trauma, cyanosis, or edema. The patient has 2+ distal pulses. Skin is warm and dry. A routine ECG is obtained on arrival at the ED.

CLINICAL CHALLENGES AND QUESTIONS

1. What does this 12-lead ECG show?

2. How would you treat this patient?

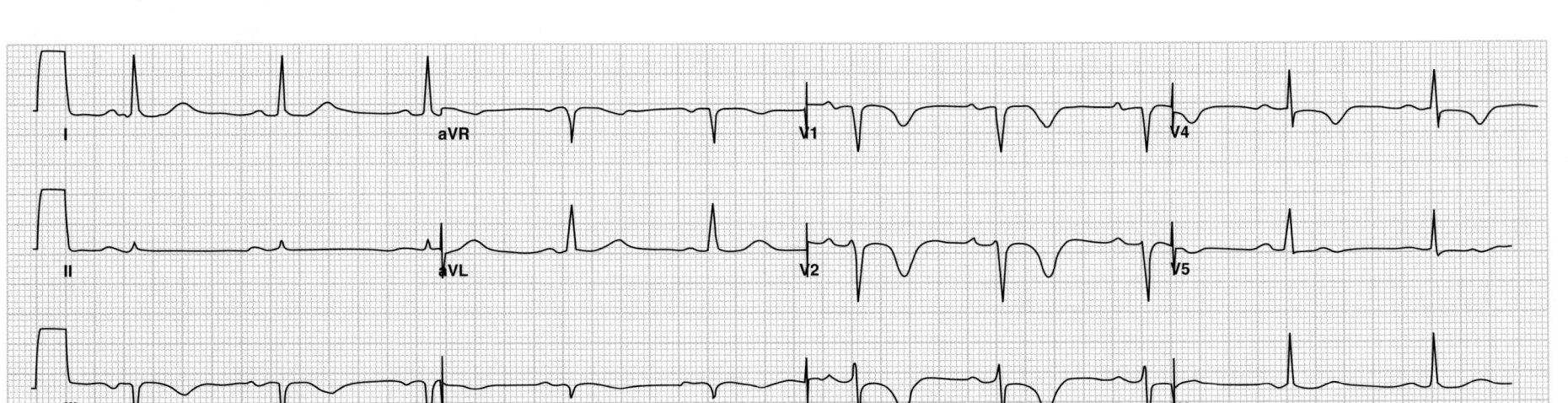

CHIEF COMPLAINT: Chest pain

HISTORY OF PRESENT ILLNESS	Advanced providers respond to a report of a 67-year-old male who is experiencing crushing chest pain. He rates the pain a 4 on a 10-point scale. He reports some mild nausea but no vomiting. He further explains that he had a similar episode the day before but that it subsided within several minutes.
PAST MEDICAL HISTORY	Hypertension, osteoporosis
MEDICATIONS	Metformin, vitamin D, calcium
ALLERGIES	None
VITAL SIGNS	BP: 110/70 mm Hg; P: 60 beats/min.; R: 16 breaths/min., nonlabored; SpO$_2$: 96%
EXAM	The patient is a well-developed, well-nourished 67-year-old male. Lung sounds are clear but diminished in all fields. He does not have any edema in the lower extremities. Distal pulses are 1+ bilaterally at the radial arteries. Skin is cool and clammy.

CLINICAL CHALLENGES AND QUESTIONS

1. What does this 12-lead ECG show?

2. How would you treat this patient?

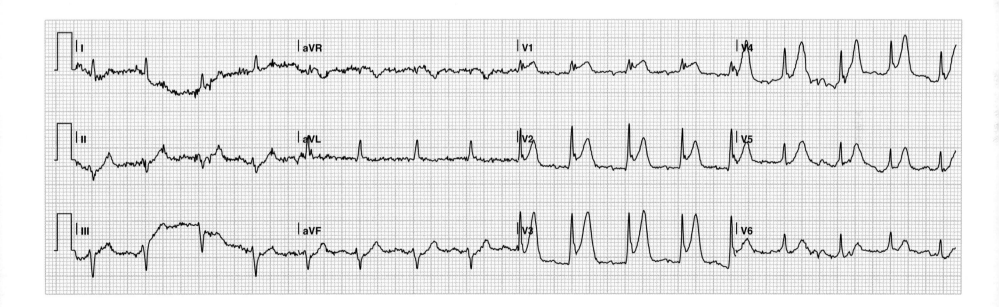

CASE 79   CHIEF COMPLAINT: Syncope

HISTORY OF PRESENT ILLNESS	Advanced providers respond to the report of a 63-year-old male who experienced a syncopal episode. He is now completely awake and apologizes for bothering you. The patient wants to decline further evaluation and treatment. He denies headache or vomiting, and admits only to slight "indigestion" and nausea.
PAST MEDICAL HISTORY	None
MEDICATIONS	None
ALLERGIES	Unknown
VITAL SIGNS	BP: 90/54 mm Hg, P: 40 beats/min., R: 20 breaths/min., SpO$_2$: 97%
EXAM	The patient is awake, alert, and oriented. Heart sounds are normal. Lung sounds are clear bilaterally. The abdomen is soft and nontender to palpation. Distal pulses are strong.

CLINICAL CHALLENGES AND QUESTIONS

1. What does this 12-lead ECG show?
2. How would you treat this patient?

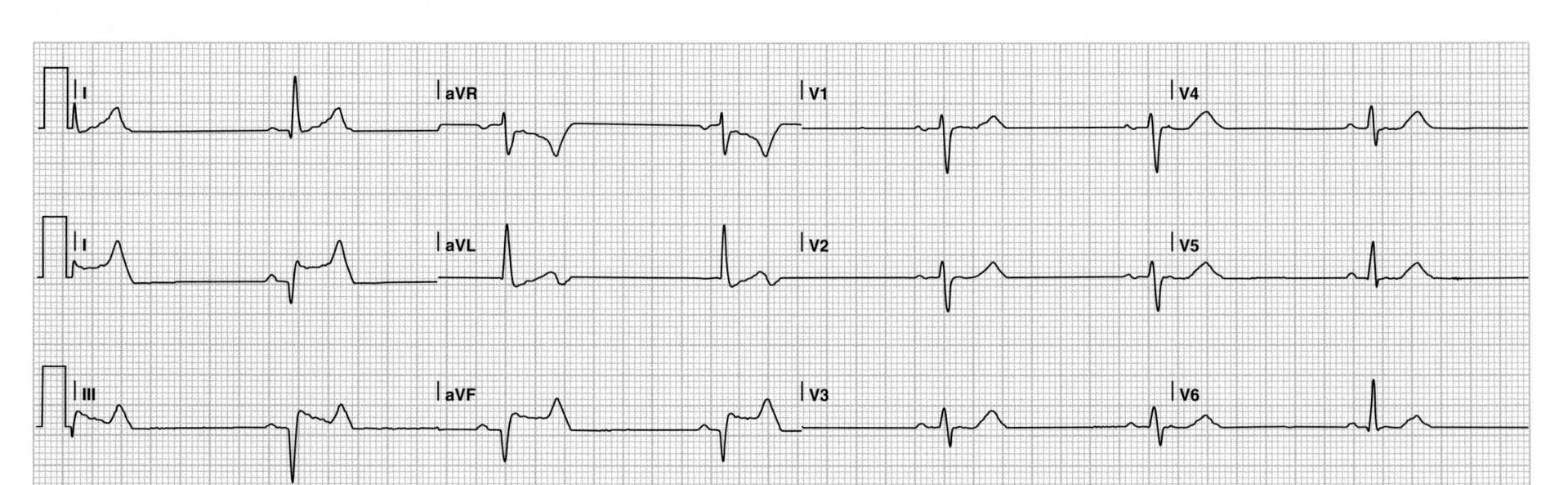

CHIEF COMPLAINT: Chest pain

HISTORY OF PRESENT ILLNESS	You arrive at the home of a 42-year-old male who has "burning in his chest." It started 2 days ago and since then has worsened progressively. The burning radiates to his back and is greatly relieved when he leans forward. The patient denies associated loss of consciousness or shortness of breath.
PAST MEDICAL HISTORY	HIV
MEDICATIONS	Lamivudine/zidovudine, enfuvirtide
ALLERGIES	None
VITAL SIGNS	T: 100.7 F, BP: 110/580 mm Hg, P: 60 beats/min., R: 18 breaths/min., SpO$_2$: 97%
EXAM	The patient is a cachectic adult male in mild to moderate distress when lying supine. He is awake, alert, and oriented. Heart sounds reveal a pericardial friction rub. Lung sounds are clear, and the abdomen is soft and nontender. Extremities are without edema. Radial pulses are strong and equal. Skin is warm and dry.

CLINICAL CHALLENGES AND QUESTIONS

1. What does this 12-lead ECG show?

2. How would you treat this patient?

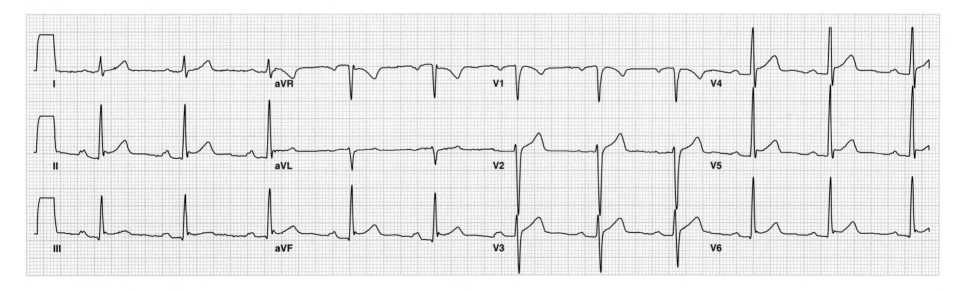

CASE 81   CHIEF COMPLAINT: Chest pain, nausea

HISTORY OF PRESENT ILLNESS	Advanced providers are transporting a 40-year-old male patient from a local cardiology office to the local community hospital for an emergent cardiac catheterization. The patient presented to his cardiologist's office approximately 30 minutes ago. He had chest pain, nausea, and diaphoresis. The cardiologist hands you the ECG shown below.
PAST MEDICAL HISTORY	Diabetes mellitus, hypertension, hyperlipidemia
MEDICATIONS	Baby aspirin, atorvastatin, atenolol, metformin
VITAL SIGNS	BP: 90/60 mm Hg, P: 60–70 beats/min., R: 20 breaths/min., SpO$_2$: 94% on nasal cannula at 2 L/min.
EXAM	The patient is ill appearing and neurologically intact. Lung sounds reveal crackles bilaterally. His abdomen is soft and nontender. No bilateral lower extremity edema. Skin is cool and wet.

CLINICAL CHALLENGES AND QUESTIONS

1. What does this 12-lead ECG show?

2. How would you treat this patient?

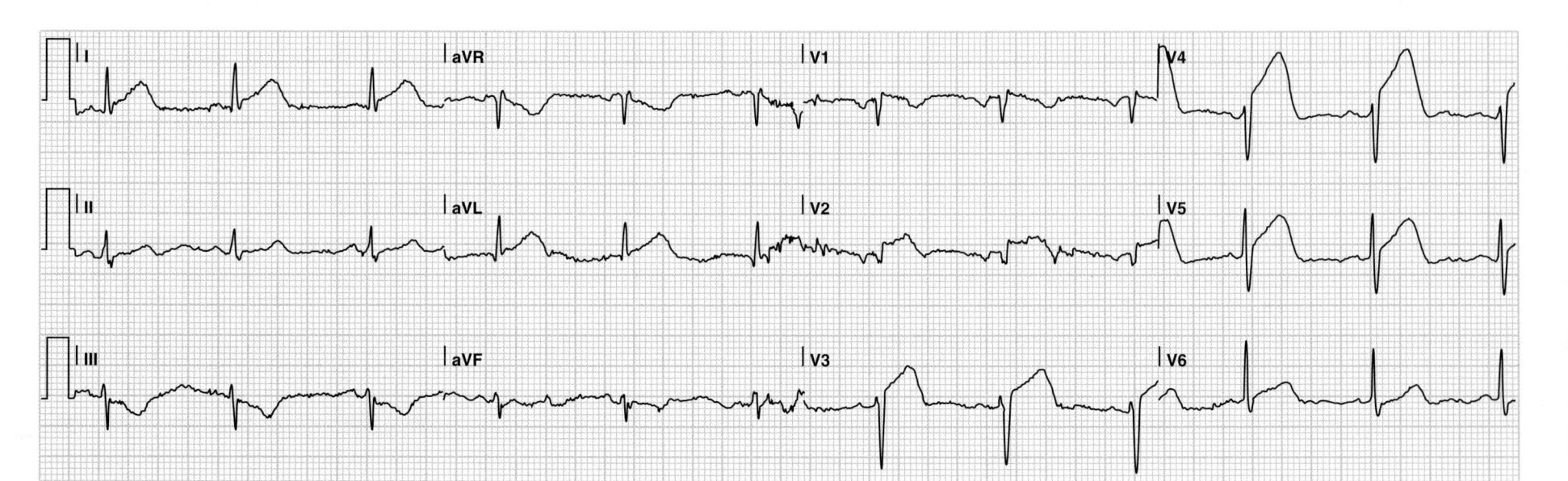

CHIEF COMPLAINT: Sharp chest pain

HISTORY OF PRESENT ILLNESS	Advanced providers arrive at a scene where a 19-year-old female reports sharp chest pain that began while she was lifting weights. The pain is currently a 6 on a 10-point scale. It gets worse with deep inspiration and localizes to the right anterior chest. The pain does not radiate to her arm, neck, or back. The patient has not experienced shortness of breath, nausea, or vomiting.
PAST MEDICAL HISTORY	None
MEDICATIONS	Oral contraceptives
ALLERGIES	None
VITAL SIGNS	BP: 118/66 mm Hg, P: 70 beats/min., R: 14 breaths/min., SpO$_2$: 97%
EXAM	The patient is an adult female in mild distress. She is alert and oriented. Heart sounds are normal. Her lung sounds are clear, and her abdomen is soft and nontender. Extremities are warm and well perfused. Upper extremity pulses are 2+ and strong. Skin is warm and dry. The patient's pain is reproducible with movement and palpation of the anterior chest wall.

CLINICAL CHALLENGES AND QUESTIONS

1. What does this 12-lead ECG show?

2. How would you treat this patient?

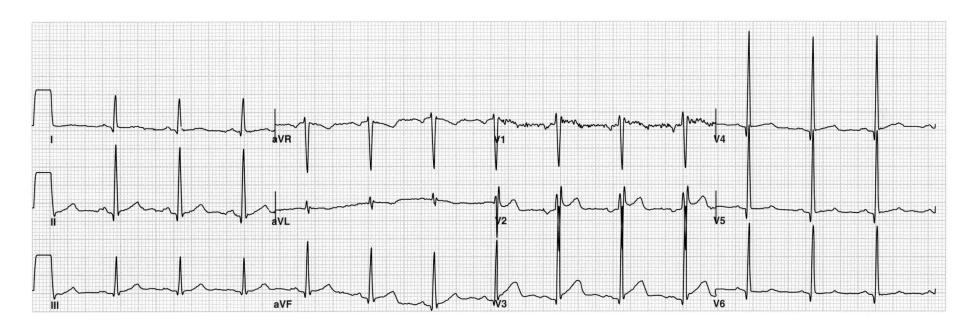

CASE 83

CHIEF COMPLAINT: Stomach burning

HISTORY OF PRESENT ILLNESS	A 40-year-old male comes to the emergency department after tripping on a curb and injuring his left shoulder. The patient has had left anterior chest wall discomfort since the injury. He denies other associated symptoms: shortness of breath, nausea, vomiting, or back pain. The patient is diagnosed with an anterior shoulder dislocation and requires a routine ECG before intravenous administration of a sedative and analgesic.
PAST MEDICAL HISTORY	Hypertension
MEDICATIONS	Atenolol
ALLERGIES	None
VITAL SIGNS	BP: 140/70 mm Hg, P: 48 beats/min., R: 12 breaths/min., SpO$_2$: 99%
EXAM	The patient is an adult male in mild distress secondary to pain. He is awake, alert, and oriented. Heart sounds are normal. He has bruising and ecchymosis localized to the left shoulder. Lung sounds are clear to auscultation bilaterally. The abdomen is nontender and nondistended. Extremities are without cyanosis or edema. There is swelling of the proximal left upper extremity with some obvious deformity. Radial pulses are 2+ and strong. Skin is warm and dry.

CLINICAL CHALLENGES AND QUESTIONS

1. What does this 12-lead ECG show?

2. How would you treat this patient?

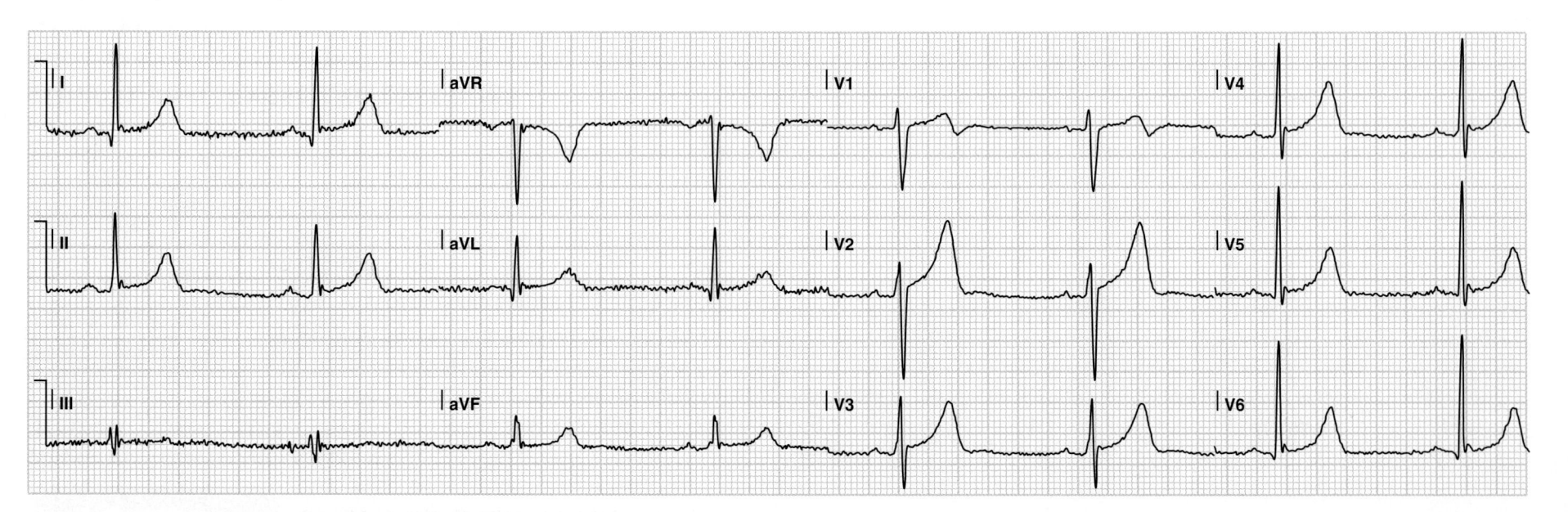

CHIEF COMPLAINT: Chest pain

HISTORY OF PRESENT ILLNESS	Advanced providers respond to the report of a 76-year-old male who is experiencing retrosternal chest pain. He recently finished shoveling snow after a storm. Despite resting on his couch for 30 minutes, he continued to experience chest pain. He also reports nausea and vomiting. He states that the pain radiates to his left arm and jaw.
PAST MEDICAL HISTORY	None, previously healthy
MEDICATIONS	None, vitamins
ALLERGIES	Seasonal allergies
VITAL SIGNS	BP: 138/82 mm Hg, P: 60s, R: 18 breaths/min., SpO$_2$, 99%
EXAM	The patient is a well-nourished male. His lung sounds are clear. The abdomen is distended. There is +1 pedal edema bilaterally. Skin is warm and dry.

CLINICAL CHALLENGES AND QUESTIONS

1. What does this 12-lead ECG show?

2. How would you treat this patient?

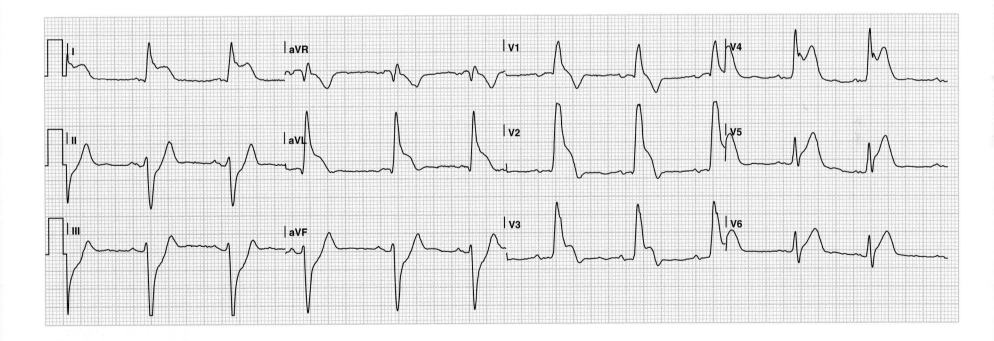

CASE 85

CHIEF COMPLAINT: Syncope

HISTORY OF PRESENT ILLNESS	You arrive at the home of an 85-year-old female who passed out after getting up from the dinner table. Between the time of the 9-1-1 call and your arrival, she recovered and now reports no illness. She denies chest pain, shortness of breath, nausea, or vomiting.
PAST MEDICAL HISTORY	None
MEDICATIONS	None
ALLERGIES	None
VITAL SIGNS	BP: 138/72 mm Hg, P: 70 beats/min., R: 12 breaths/min., SpO$_2$: 96%
EXAM	The patient is an elderly female who is awake, alert, and oriented. She responds appropriately to all questions. There are no obvious signs of trauma. Heart sounds are normal; lung sounds are clear to auscultation bilaterally. The abdomen is soft and nontender. Extremities are warm and well perfused. Strong distal pulses are present bilaterally. Skin is warm and dry.

CLINICAL CHALLENGES AND QUESTIONS

1. What does this 12-lead ECG show?

2. How would you treat this patient?

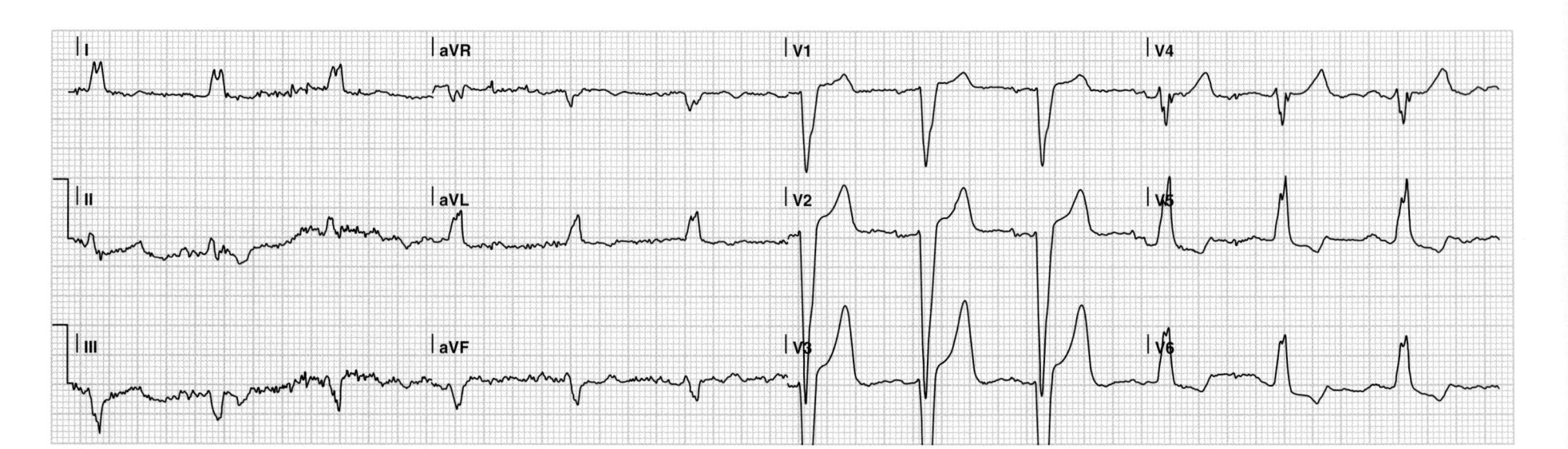

CHIEF COMPLAINT: Shortness of breath

HISTORY OF PRESENT ILLNESS	You are triaging a 40-year-old female who was brought in by ambulance. She reports mild shortness of breath and general malaise. She denies nausea, vomiting, sweating, or loss of consciousness.
PAST MEDICAL HISTORY	None
MEDICATIONS	Multivitamin
ALLERGIES	None
VITAL SIGNS	BP: 138/74 mm Hg, P: 60 beats/min., R: 18 breaths/min., SpO$_2$: 97%
EXAM	The patient is awake and alert. Heart sounds are normal. Lung sounds are clear bilaterally. The radial pulses are strong and equal. Skin is well perfused.

CLINICAL CHALLENGES AND QUESTIONS

1. What does this 12-lead ECG show?

2. How would you treat this patient?

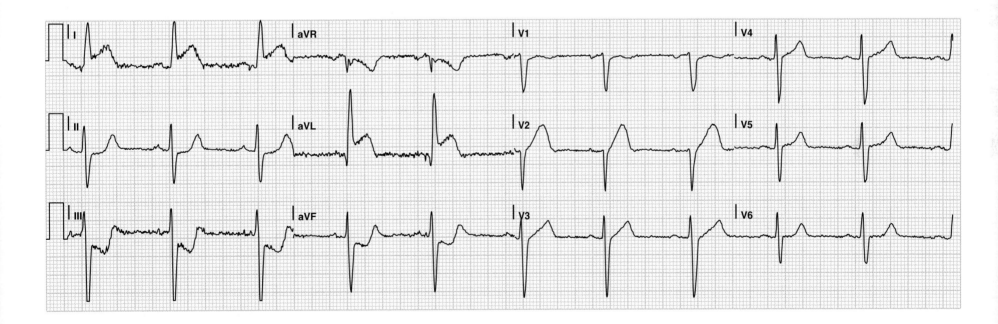

CASE 87

CHIEF COMPLAINT: Difficulty breathing

HISTORY OF PRESENT ILLNESS	Advanced providers arrive on the scene of an 84-year-old male experiencing shortness of breath.
PAST MEDICAL HISTORY	Chronic obstructive pulmonary disease
MEDICATIONS	Inhalers
ALLERGIES	None
VITAL SIGNS	BP: 108/74 mm Hg, P: 150s, R: 28 breaths/min., SpO$_2$: 93%
EXAM	The patient appears to be experiencing moderate respiratory distress. Heart sounds are irregular. Lung sounds are diminished with wheezes. Radial pulses are equal. The skin is cool and clammy.

CLINICAL CHALLENGES AND QUESTIONS

1. What does this rhythm strip show?

2. How would you treat this patient?

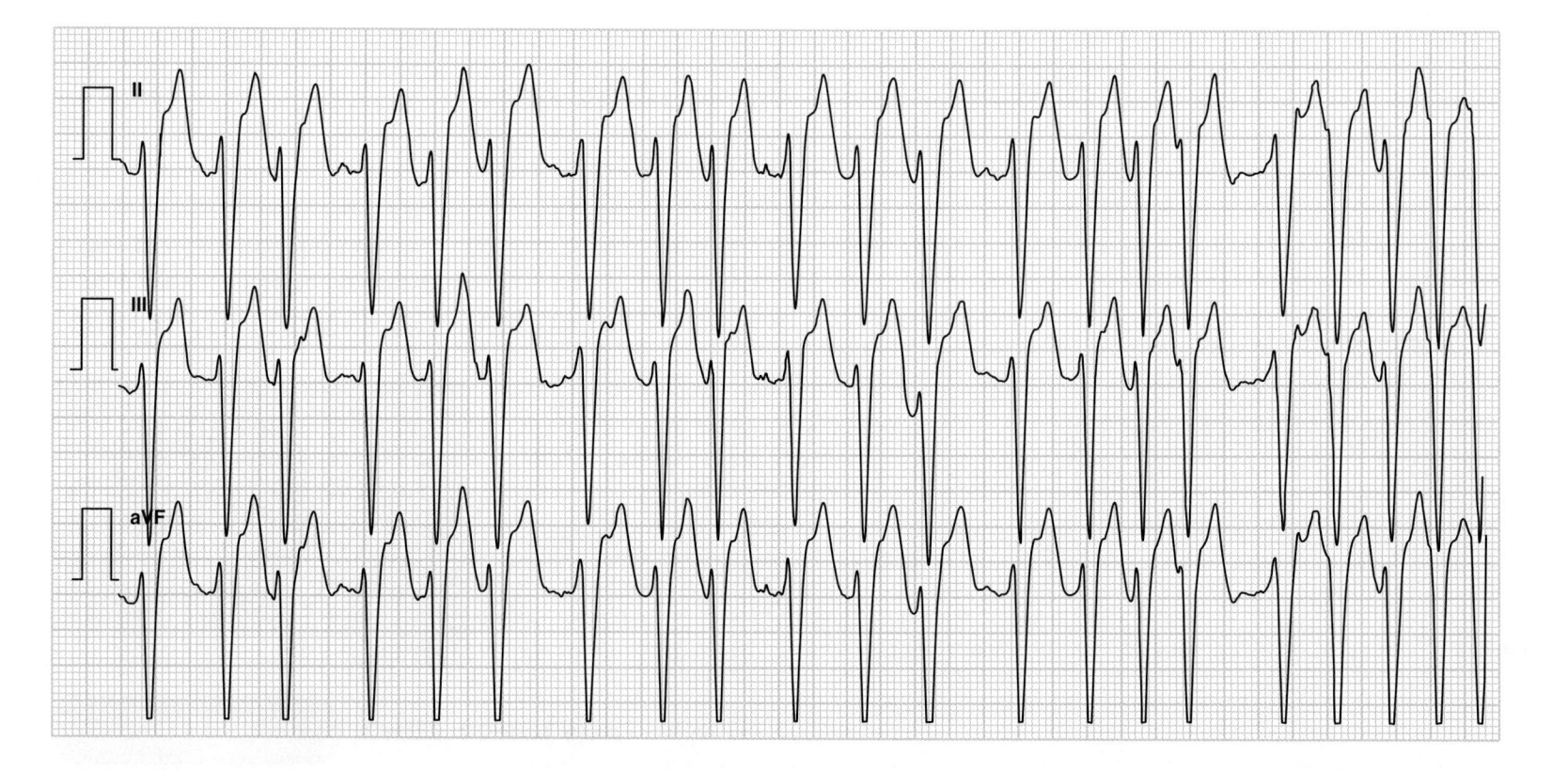

CHIEF COMPLAINT: Dizziness

HISTORY OF PRESENT ILLNESS	A 37-year-old male calls emergency medical services and reports lightheadedness that occurred while he was doing yard work. His symptoms went away after sitting down for approximately 5 minutes. He denies any chest pain, blurry vision, shortness of breath, diaphoresis, or loss of consciousness. He states that he has experienced similar symptoms in the past, but never this severe. He is feeling much better now, and does not want to go the hospital.
PAST MEDICAL HISTORY	None
MEDICATIONS	None
ALLERGIES	None
VITAL SIGNS	BP: 125/80 mm Hg, P: 40 beats/min., R: 18 breaths/min, SpO$_2$: 98%
EXAM	The patient is a young-appearing male, in no acute respiratory distress. He is alert and oriented. Heart sounds are normal. The abdomen is soft and nontender. Extremities are without cyanosis, clubbing, or edema. Radial and dorsalis pedis pulses are equal but irregular to palpation. Skin is warm and dry.

CLINICAL CHALLENGES AND QUESTIONS

1. What does this 12-lead ECG show?

2. How would you treat this patient?

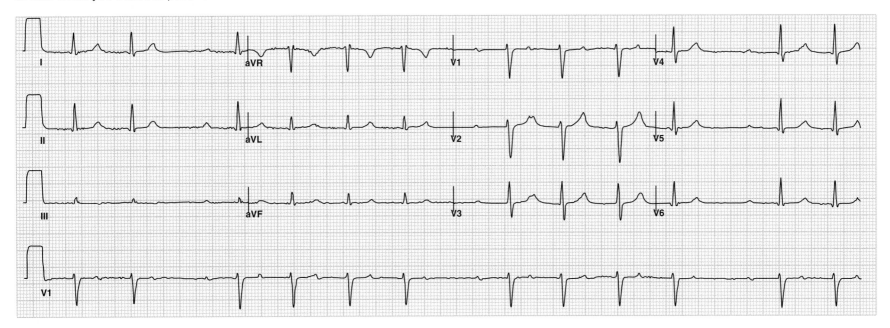

CASE 89   CHIEF COMPLAINT: Chest pain

HISTORY OF PRESENT ILLNESS	A 67-year-old male calls emergency medical services and reports that he has had constant substernal chest pain for 45 minutes. He describes the pain as a "heaviness," which he associates with lingering discomfort in the right shoulder. The patient feels somewhat anxious and appears diaphoretic. He denies nausea, vomiting, or shortness of breath. Further questions about the man's medical history reveal 3 days of intermittent chest pain and shortness of breath related to minimal exertion and relieved after 15–20 minutes of rest. The patient has not previously experienced these symptoms.
PAST MEDICAL HISTORY	Hypertension, hyperlipidemia
MEDICATIONS	HCTZ, simvastatin
ALLERGIES	None
VITAL SIGNS	BP: 180/90mm Hg, P: 80 beats/min, R: 24 breaths/min., SpO$_2$: 98%
EXAM	The patient is an anxious-appearing male in no acute respiratory distress. He is alert and oriented. Heart sounds are normal. Radial and dorsalis pedis pulses are equal throughout. Lungs are clear; chest wall is without retraction or tenderness. Abdomen is soft and nontender. Extremities are without cyanosis or clubbing. There is no lower extremity edema or calf tenderness. Strong distal pulses are present, and the skin is well perfused.

CLINICAL CHALLENGES AND QUESTIONS

1. What does this 12-lead ECG show?
2. How would you treat this patient?

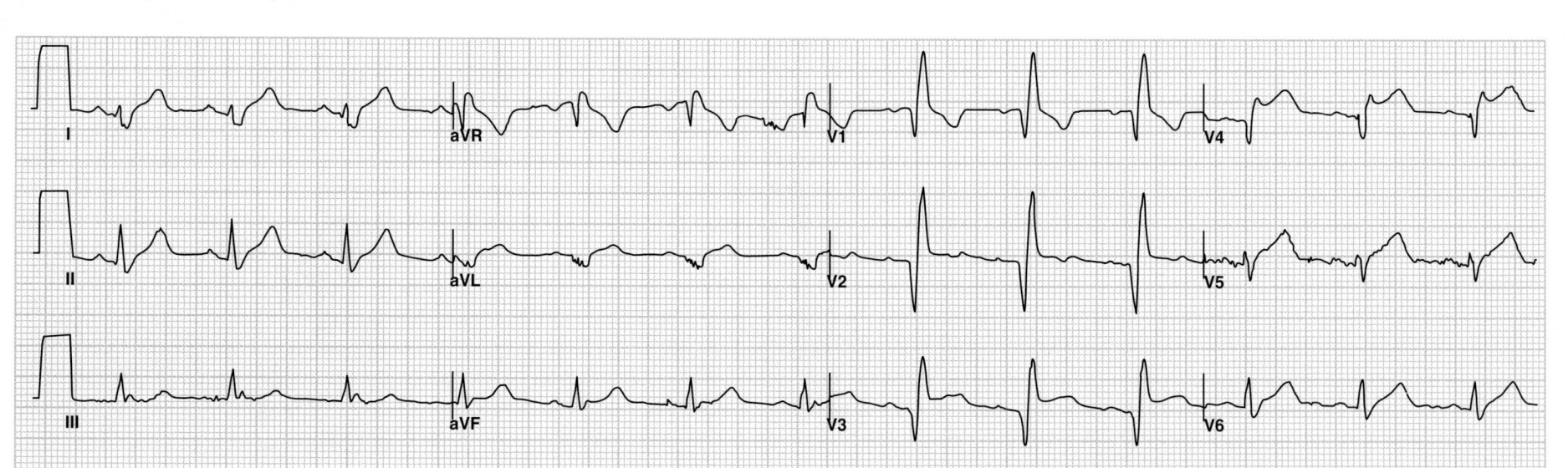

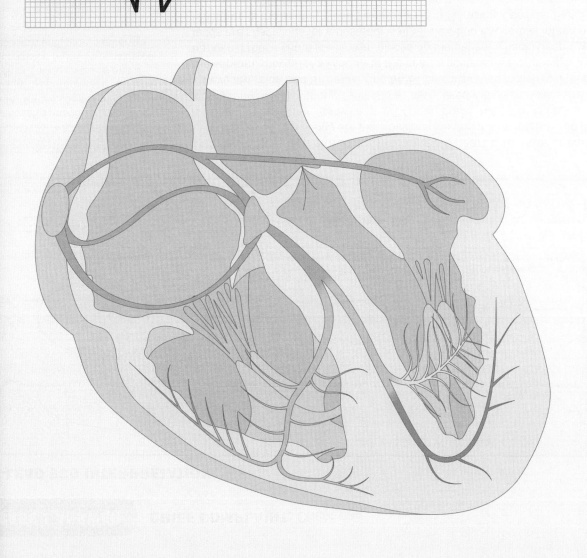

ECG Answers

CASE 1 ANSWER   CHIEF COMPLAINT: Chest pain

12-LEAD ECG INTERPRETATION

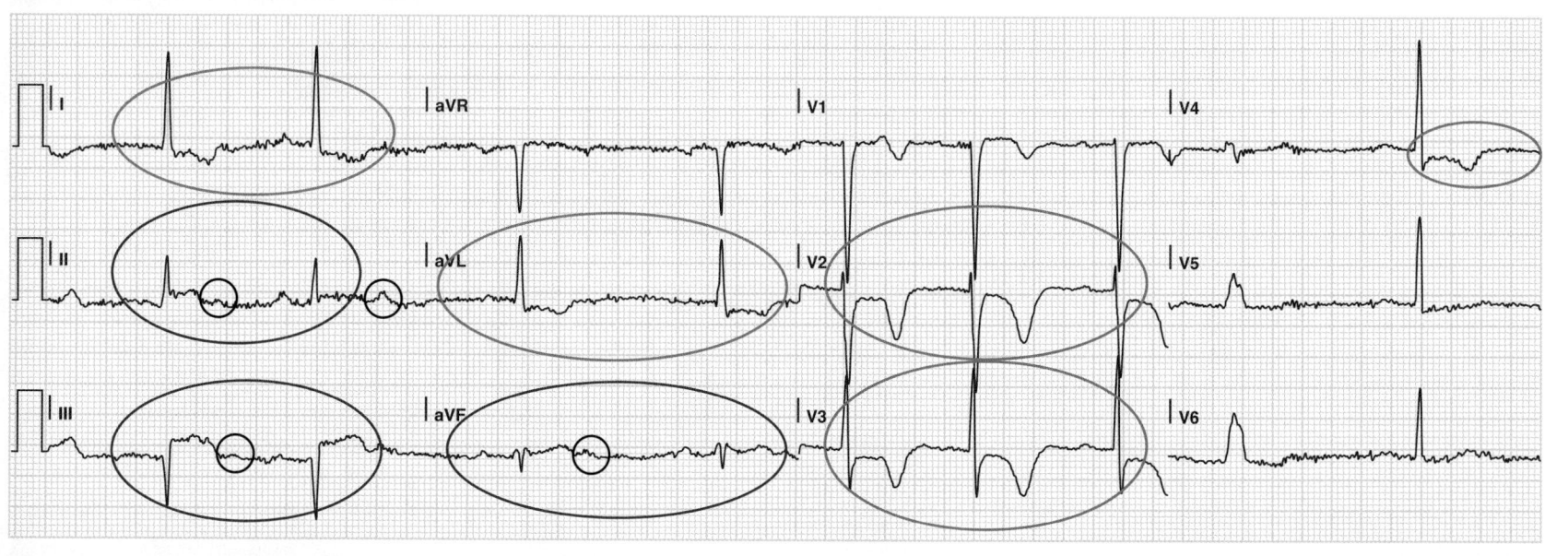

Undetermined (non-sinus) rhythm, variable heart rate, inferior wall STEMI with possible posterior wall extension.

In this case, ST elevations are most obvious in inferior limb leads II and III, and minimally in aVF (*red ovals*). The expected reciprocal changes appear in leads I and aVL (*green ovals*). Note that leads V_2, V_3, and V_4 demonstrate T wave inversion and ST depression (*green ovals*). Although sometimes associated with "ventricular strain" in the setting of hypertrophy, the combination of T wave inversion and ST depression MUST be considered ischemic until proved otherwise. Because V_2 and V_3 are situated over the septum, they offer a window to the heart's posterior wall. Although V_2 and V_3 clearly show ST depression, imagine what would happen if those same leads were placed on the patient's back. Deep T wave inversions with concurrent depression in the septal leads are suspicious for a posterior wall ST elevation myocardial infarction (STEMI)! Without question, the most important point to recognize is the acutely ischemic-appearing ECG tracing. Consider that ST depression in septal and precordial leads (V_1 through V_3) may actually represent ST elevation on the heart's posterior surface. An accurate assessment of the underlying rhythm is not possible without an additional rhythm strip. Hospital personnel might acquire a posterior ECG by placing the V_1 and V_2 leads on the patient's back. This patient requires rapid transport to the cardiac catheterization lab.

A detailed examination of the inferior leads reveals the presence of nonconducted P waves (*black circles*). Sinus rhythm, by definition, exhibits a 1:1 P-to-QRS ratio in addition to a constant P-R interval. Of greater importance to the prehospital provider is the identification of acute infarction.

The emergency department paramedic expedites this patient's transfer to the acute care area. While awaiting the arrival of the interventional cardiology team, the paramedic starts two large-bore intravenous lines, obtains a portable chest film, and administers 162 mg of chewable aspirin. Nitroglycerin is administered for ischemic chest pain, and the patient receives one dose of fentanyl for continuing discomfort.

12-LEAD ECG INTERPRETATION

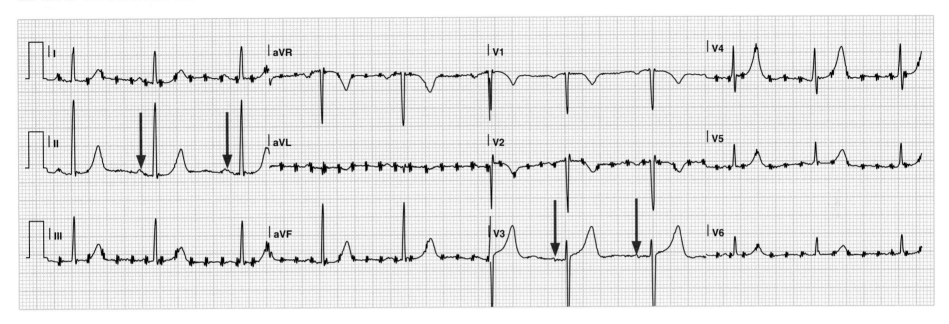

CLINICAL PEARL

Transcutaneous electrical nerve stimulation devices, audio equipment, and cellular phones have all been reported to cause ECG artifacts.

Sinus rhythm, heart rate: 60 beats/min., artifact resembling pacemaker spikes.

"Spikes" are noted on the tracing and occur at a rate of approximately 300 beats/min. Close inspection of leads II, V_1, and V_3 (*red arrows*) reveals normal P waves. The QRS and T wave morphology are also normal and suggest an interpretation of sinus rhythm. Spikes are often indicative of a functioning implanted pacemaker. However, other sources of electromagnetic interference can create artifacts resembling pacemaker spikes on the ECG. In this case, the artifact was determined to originate from the patient's cell phone. Transcutaneous electrical nerve stimulation devices, audio equipment, and cellular phones have all been reported to cause ECG artifacts. Remember to challenge unexpected findings on ECGs, especially if the findings are inconsistent with the clinical context.

CASE 3 ANSWER   CHIEF COMPLAINT: Unresponsiveness

12-LEAD ECG INTERPRETATION

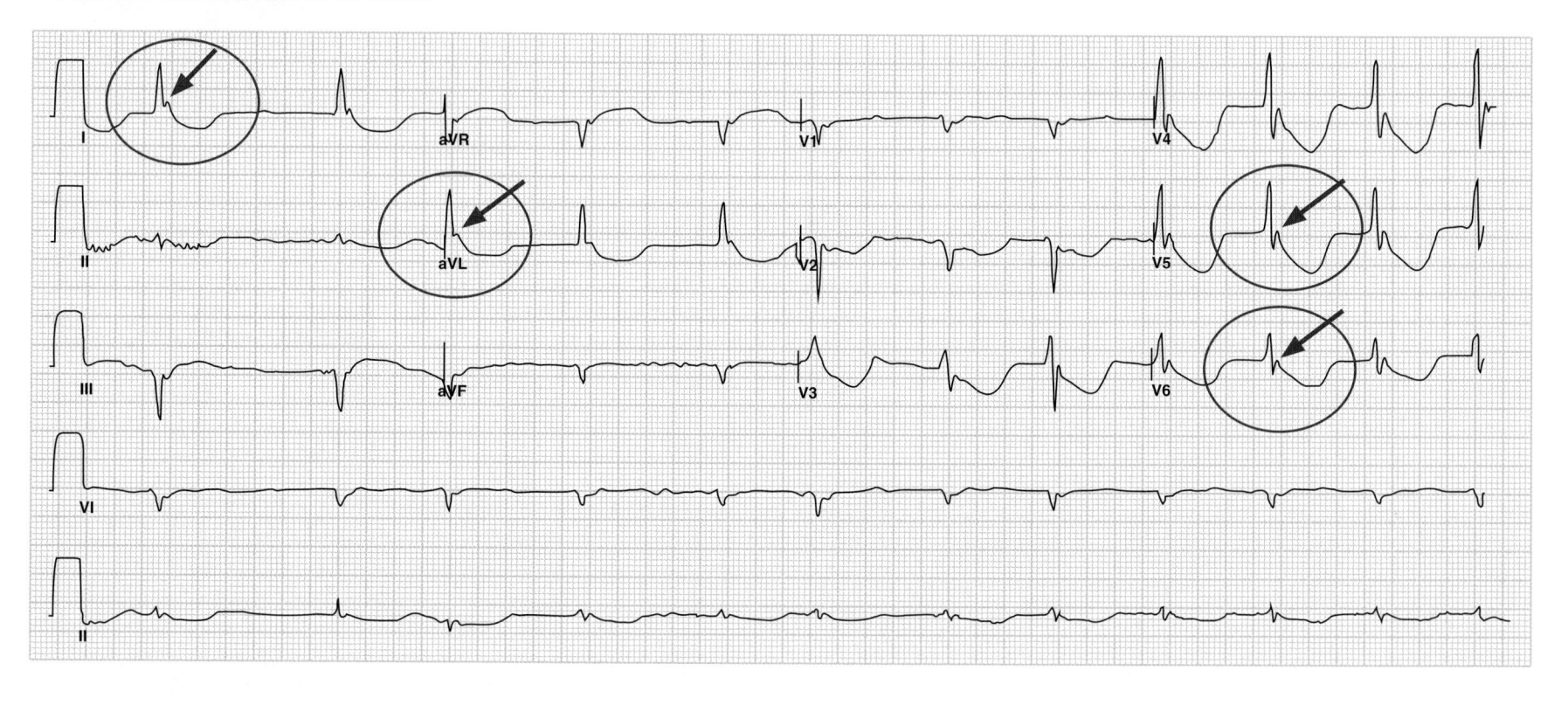

Atrial fibrillation, heart rate: 60–69 beats/min., prolonged QT interval, presence of Osborn waves, ECG consistent with hypothermia.
There are no clearly defined P waves; the rhythm is irregular and the baseline appears to show fine (low-amplitude) atrial fibrillation. The atrial fibrillation with a relatively slow ventricular response, the long QT segment, and the presence of Osborn waves (*arrows*) confirm the electrocardiographic diagnosis of hypothermia. QT intervals longer than 500 ms predispose patients to dysrhythmias. Because hypothermia can prolong cardiac repolarization, it is important to minimize stimuli and interventions. The Osborn wave is the "hump" that appears after the QRS complex. It is usually a small positive deflection highly suggestive of hypothermia. Hypothermia causes many types of electrocardiographic abnormalities, including atrial fibrillation with a slow ventricular response, slow junctional rhythms, and prolongation of all intervals. Tachy-cardia can develop during rewarming. The diagnosis is best confirmed through measurement of core body temperature.

Because this patient has a palpable pulse, you opt for conservative treatment. The myocardium is susceptible to dysrhythmias, so patients should be handled gently. You remove the wet clothes, apply warm blankets, and drive cautiously to the emergency department. On arrival, the patient's core temperature measures 85°F. Several liters of warmed intravenous fluids are administered, as well as warmed, humidified oxygen via mask. The patient is placed on a warming blanket, and a Foley catheter is inserted to measure urine output. Hypothermia may induce cold diuresis, so patients are often volume depleted.

12-LEAD ECG INTERPRETATION

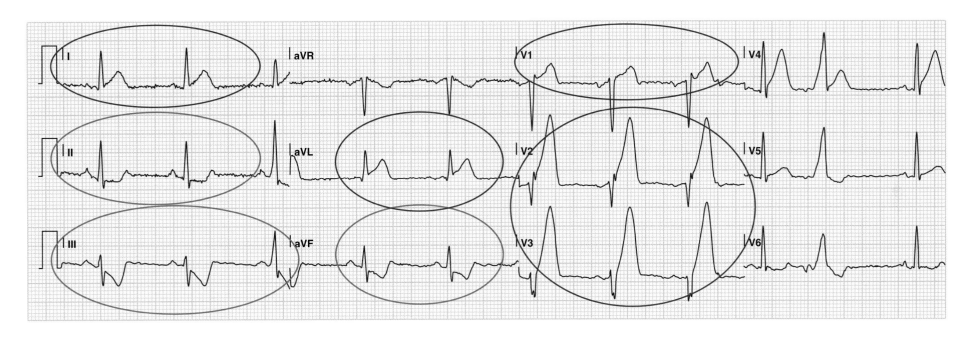

CLINICAL PEARL

Although they are often a sign of hyperkalemia, tall ("hyperacute") T waves are also commonly seen in patients with early ischemia after MI.

Sinus rhythm, heart rate: 60–70 beats/min., anterior lateral wall STEMI.

The ECG indicates an anterior lateral wall myocardial infarction. The characteristic ST elevation typical of left anterior descending (LAD) artery occlusion is present. ST elevation is noted in V_1 (*red oval*), and in V_2 and V_3 (*red circle*), consistent with anterior wall infarction, and in leads I and aVL (*red oval*), consistent with lateral wall infarction. Reciprocal changes are present in the inferior leads II, III, and aVF (*green ovals*). The T waves in V_2 and V_3 are disproportionately large and peaked. Although often a sign of hyperkalemia, tall ("hyperacute") T waves are also commonly seen in patients with early ischemia after myocardial infarction (MI) (see the appendix " Comparison of T Wave Morphology in Hyperkalemia and in AMI"). In this case, the alert emergency department triage medic expedited the patient's transfer to the cardiac catheterization laboratory.

CASE 5 ANSWER   CHIEF COMPLAINT: Syncope

12-LEAD ECG INTERPRETATION

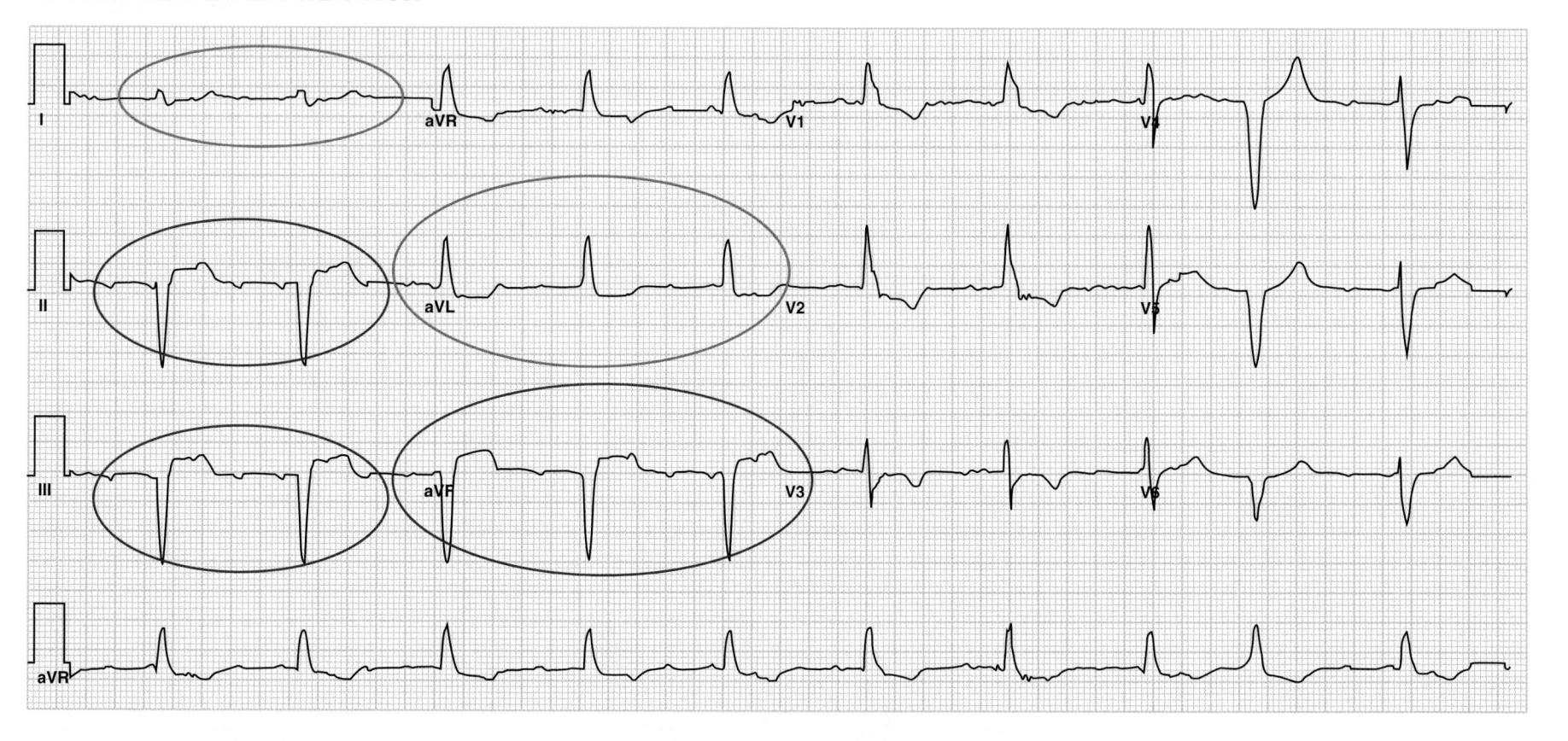

Third-degree heart block, heart rate: approximately 60 beats/min., inferior wall STEMI.

This patient's ECG demonstrates several troubling findings. It is clear that the underlying rhythm is no longer sinus in origin. The R-R intervals are regular, but there is no consistent PR interval. You are appropriately concerned about the development of a third-degree block. Furthermore, ST elevations are present in the inferior limb leads II, III, and aVF (*red ovals*). Reciprocal changes are present in leads I and aVL (*green ovals*). Subtle ST depression begins in V_2, and there is an ischemic, inverted T wave in V_3. These ominous changes also raise the possibility of right ventricular or posterior wall involvement. The patient has the potential to become hemodynamically unstable and to deteriorate during transport. Although the patient cannot remain in a free-standing emergency department, certain interventions should be considered before transport.

Because the patient remains awake, alert, and oriented, the emergency department physician decides against insertion of a transvenous pacer. Pacer pads are applied prophylactically to the patient's chest, and a bolus of heparin is administered as you move the patient onto the transport stretcher. A second large-bore intravenous line is established in anticipation of the hypotension that may accompany an inferior wall myocardial infarction. The emergency department physician communicates the change in patient status to the receiving facility, and your crew is instructed to proceed directly to the catheterization lab. The patient is found to have diffuse coronary artery disease with a new, nearly complete occlusion of the right coronary artery.

12-LEAD ECG INTERPRETATION

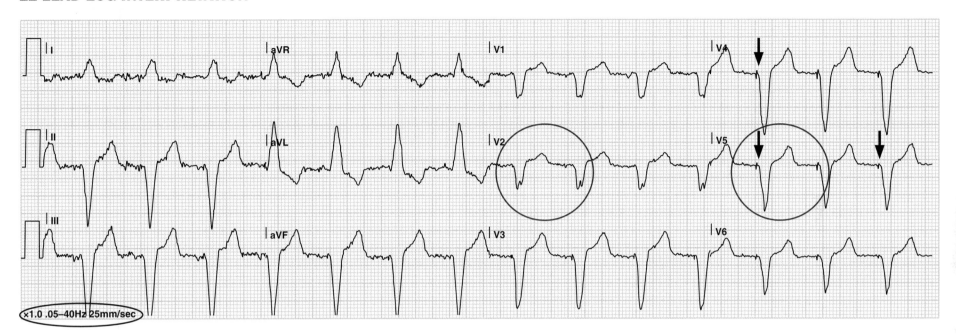

×1.0 .05–40Hz 25mm/sec

Paced ventricular rhythm, heart rate: 80 beats/min.

The ECG reveals a paced ventricular rhythm. Pacemaker "spikes" are often difficult to see. The average pacemaker signal frequency is in the range of 150–250 Hz. The ECG shown above reflects signals between 0.05 and 40 Hz (*black oval*), so the higher-frequency signals of the pacemaker are "missed." Close inspection of the left precordial leads reveals small spikes just before the QRS complex (*black arrows*). Note the direction of the QRS complexes in the precordial leads: all six leads exhibit a pattern of QRS concordance (i.e., all QRS complexes are deflected in the same direction) (*red circles*). This is highly suggestive of a ventricular rhythm (in this case, an artificially initiated ventricular rhythm). The QRS complexes and T waves exhibit a pattern of discordance (T waves are deflected in an opposite direction from the QRS complex).

Paced ventricular rhythms are considered STEMI mimics because they alter the appearance of the ST segment and pose challenges to the diagnosis of acute cardiac ischemia. In patients with troubling presentations or symptoms, always consider ST elevation as a presentation of ischemia until proved otherwise.

This patient is transported to the closest emergency department. Previous ECGs on file at the hospital reveal no change in interval.

CASE 7 ANSWER   CHIEF COMPLAINT: Syncope

12-LEAD ECG INTERPRETATION

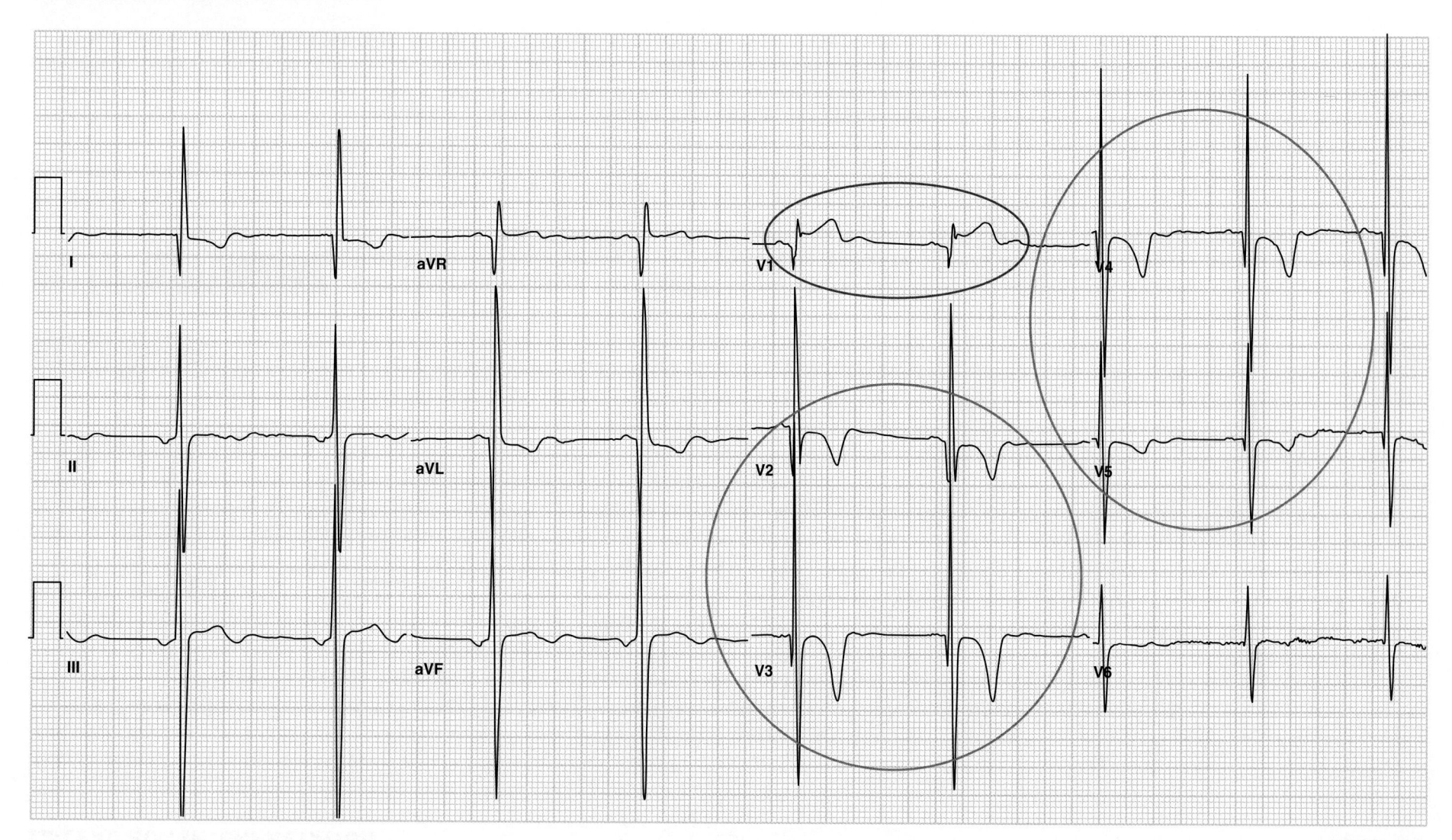

(Continued)

CHIEF COMPLAINT: Syncope

Sinus rhythm, heart rate: 50–60 beats/min., ST elevation in lead V$_1$ with ST depression and T wave inversions in leads V$_2$–V$_5$.

The ECG reveals a sinus rhythm. Isolated ST elevation is seen in lead V$_1$ (*red oval*). T wave inversions and ST segment depressions are visible across the precordium (*green circles*). These findings suggest active ischemia until proved otherwise, even though coronary artery disease is unlikely in a young man without comorbidities, such as diabetes or hypertension. The presence of syncope coupled with the electrocardiographic changes should always prompt rapid treatment and transport.

The deep, narrow Q waves in leads I and aVL, the high ventricular voltage, and the ST segment changes suggest hypertrophic cardiomyopathy (HCM). The condition causes septal wall thickening and enlargement of the left ventricle. The most devastating presentation of HCM is sudden cardiac death. Patients presenting with syncopal symptoms are at great risk for lethal dysrhythmia. Patients with HCM are generally diagnosed in their 30s and may present with chest pain, dyspnea on exertion, and other angina-like symptoms. This patient's presentation is particularly worrisome because the syncopal episode may have been secondary to ventricular tachycardia.

The patient is currently symptom free. You apply ECG leads, administer oxygen, and transport him to a cardiac receiving center. In the hospital, a two-dimensional echocardiogram confirms the diagnosis of ventricular hypertrophy. This patient receives a pacemaker-defibrillator during his hospital stay.

Hypertrophic cardiomyopathy may alter P-wave morphology as well as ST-T segment appearance. ECG changes associated with HCM include shortening of the P-R interval, the presence of etopic atrial rhythms, and sinus bradycardia.

CASE 8 ANSWER   **CHIEF COMPLAINT:** Chest pain

12-LEAD ECG INTERPRETATION

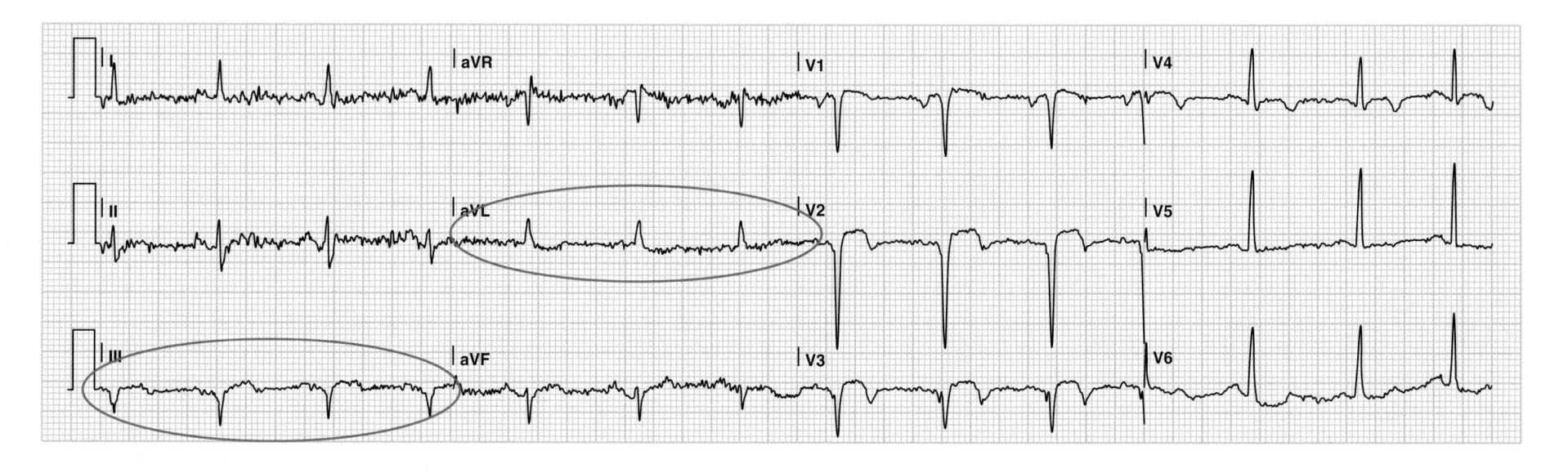

Sinus rhythm, heart rate: 80 beats/min., ST elevation in leads V$_2$–V$_3$, T wave inversion in anterior and lateral leads.
This ECG's findings are subtle but important. The ECG does not meet the strict criteria for diagnosis of an ST elevation myocardial infarction (STEMI). To diagnose STEMI, you must have at least 2 mm of elevation in the precordial leads and at least 1 mm of elevation in the limb leads. A pathologic Q wave is present in lead III (*green oval*), and a downsloping ST segment is present in aVL (*green oval*). Baseline artifact interferes with more detailed analysis.

The ST elevation in V$_2$ is horizontal in appearance. Minimal ST elevation is present in V$_3$, as is terminal T wave inversion. The constellation of ECG abnormalities, in conjunction with the patient's appearance, prompts you to transmit the ECG and contact medical control.

Medical control agrees with the decision to transport the patient to a cardiac referral center. The patient undergoes emergent coronary angiography and is found to have an acute occlusion of the left anterior descending coronary artery.

CHIEF COMPLAINT: Chest pain

12-LEAD ECG INTERPRETATION

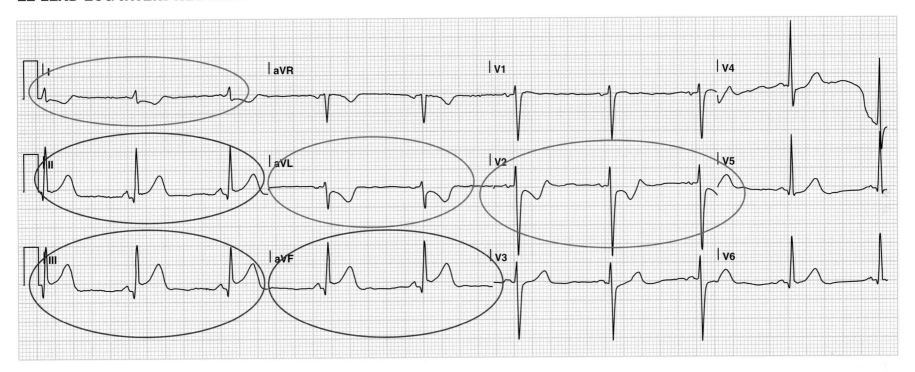

Sinus rhythm, heart rate: 50–60 beats/min., inferior wall STEMI.

ST elevations are demonstrated in leads II, III, and aVF (*red ovals*). Reciprocal changes are noted in leads I, aVL, and V$_2$ (*green ovals*). This ECG is consistent with an inferior wall ST elevation myocardial infarction (STEMI). Also note the ST segment and T wave changes in lead V$_2$. The isolated changes in lead V$_2$ may be caused by posterior wall involvement or reciprocal change associated with the inferior wall STEMI.

(*Continued*)

CASE 9 ANSWER   CHIEF COMPLAINT: Chest pain

You expeditiously transport the patient to the regional cardiac referral center. En route, you administer oxygen and record another 12-lead ECG (see below).

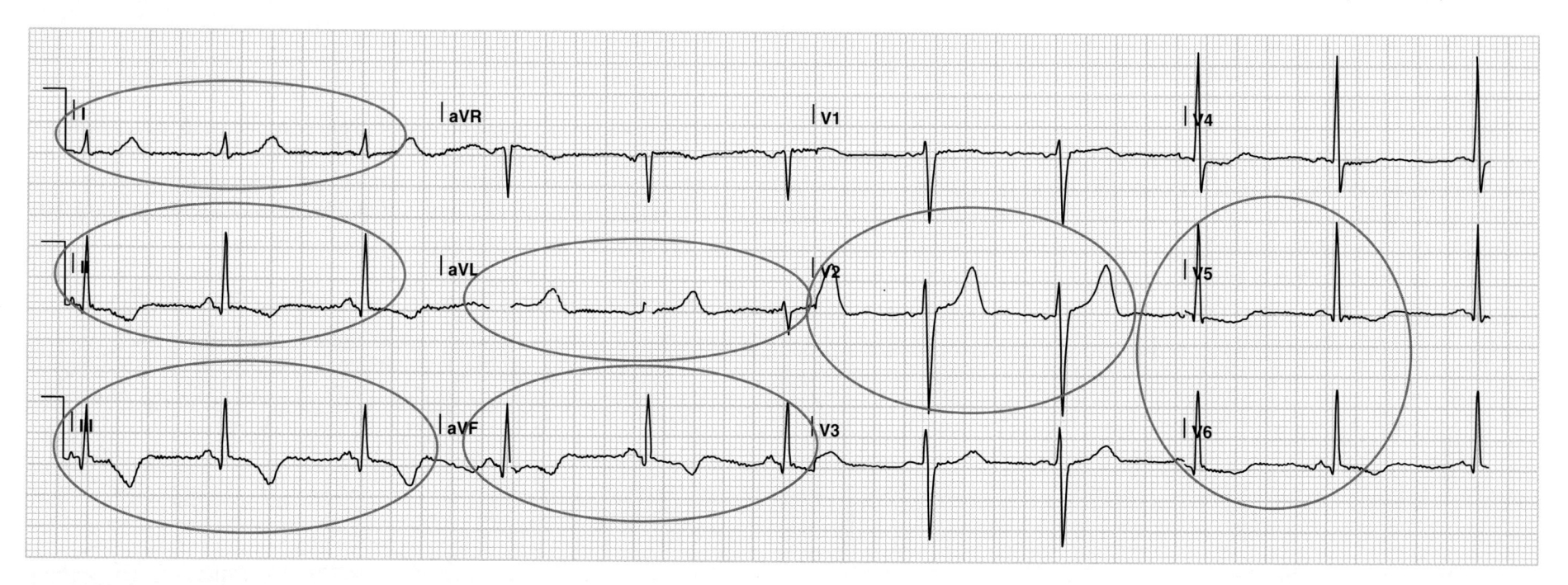

The repeat ECG reveals ST depression and T wave inversion in the inferior leads. All ST segment elevation seems to have completely resolved during transport. ST depression and T wave inversion previously seen in leads I, aVL, and V_2 also seem to have normalized. The patient reports the chest pain has eased and rates the current pain as 2 on a 10-point scale. This case illustrates the importance of recording serial ECGs throughout transport. It also demonstrates the importance of recording a 12-lead ECG during the initial minutes of patient contact. Had the crew waited 10–15 minutes to record the initial ECG, the STEMI would have been missed completely!

Vasospasm and constriction can induce ST segment changes. The persistent ST depression in the inferior leads is suggestive of ongoing ischemia. This patient undergoes emergent cardiac catheterization at the receiving facility. The patient is diagnosed with an occlusion of the right coronary artery.

RHYTHM STRIP INTERPRETATION

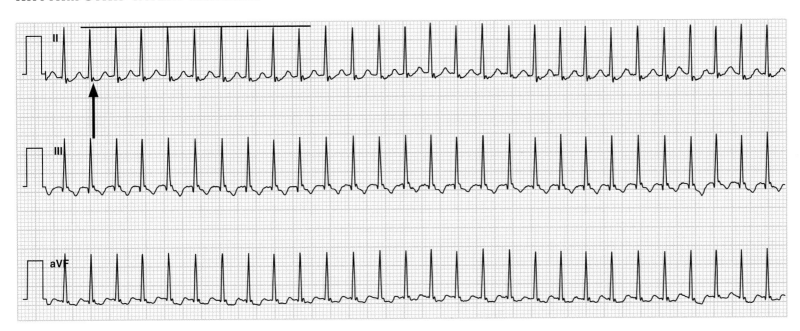

Supraventricular tachycardia, heart rate in the 210s.

A narrow complex, supraventricular tachycardia (SVT) is noted on the rhythm strip. Close inspection reveals P waves immediately following the QRS complex, which is suggestive of a specific type of SVT called atrioventricular nodal reentry tachycardia (AVNRT). The atrioventricular (AV) node is designed to allow electrical messages to be transmitted only from the atria to the ventricles. Pathology of the AV node can alter the flow of electricity, allowing transmission of impulses from the ventricles to the atria. When messages re-enter and depolarize the atria, a retrograde P wave (*black arrow*) appears on the rhythm strip. Another finding that favors the diagnosis of AVNRT is the presence of electrical alternans. Electrical alternans is characterized by alternating QRS complex amplitude (*horizontal black line*). In this case, the alternating amplitudes were caused by cardiac motion and were essentially artifacts generated as the heart swung inside the chest. Management of SVT depends on the patient's clinical presentation. Patients with unstable vital signs or changes in mental status are candidates for electrical cardioversion. Hemodynamically stable patients may benefit from vagal maneuvers or the administration of AV nodal blocking agents such as adenosine.

CASE 11 ANSWER   CHIEF COMPLAINT: Chest pain

12-LEAD ECG INTERPRETATION

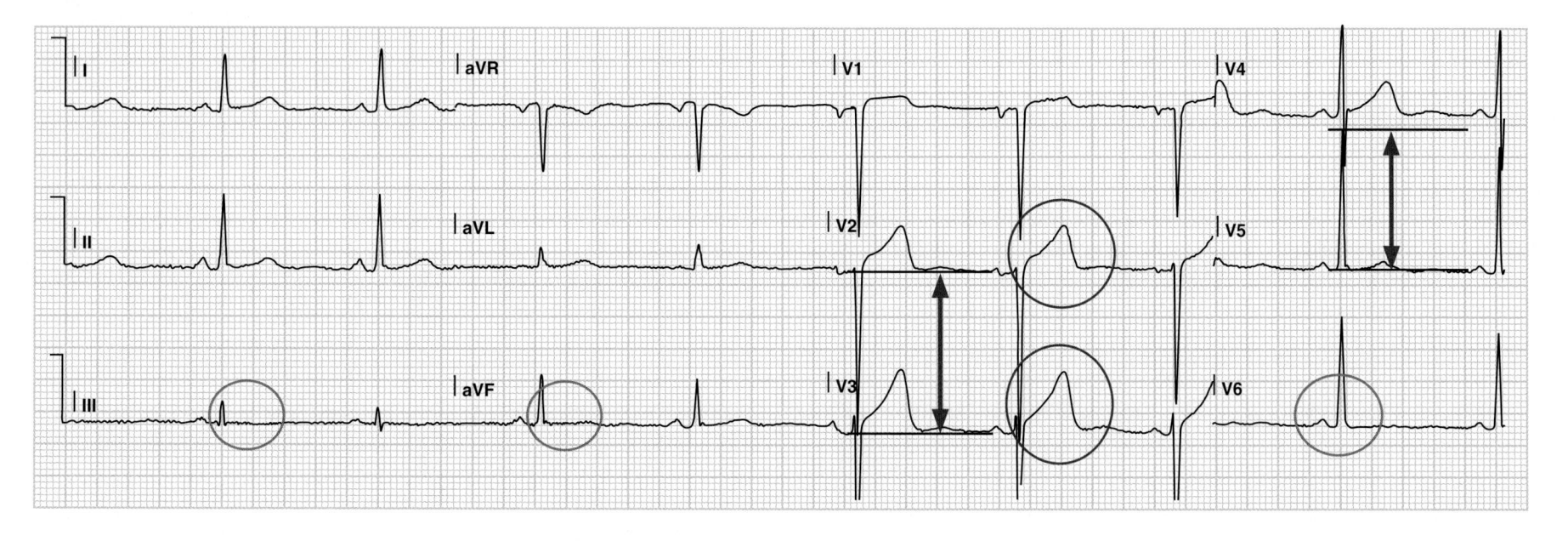

Sinus rhythm, heart rate: 60 beats/min., left ventricular hypertrophy.

Voltage criteria for left ventricular hypertrophy (LVH) are seen in this example (see the appendix "Diagnostic Criteria for Sgarbossa, LVH, and LBBB"). Note the large discordant ST elevation and upright T waves in V_2 and V_3 (*red circles*), which are characteristic repolarization abnormalities found in LVH. The tall R and deep S waves (*red arrows*) represent high left ventricular voltage. Flat ST segments are seen in the inferior and lateral leads (*green circles*). Although commonly thought of as a "non-specific" change, diffuse ST segment flattening may occur in the setting of ischemia. Approximately 40% of initial ECGs in patients with acute coronary syndromes are interpreted as either normal or nonspecific.

You consult medical control and begin transport. En route to the hospital, you administer aspirin, nitroglycerin, and oxygen. A repeat ECG performed in the ambulance reveals no ST or T wave changes. The patient is admitted to the hospital for further diagnostic testing.

12-LEAD ECG INTERPRETATION

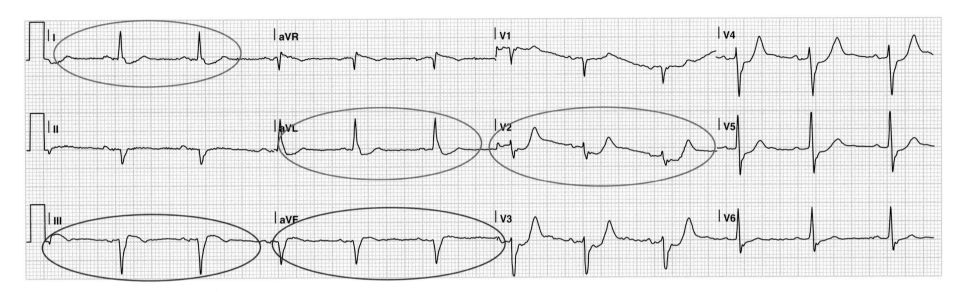

Sinus rhythm, heart rate: 60–70 beats/min., inferior wall STEMI with possible posterior wall extension.

This ECG demonstrates mild ST elevation in leads III and aVF (*red ovals*). Deep Q waves also appear in these inferior leads. Reciprocal changes are present in leads I and aVL (*green ovals*). ST depression is evident in V_1 and V_2. These might be reciprocal changes, but they might also represent signs of posterior infarction. If a posterior ECG was performed by placing leads on the patient's left mid-back, they would demonstrate ST elevation. Posterior extension is a complication of an inferior wall injury and may also prompt the advanced provider to consider obtaining a right-sided 12-lead ECG.

The medic unit notifies medical command of the ST elevation myocardial infarction (STEMI). The providers administer aspirin and start a large bore peripheral intravenous line. Nitroglycerin is administered as per protocol. After the second sublingual dose, the patient experiences a precipitous drop in blood pressure and nearly loses consciousness. Further doses are withheld and the patient is resuscitated with one liter of normal saline administered intravenously.

CLINICAL PEARL

Consider the possibility of a posterior wall myocardial infarction when the following inferior wall ST segment changes are present:
- ST segment depression in V_1 through V_3
- Upright T waves in V_1 through V_3
- Tall R waves

CASE 13 ANSWER   CHIEF COMPLAINT: Fever, change in mental status

12-LEAD ECG INTERPRETATION

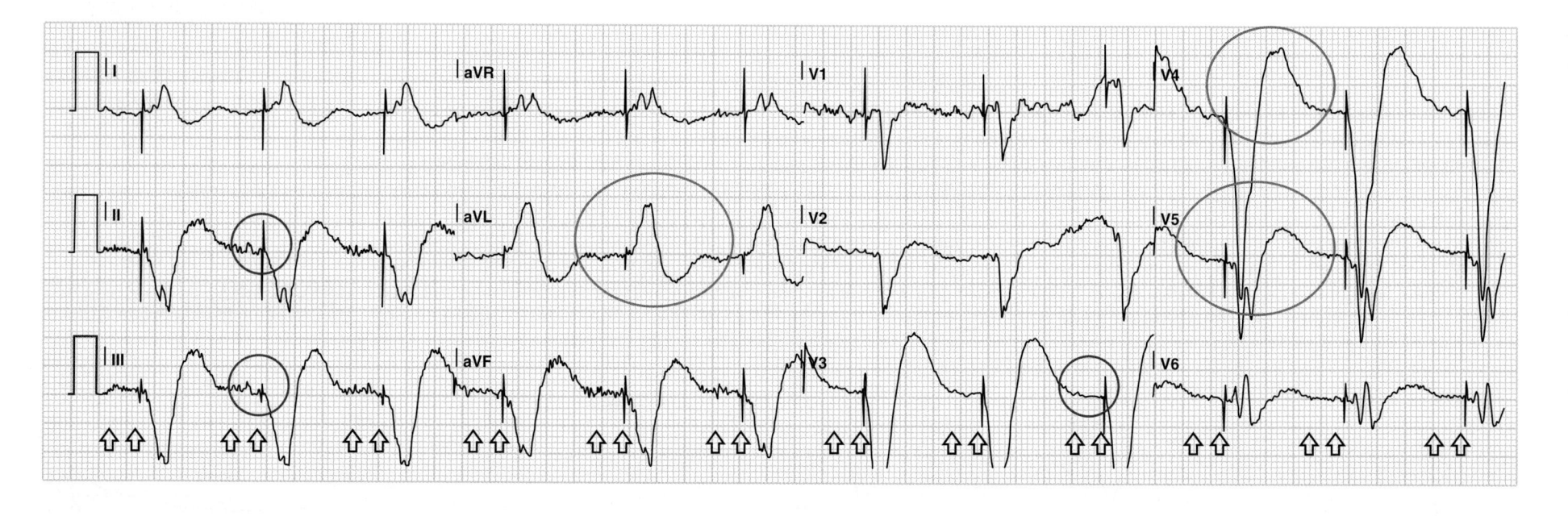

A-V sequential pacemaker, heart rate: 70 beats/min.

The ECG reveals large, extremely wide QRS complexes, QRS concordance in the precordial leads, and QRS/ST discordance throughout, resulting in ST elevation (*green circles*). These findings are consistent with a paced ventricular rhythm. P waves can be seen clearly in leads II, III, and V$_3$ (*red circles*). The atrial pacemaker spikes are not visible because of their low amplitude. This ECG machine places indicator arrows at the bottom of the tracing to show the "invisible" pacemaker activity.

The presence of fever, altered mental status, and dark urine suggests an acute systemic infection. The advanced providers administer an intravenous bolus of normal saline. The patient's temperature is 101°F by rectum. Acetaminophen is administered by gastric tube. Given the patient's respiratory distress, the senior provider elects to place the patient on the transport ventilator while en route to the local hospital. The patient requires intravenous antibiotics, aggressive rehydration, mechanical ventilatory support, and admission to an intensive care unit.

CHIEF COMPLAINT: Acute pericarditis

12-LEAD ECG INTERPRETATION

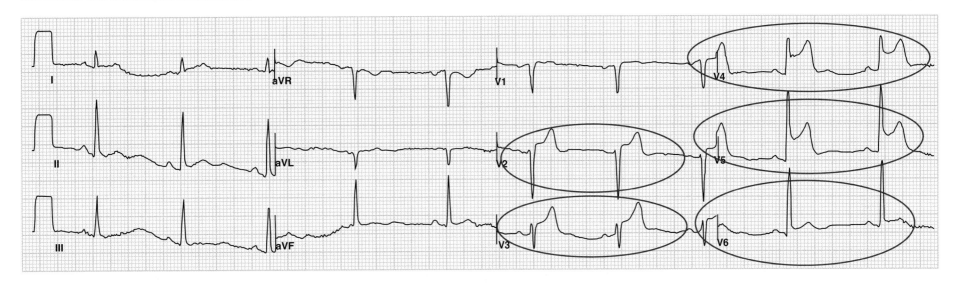

Sinus rhythm, heart rate: approximately 60 beats/min., anterior wall STEMI.

ST elevations occur in precordial leads V_2 through V_6 (*red ovals*). There are no obvious reciprocal ST segment changes. T wave flattening is noted in leads III and aVF. These "nonspecific" changes warrant concern considering the patient's presentation. Recall that nondiagnostic and nonspecific ECG changes are common presentations of acute coronary syndrome.

You clearly recognize ST changes associated with acute myocardial infarction. In contrast to the widespread and diffuse changes of pericarditis, these ST elevations occur in an anatomic distribution (anterior wall), which weighs against pericarditis. Furthermore, pericarditis rarely produces ST elevation ≥ 5 mm, as noted here in leads V_4 and V_5.

Diabetics are at risk for an atypical presentation of acute coronary syndrome. In a minority of patients, atypical presentation includes chest discomfort that is reproducible with movement or palpation. You alert the emergency department nurse and the attending physician to this patient's ECG findings.

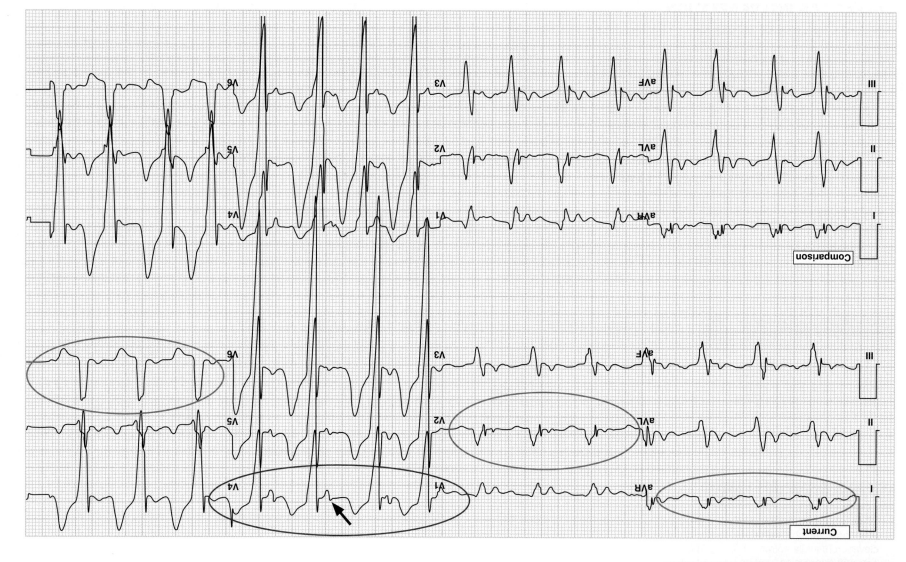

12-LEAD ECG INTERPRETATION

CASE 15 ANSWER **CHIEF COMPLAINT:** Shortness of breath

CHIEF COMPLAINT: Shortness of breath

Sinus rhythm, heart rate: approximately 100 beats/min., old left bundle branch block pattern, indeterminate for ischemia.

Given this patient's reported symptoms and abnormal vital signs, he is brought back to the emergency department treatment area for evaluation. His ECG illustrates several abnormalities. Fortunately, you have an old ECG for comparison. First, there is a baseline sinus rhythm. Large biphasic P waves (*black arrow*) indicate atrial enlargement. P-wave abnormalities are rarely associated with ischemia. A left bundle branch block pattern is present, indicated by a QRS complex >0.12s in lead V_1 (*red oval*); large S waves in the right precordial leads; large monophasic R waves in lateral leads I, aVL, and V_6 (*green ovals*); and discordance between the QRS complexes and the ST segments (see the appendix "Diagnostic Criteria for Sgarbossa, LVH, and LBBB").

The finding of a new or presumably new left bundle branch block in combination with anginal symptoms should prompt consultation with a cardiac center. In many cases, the emergency physician or cardiologist will activate the catheterization lab. A new left bundle branch block may be associated with acute ischemia. Because old ECGs are almost never available in the field, an advanced provider should err on the side of caution and transport patients with these electrocardiographic readings expeditiously. Left bundle branch blocks might obscure typical signs of acute myocardial infarction, such as ST elevation. To support a diagnosis of a myocardial infarction, elicit a careful patient history and scrutinize the ECG for (1) ST elevation >5 mm and (2) reciprocal changes.

CASE 16 ANSWER   CHIEF COMPLAINT: Syncope

3-LEAD ECG INTERPRETATION

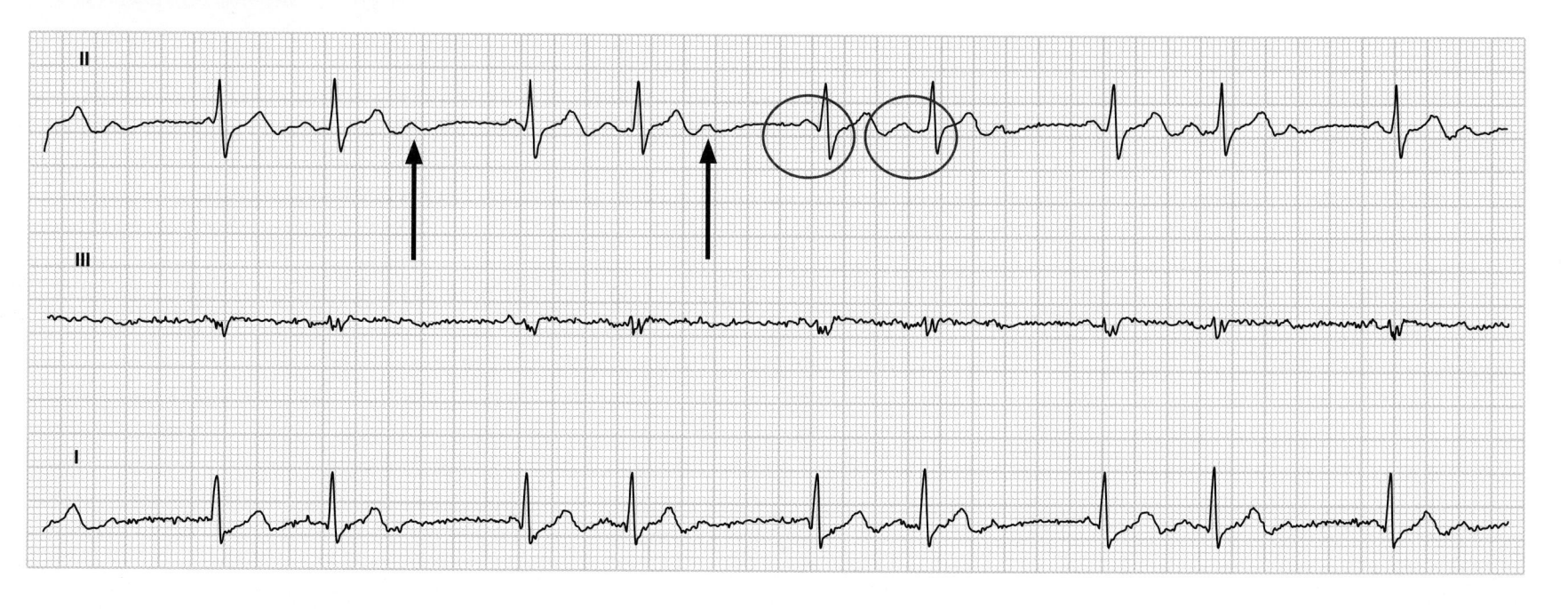

Second-degree type I heart block, heart rate in the 70s.

Second-degree type I heart block is characterized by a progressively increasing P-R interval (*red circles*) and eventual loss of conduction to the ventricles resulting in a dropped QRS complex (*black arrows*). Causes of second-degree type I heart block include strong vagal tone (as in the case of a well-conditioned athlete), hypoxia, and certain medications, including digoxin, calcium-channel blockers, and beta-blocking agents.

After arriving at the emergency department, the ECG tracing above was compared with a previously acquired tracing and determined to be the patient's normal heart rhythm. The patient was diagnosed with dehydration and received several liters of normal saline.

Intravenous atropine and transcutaneous pacing may be indicated for patients who remain symptomatic or hypotensive. Second-degree heart block may result from coronary artery disease. Initiate intravenous access and transport patients expeditiously.

12-LEAD ECG INTERPRETATION

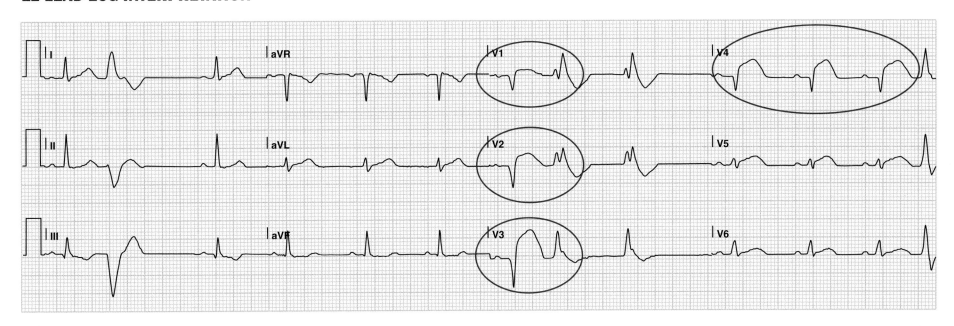

Sinus rhythm with premature ventricular contractions, heart rate: 70–80 beats/min., anterior wall STEMI.

This patient's ECG is diagnostic for acute anterior wall ST elevation myocardial infarction (STEMI). ST elevations are present in leads V_1 through V_4 (*red ovals*). This ECG is particularly interesting because aberrantly conducted beats appear in leads V_1 through V_3, almost completely masking the "normal" beats and ST elevation. Furthermore, this ECG reveals an absence of the expected reciprocal changes in the inferior leads: II, III, and aVF. This case illustrates the importance of recording several ECGs in patients presenting with acute coronary syndrome, even if transport times are short.

Transmission of the prehospital ECG resulted in activation of the STEMI team, and the patient was transferred to the cardiac catheterization lab for urgent angioplasty.

CASE 18 ANSWER   CHIEF COMPLAINT: Chest pain

12-LEAD ECG INTERPRETATION

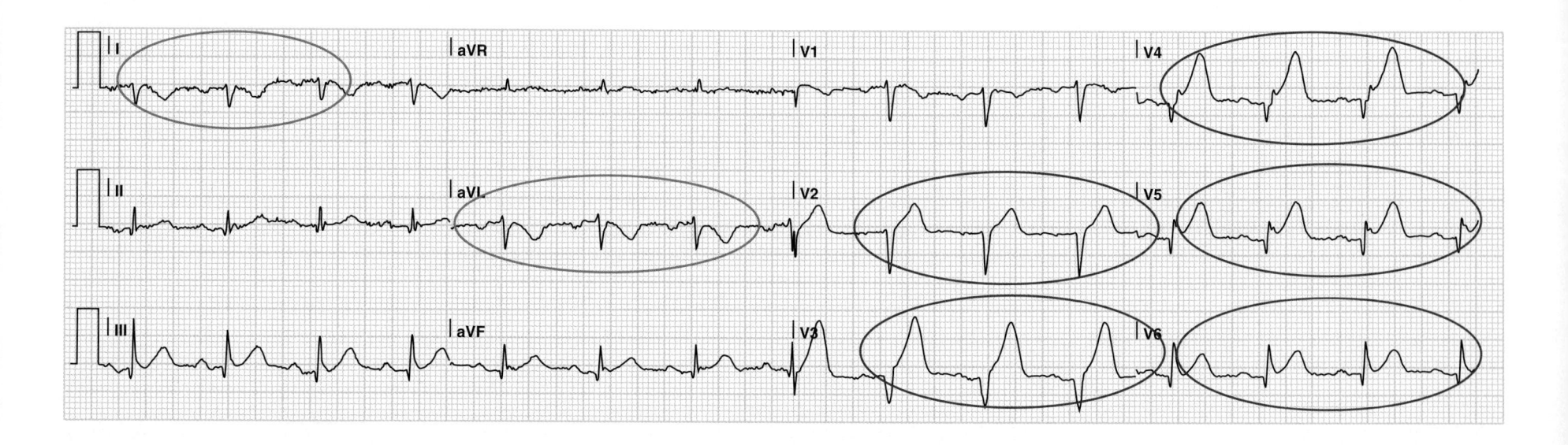

CLINICAL PEARL

Patients experiencing massive myocardial infarctions are at risk for the development of cardiogenic shock. Cardiogenic shock occurs when a large portion of the myocardial muscle mass is damaged or stunned.

Sinus rhythm, heart rate: 80–89 beats/min., anterior inferior wall STEMI.

The ST elevation in many of the precordial leads (*red ovals*) of this patient's ECG is characteristic of an anterior wall myocardial infarction (MI). The normal progression of R wave development has been lost, as occurs in patients with acute or previous anterior wall infarctions. T wave inversions in leads I and aVL (*green ovals*) corroborate the field impression of ischemia and indicate reciprocal change.

This patient would benefit from rapid transport to a facility capable of percutaneous coronary intervention.

12-LEAD ECG INTERPRETATION

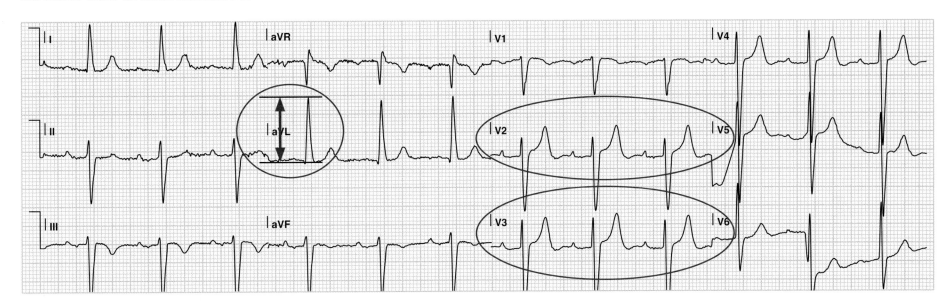

Sinus rhythm, heart rate: 80 beats/min., first-degree AV block, left ventricular hypertrophy.

The ECG reveals a left anterior hemiblock (LAHB) and left ventricular hypertrophy. LAHB is indicated by the presence of a QRS complex of <120 ms; left axis deviation in the frontal ECG plane; Q-R complexes in leads I and aVL; and rS complexes in leads II, III, and aVF. As an isolated electrocardiographic finding, LAHB rarely suggests active ischemia. The voltage criteria for left ventricular hypertrophy (LVH) are altered slightly in the presence of LAHB. One voltage criterion that is generally accepted for LVH includes R wave amplitude in excess of 11 mm in lead aVL. The R wave in this tracing is estimated at approximately 15 mm (*red circle/ arrow*), which is consistent with established voltage criteria. For a more comprehensive description of electrocardiographic findings in LVH, please see the appendix "Diagnostic Criteria for Sgarbossa, LVH, and LBBB".

In this case, the absence of associated symptoms argues against cardiogenic chest pain. Though this patient's clinical picture is reassuring, it is impossible to eliminate acute coronary syndromes on the basis of a single ECG. The electrocardiographic findings are likely a result of physiologic hypertrophy related to the patient's cardiovascular conditioning.

The electrocardiographic changes in this ECG are subtle. You initiate intravenous access and transport the patient to the receiving hospital for further diagnostics. The diagnosis of reflux is one of exclusion and may even coexist with ischemic presentations. Always consider the most life-threatening diagnosis when evaluating patients with chest pain.

CLINICAL PEARL

Gastroesophageal reflux is not a common prehospital or emergency department diagnosis! The presence of "reflux" does not exclude ischemia. An inferior wall acute coronary syndrome may present with "gastrointestinal" symptoms such as nausea, vomiting, and indigestion.

CASE 20 ANSWER   CHIEF COMPLAINT: Weakness

12-LEAD ECG INTERPRETATION

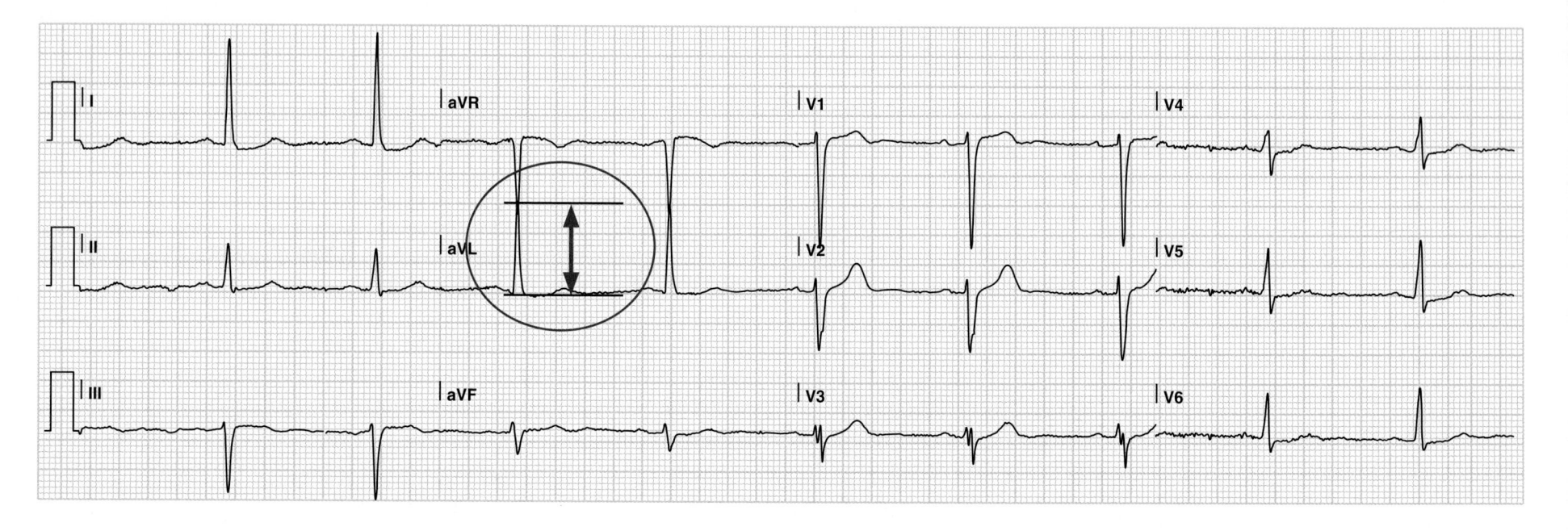

Sinus rhythm, heart rate: 60 beats/min., left ventricular hypertrophy.

The ECG reveals a regular sinus rhythm as well as an indication of left ventricular hypertrophy (LVH): the presence of an R wave > 11 mm in amplitude in lead aVL (*red circle*). Additional electrocardiographic signs of LVH (not evident in this patient's ECG) are repolarization abnormalities (ST depression or elevation, T wave inversion), tall R waves, and deep S waves. Although a variety of "ECG voltage" criteria suggest the presence of LVH (see the appendix "Diagnostic Criteria for Sgarbossa, LVH, and LBBB"), the definitive diagnosis is made by echocardiogram. Because LVH can cause ST elevation and changes in T wave morphology, it is considered an electrocardiographic mimic of ischemia.

This particular ECG does not meet criteria for the diagnosis of ST elevation myocardial infarction. However, weakness reported by elder patients is of concern because it can be associated with concurrent cardiac ischemia. The patient is transported to the hospital for further diagnostic testing.

12-LEAD ECG INTERPRETATION

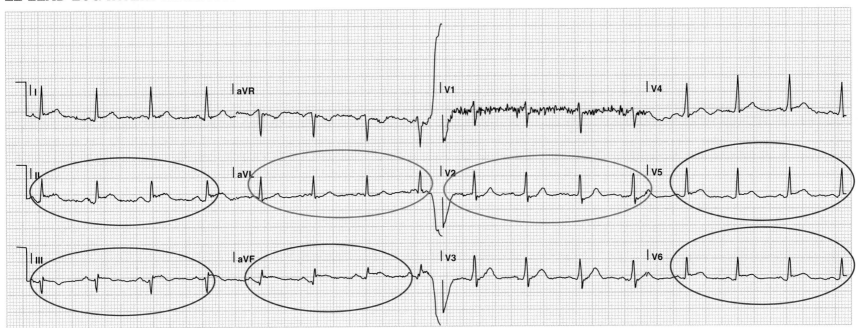

Sinus rhythm, heart rate: 90–100 beats/min., inferior lateral wall STEMI.

CLINICAL PEARL

ST segment shape also suggests underlying illness. A horizontal or "convex upward" segment shape is usually associated with ischemia

CLINICAL PEARL

Shortness of breath and atypical presentations are common in elderly, female, and immunosuppressed patient populations. Many of these patients suffering from an acute coronary syndrome might present without pain.

Based on this ECG, this patient could easily be misdiagnosed as having acute pericarditis. The ECG shows ST elevation in multiple leads (*red ovals*). There is a slight PR segment depression in many of those leads, and PR segment elevation in lead aVR, both of which are highly suggestive of acute pericarditis. However, it is important to understand that these PR segment changes are not pathognomonic for acute pericarditis. The ECG does demonstrate reciprocal ST depression in leads aVL and V$_2$ (*green ovals*), which indicates acute myocardial infarction (MI)—the presence of any ST depression in leads other than V$_1$ or aVR virtually excludes a diagnosis of acute pericarditis. Additionally, leads III and aVF demonstrate horizontal ST elevation, which also excludes acute pericarditis. The ST elevation morphology of acute pericarditis is always concave upward (like a cup holding water); horizontal or convex upward (i.e., tombstone morphology) ST elevation is associated with acute MI (see the appendix "The Many Faces of Ischemia"). The deep Q waves in leads III and aVF suggest that the patient's ischemia may have been present for quite some time before presentation. Pathologic Q waves (i.e., greater than one-third the height of the R wave, or more than 0.04 seconds wide) may also indicate previous MI.

This case also illustrates some important diagnostic pearls. Advanced age, diabetes, and female gender are all factors associated with an atypical clinical presentation. Elderly patients may present with only shortness of breath or fatigue. The presence of diabetes further confounds the history of present illness. Maintain a low threshold for (1) transporting elderly patients and (2) obtaining a 12-lead ECG.

The advanced provider initiated the emergency department's ST elevation myocardial infarction (STEMI) protocol. The patient received aspirin and was expeditiously transported to the catheterization laboratory for intervention.

CASE 22 ANSWER   CHIEF COMPLAINT: Chest pain, weakness

12-LEAD ECG INTERPRETATION

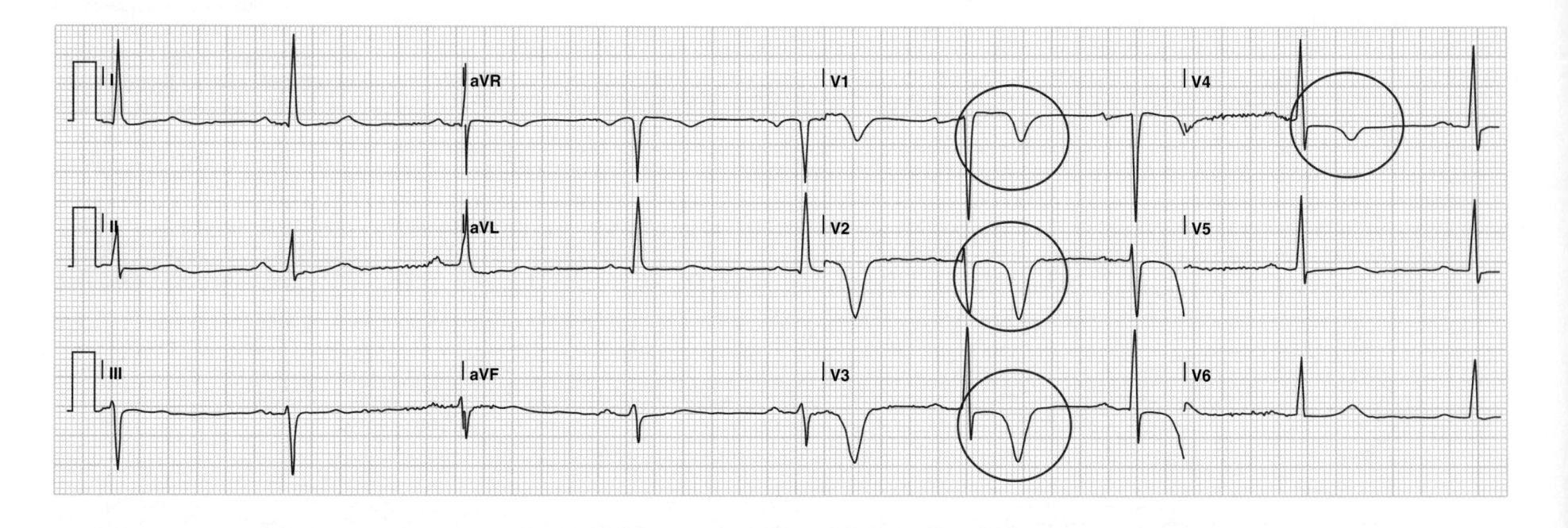

Sinus bradycardia, heart rate: 50–60 beats/min., anterior ischemia.

The ECG reveals sinus bradycardia. Also note the deeply inverted, symmetric T waves in V$_1$ through V$_4$ (*red circles*). Weakness and syncope are of extreme concern in elderly patients, and dyspnea and fatigue are common "angina equivalents" in these patients. The patient received an extensive workup in the emergency department and was admitted for further diagnostic testing. Cardiac enzymes were negative for obvious myocardial infarction. Providers should have a low threshold for the treatment of elderly patients presenting with respiratory symptoms or complaints of weakness. Deeply inverted and symmetric T wave morphology can herald an ischemic event. Prehospital treatment priorities include obtaining a thorough history, a complete set of vital signs, and a 12-lead ECG.

(Continued)

Two weeks later, the patient called 9-1-1 with a similar complaint. He had experienced an episode of chest pain and associated weakness that had resolved by the time the paramedic arrived. The patient was transported to the emergency department, where his evaluation included an ECG (*shown below*). Note the same findings of deeply inverted, symmetric T waves in the anterior leads (*red ovals*). This time, the patient was diagnosed with Wellens' syndrome and sent for urgent cardiac catheterization. The angiogram revealed a critical obstruction in the proximal left anterior descending artery (LAD), which required stent placement.

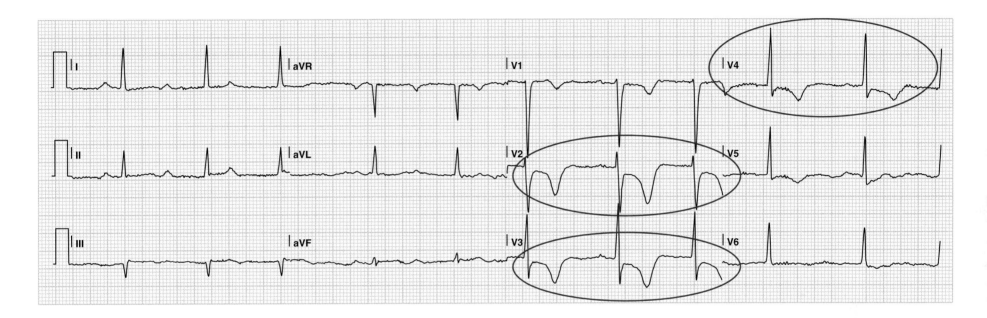

Wellens' syndrome is a pattern of changes in leads V_2 through V_4 characterized by deeply inverted, symmetric T waves. Biphasic T waves might also appear in the anterior precordial leads.

Wellens' syndrome is a pattern of changes in V_2 through V_4 (*red ovals*) characterized by deeply inverted, symmetric T waves. The patient is usually symptom-free but is at high risk for anterior MI and death. Cardiac enzyme measurements are often normal (as was the case during this patient's first emergency department visit). Medical management alone is ineffective in these patients. Early cardiac catheterization is critical in the detection of and intervention for LAD obstruction.

CASE 23 ANSWER   **CHIEF COMPLAINT:** Chest pain

12-LEAD ECG INTERPRETATION

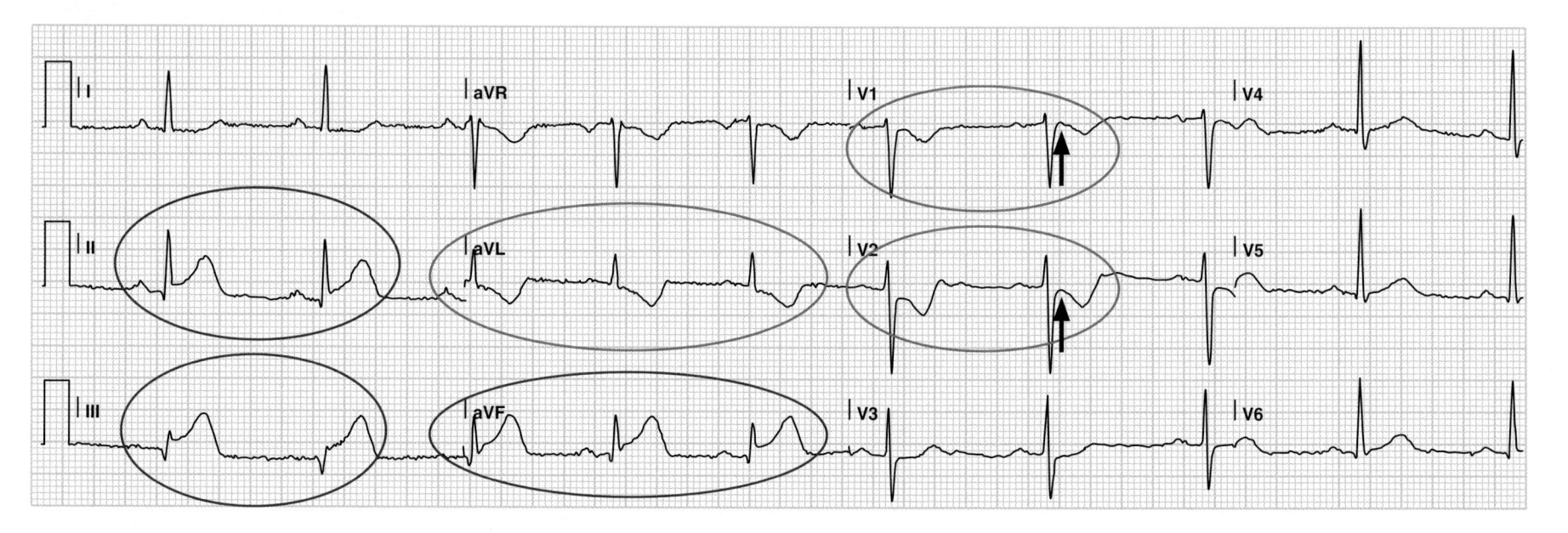

Sinus rhythm, heart rate: 60 beats/min., inferior wall STEMI with possible posterior wall extension.

This ECG illustrates clear ST elevation in leads II, III, and aVF (*red ovals*). Reciprocal changes are present in aVL, V_1, and V_2 (*green ovals*). Although the ST depression in V_1 and V_2 (*arrows*) might also represent reciprocal changes, they could also signify extension of the infarct into the heart's posterior wall. A simple method for determining if these changes represent reciprocal changes rather than posterior infarction is to repeat the ECG with posterior leads (i.e., two leads placed in the left mid-back area). If the posterior leads demonstrate ST elevation, then posterior wall infarction is confirmed. Posterior extension is a typical complication of an inferior wall injury.

The advanced providers notify the receiving hospital of the ST elevation myocardial infarction (STEMI), and they administer aspirin. A large-bore peripheral intravenous line is started, and nitroglycerin is administered according to protocol.

12-LEAD ECG INTERPRETATION

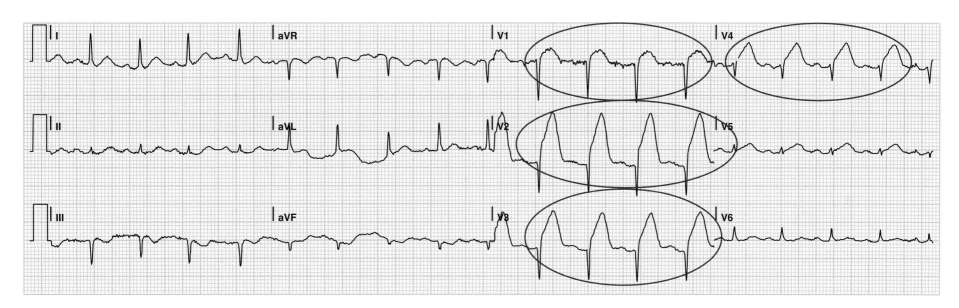

CLINICAL PEARL

Approximately one-third of patients with acute coronary syndromes present without pain, and among them, neurologic complaints such as syncope are common "anginal equivalents."

Sinus tachycardia, heart rate: 100 beats/min., anterior wall STEMI.

This ECG illustrates ST elevation across the precordial leads V_1 through V_4 (*red ovals*). Lead V_5 shows hyperacute (broad based and relatively large in comparison with the QRS complex) T waves—a finding consistent with acute anterior wall injury. Note that the typical reciprocal changes are not immediately evident in the patient's limb leads. Have a low threshold for obtaining 12-lead ECGs in diabetics and patients who recover from a syncopal episode. Approximately one-third of patients with acute coronary syndromes present without pain, and among them, neurologic complaints such as syncope are common "anginal equivalents." Anterior wall myocardial infarctions (MIs) are commonly caused by occlusion of the left anterior descending artery, which supplies a large area of the left ventricle. As a result, patients with this condition are at high risk for early development of congestive heart failure, malignant dysrhythmias, and cardiogenic shock. The syncopal episode may have resulted from a brief episode of ventricular tachycardia.

In this case, advanced providers obtain a 12-lead ECG and alert the receiving facility to the possibility of an ST elevation myocardial infarction (STEMI). The patient is given 162 mg of baby aspirin, and a large-bore peripheral intravenous line is established. The patient is placed on oxygen and transported to a waiting catheterization lab.

CASE 25 ANSWER   **CHIEF COMPLAINT:** Unresponsiveness

12-LEAD ECG INTERPRETATION

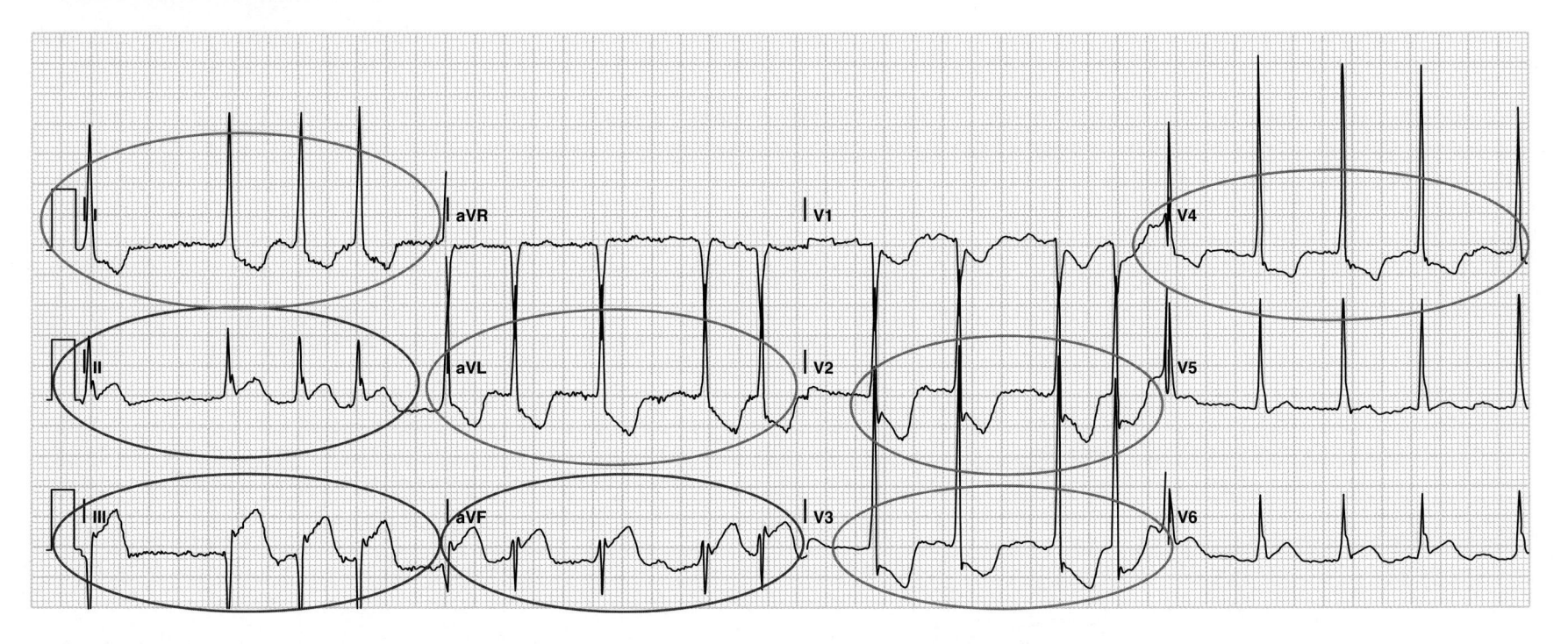

Atrial fibrillation with a rapid ventricular response, heart rate: 100–130 beats/min., inferior wall STEMI.

ST elevations are present in the inferior wall region (*red ovals*), which indicates an ongoing infarction. Leads V_2 through V_4 demonstrate ST depression with prominent R waves (*green ovals*), which is highly suggestive of extension of the infarct into the posterior wall. Reciprocal changes are evident in limb leads I and aVL (*green ovals*).

This patient became unresponsive and hypotensive after administration of nitroglycerin (NTG). You start high-flow oxygen and prepare the patient for rapid transport. The patient's lungs are clear, and the SpO_2 improves with gentle airway repositioning and high-flow oxygen. You administer a bolus of normal saline wide open; you give no further doses of NTG. The student provider asks to start dopamine at 5 mcg/kg/min, but the patient's BP increases to 90 mm Hg after 1.5 L of normal saline is administered, so an infusion of dopamine is not required. The patient becomes more alert and cooperative. The student provider then administers 324 mg of chewable aspirin and requests activation of the local PCI center. You obtain a right-sided ECG en route to the hospital and confirm the presence of right ventricular involvement (i.e., ST elevation in leads V_4R through V_6R).

12-LEAD ECG INTERPRETATION

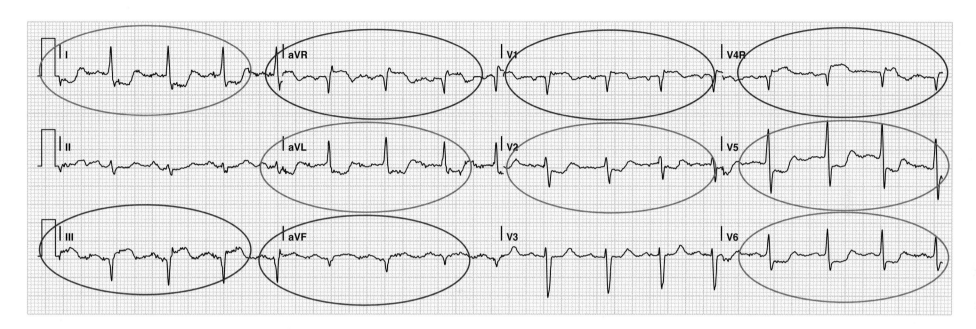

CLINICAL PEARL

Suspect right ventricular wall infarction in patients who present with:

- Hypotension
- Ischemic changes in inferior leads
- ST elevation in V_4R

Sinus tachycardia, heart rate: 100–110 beats/min., inferior wall STEMI, right ventricular infarction.

This ECG reveals ST elevation in leads III and aVF (*red ovals*). Reciprocal ST depression is seen in leads I and aVL (*green ovals*). Also note the ST depression in lead V_2 (*green ovals*). Findings of ST elevation in inferior leads (III and aVF) and hypotension are suggestive of right ventricular infarction (RVI). In this case, the paramedic recorded lead V_4R to confirm the RVI. Note the convex ST segment morphology and ST elevation in lead V_4R (*red oval*), confirming the diagnosis of RVI.

ST elevation is also evident in leads aVR and V_1. Although these changes might be seen in association with RVI, ST elevation in lead aVR can indicate disease of the left main coronary artery. The patient's presentation and ECG findings are extremely concerning and require aggressive treatment with intravenous fluid and percutaneous coronary intervention.

CASE 27 ANSWER   CHIEF COMPLAINT: Myocardial infarction

12-LEAD ECG INTERPRETATION

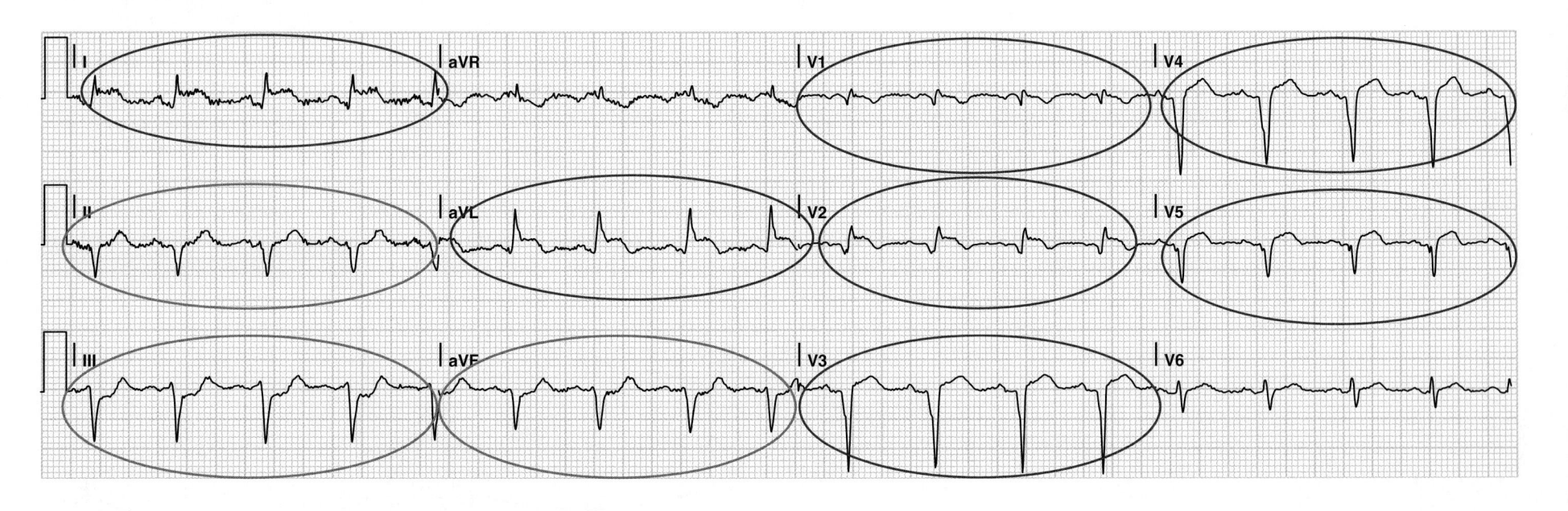

Sinus tachycardia, heart rate: 100 beats/min., anterolateral wall STEMI.
ST elevation is demonstrated in leads V_1 though V_5, and in leads I and aVL (*red ovals*). Reciprocal ST depression is noted in the inferior leads (*green ovals*). This ECG is consistent with an anterolateral wall ST elevation myocardial infarction (STEMI). The loss of R wave amplitude across the precordial leads is consistent with infarction of the heart's anterior wall. In non-ischemic ECGs, the R wave is usually greater than 2–3 mm in lead V_3. The only positive precordial R wave deflection in this tracing appears in lead V_6. The patient developed pulmonary edema during the interfacility transfer, and paramedics initiated continuous positive airway pressure and increased the NTG infusion. Medical control advised the crew to continue the maximal medical therapy and transport the patient directly to a waiting cardiac catheterization laboratory.

12-LEAD ECG INTERPRETATION

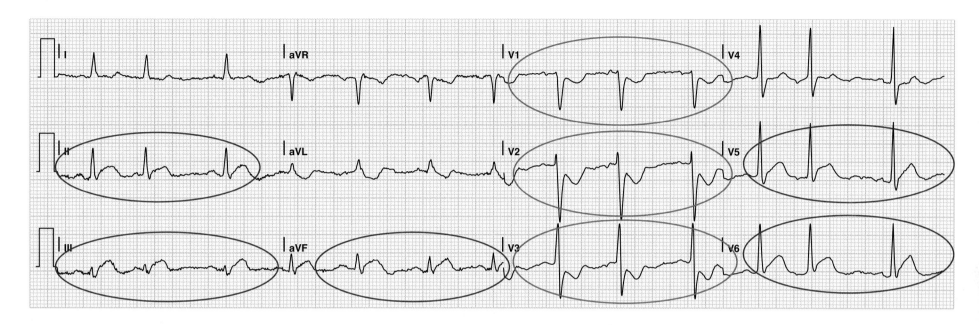

Sinus rhythm, heart rate: 80 beats/min., acute inferior lateral ischemia, probable acute posterior wall myocardial infarction.

The changes seen in this patient's ECG are consistent with acute myocardial infarction (MI). Convex ST segment morphology and broad-based T waves are present in the inferolateral leads (*red ovals*). Furthermore, close inspection of the inferior lead ST segments reveals minimal ST segment elevation. Reciprocal change, in the form of ST segment depression in lead aVL, is also diagnostic of infarction. The taller-than-normal R wave in V_3 coupled with ST depression in leads V_1 through V_3 suggest posterior extension of the infarction (*green ovals*). If leads were placed directly opposite to V_2 and V_3 on the patient's left mid-back (posterior leads), they would probably display ST elevation. The presence of posterior involvement indicates a larger territory of infarction and a worse prognosis. Posterior wall infarction is a condition that benefits from percutaneous coronary intervention. It rarely occurs in isolation and can be seen concurrently with infarction of the heart's inferior wall. The patient is prepped for an emergent cardiac catheterization.

Premature supraventricular contractions are seen throughout this tracing. The remainder of the beats, however, illustrate similar PR ratios and P wave morphology. The underlying rhythm is likely sinus in origin.

CLINICAL PEARL

Clues to diagnosis of a posterior wall infarction:
- ST depression in leads V_1 through V_3
- Tall R wave in leads V_1 through V_3
- R/S wave ratio of > 1.0 in lead V_2

CASE 29 ANSWER   CHIEF COMPLAINT: Shortness of breath

12-LEAD ECG INTERPRETATION

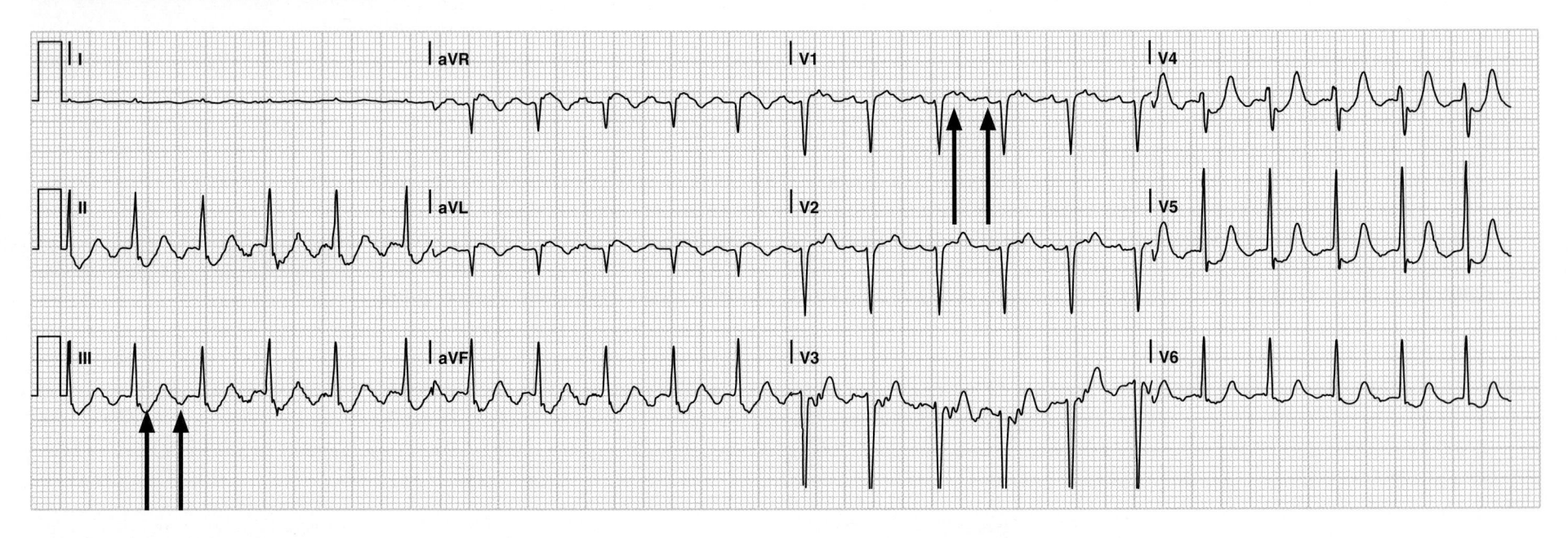

CLINICAL PEARL

Atrial flutter is often misdiagnosed as sinus tachycardia or
SVT, usually because of a failure
to scrutinize the ECG for the atrial
activity.

Atrial flutter with 2:1 conduction, heart rate: 130 beats/min.

The ECG reveals a regular narrow complex tachycardia. Differential diagnosis of narrow complex tachycardia includes sinus
tachycardia, supraventricular tachycardia (SVT), and atrial flutter. Sinus tachycardia is excluded here because there is no 1:1
relationship of P waves to QRS complexes. Instead, flutter waves create what is commonly described as a "sawtooth pattern"
(*black arrows*) in the inferior leads and lead V$_1$. It is helpful to hold the ECG tracing upside down to visualize the flutter waves more
clearly. Atrial flutter is often misdiagnosed as sinus tachycardia or SVT, usually because of a failure to scrutinize the ECG for the
atrial activity.

12-LEAD ECG INTERPRETATION

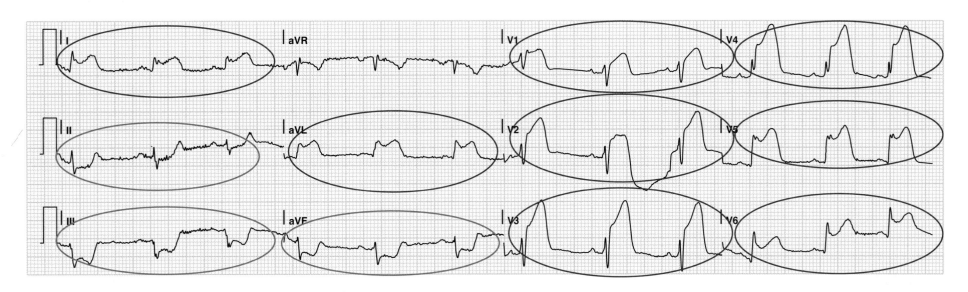

Sinus rhythm, heart rate: 70 beats/min., anterior and lateral wall STEMI.

This ECG demonstrates ST elevation across the entire precordium (represented by leads V_1 through V_6), and in leads I and aVL (*red ovals*). These changes are consistent with extensive anterior and high lateral wall injury. Reciprocal ST depression and T wave inversion is noted in the inferior leads (*green ovals*).

Advanced providers transmit the ECG to the receiving facility and begin transport. They administer 162 mg of baby aspirin en route and initiate a large-bore peripheral intravenous line. The patient is transferred to the waiting cardiac catheterization team. A massive anterior wall ST elevation myocardial infarction (STEMI) is a risk factor for the development of pulmonary edema and ventricular dysrhythmia.

CASE 31 ANSWER   CHIEF COMPLAINT: Syncope

12-LEAD ECG INTERPRETATION

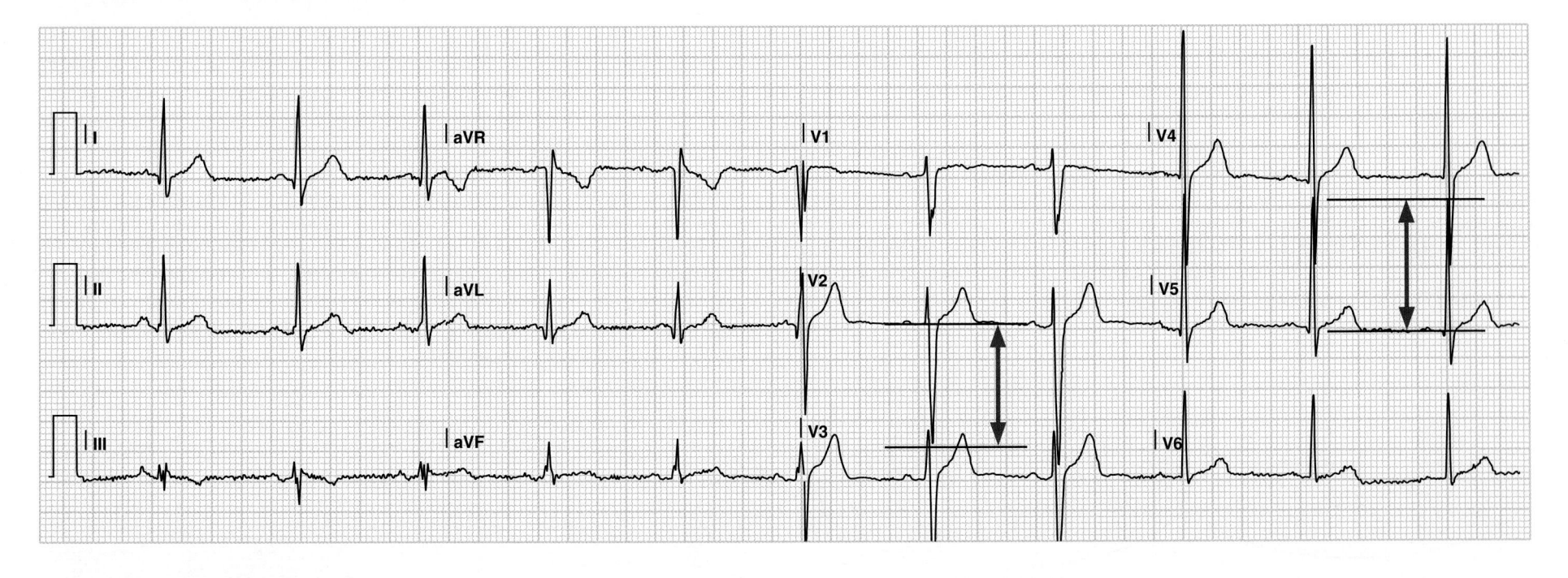

CLINICAL PEARL

One method of diagnosing LVH is to look at the precordial leads, find the deepest S wave in V_1 or V_2, the tallest R wave in V_5 or V_6, and add the two measurements together (*arrows*). If the sum of the two values exceeds 35 mm, the ECG meets the voltage criteria for LVH.

Sinus rhythm, heart rate: 70 beats/min., left ventricular hypertrophy.

The ECG reveals a sinus rhythm and voltage criteria consistent with left ventricular hypertrophy (LVH). One method of diagnosing LVH is to look at the precordial leads, find the deepest S wave in V_1 or V_2, the tallest R wave in V_5 or V_6, and add the two measurements together (*arrows*). If the sum of the two values exceeds 35 mm, the ECG meets the voltage criteria for LVH (see the appendix "Diagnostic Criteria for Sgarbossa, LVH, and LBBB"). In this ECG, the S wave in V_2 is 19 mm and the R wave in V_5 is 21 mm. The sum of 40 mm meets the electrical criteria for LVH. A definitive diagnosis of LVH must be made by echocardiogram.

A syncopal episode should prompt advanced providers to investigate potentially reversible and life-threatening causes. A thorough prehospital assessment of these patients includes vital signs, blood glucose measurement, and a 12-lead ECG.

12-LEAD ECG INTERPRETATION

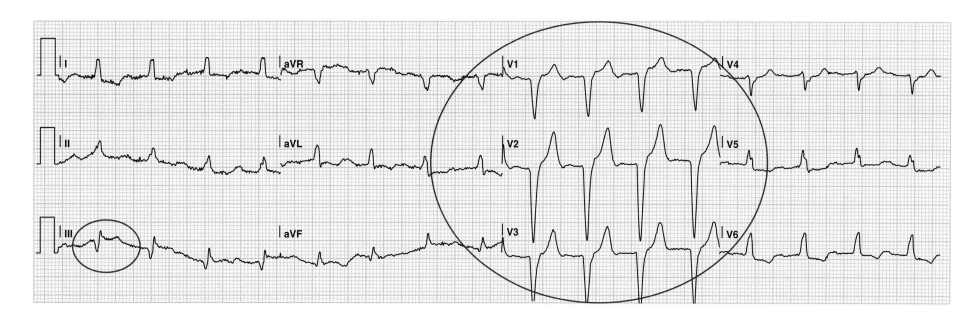

Sinus rhythm, first-degree heart block, heart rate: 90 beats/min., left bundle branch block.

Left bundle branch block (LBBB) is the obvious finding: there are wide negative QRS complexes (> 120 ms); deep, wide S waves in leads V_1 through V_3; terminal R waves in leads I, aVL, and V_6; and QRS complex/T wave discordance across the ECG. A single, deep Q wave along with ST elevation is present in lead III (*small red oval*) (see the appendix "Pathologic Q Wave"). ST elevation is also present in leads V_1 through V_3 (*large red oval*). This particular ECG does not meet strict ST elevation myocardial infarction criteria (i.e., ST elevation > 2 mm in two contiguous precordial leads). However, this finding and the LBBB, along with the patient's shortness of breath, suggest the possibility of acute cardiac ischemia. You should obtain medical consultation and transport the patient to a facility capable of percutaneous coronary intervention.

Medical control agrees that the patient's medical history and current findings are indicative of an acute event. The presence of acute-onset dyspnea, diaphoresis, and a presumably new LBBB prompts the emergency department to alert cardiology to this patient's arrival. En route to the hospital, you start an intravenous line and administer 162 mg of chewable baby aspirin. The patient is transported expeditiously to the cardiac catheterization suite.

CASE 33 ANSWER   **CHIEF COMPLAINT:** Syncope

12-LEAD ECG INTERPRETATION

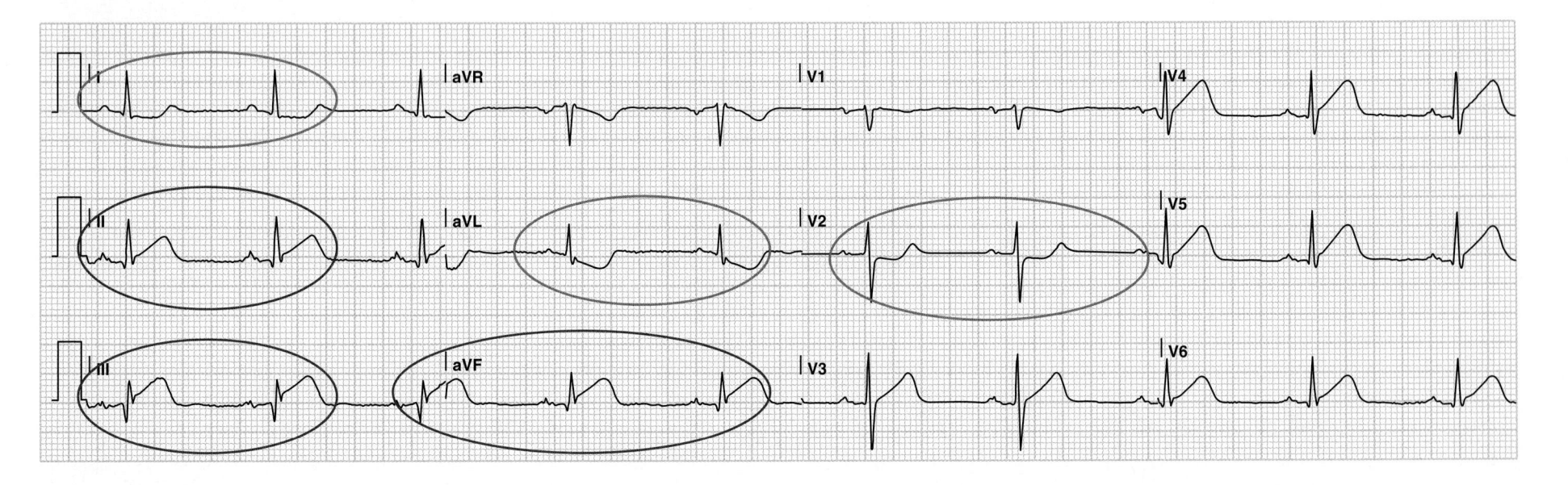

Sinus bradycardia, heart rate: 55 beats/min., inferior wall STEMI. Probable acute lateral wall ischemia.
ST elevation is present in leads II, III, and aVF (*red ovals*). Reciprocal ST depressions appear in leads V_2, I, and aVL (*green ovals*). These findings are consistent with acute inferior wall myocardial infarction (MI). Slight ST elevation is noted in the lateral precordial leads V_4 through V_6. These findings, combined with the broad-based and symmetric T waves in V_4 through V_6 suggest concurrent lateral wall myocardial infarction.

A borderline first-degree atrioventricular (AV) block is present, marked by a P-R interval measuring 0.2 seconds. This finding, combined with the inferior wall ST eleva-tion, suggests ischemia of the heart's pacemaker (sinoatrial node). Apply external pacer pads to patients presenting with symptomatic bradycardia. Close monitoring of vital signs, and administration of oxygen, aspirin, and fluid are of prime importance. Transport the patient to a cardiac center.

12-LEAD ECG INTERPRETATION

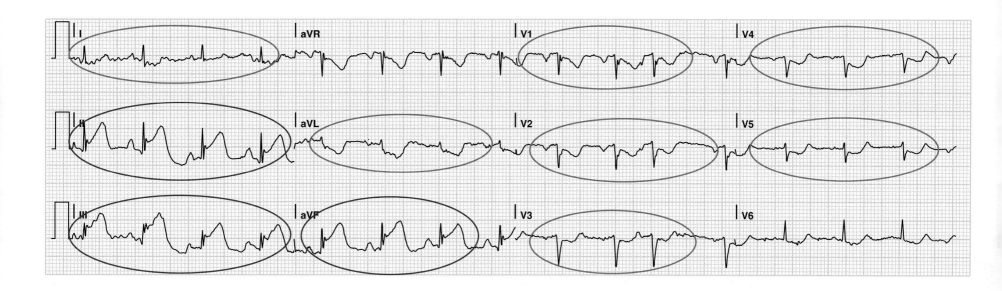

CLINICAL PEARL

- One-third of inferior STEMIs extend to the posterior wall, and one-third extend to the right ventricle. Although posterior extension does not mandate a change in management, right ventricular extension does: patients with right ventricular infarction are prone to hypotension, especially when NTG is given, and they often require intravenous fluids to maintain their BP.
- A sizeable percentage of patients with acute coronary syndrome present atypically.
- Patients experiencing "heart attack" may report nausea, vomiting, and other gastrointestinal symptoms, especially when the ischemia or infarction involves the inferior wall.

Sinus rhythm, heart rate: 90 beats/min., inferior wall STEMI.

ST elevations are present in leads II, III, and aVF (*red ovals*). Reciprocal changes in the anterolateral leads (*green ovals*) suggest inferior wall myocardial infarction. Although the ST depressions in the right precordial leads (V_1 and V_2) could possibly represent posterior extension of the inferior ST elevation myocardial infarction (STEMI), the absence of large R waves in these leads makes this less likely and is more suggestive of reciprocal ST depression.

    The patient is alarmed and surprised when he is informed of his electrocardiographic findings. He requests some antacid medicine and asks if he could "see if it works." The advanced providers emphasize that many heart attacks mimic benign heartburn, that his current symptoms are indeed those of a heart attack, and that time is of extreme importance when treating cardiac ischemia. The patient agrees to be transported. The providers administer aspirin and consider nitroglycerin (NTG) after an infusion of normal saline. A right-sided ECG confirms ST elevation in leads V_4R through V_6R, and this information is relayed to the cardiac receiving center via an updated patient care report.

CASE 35 ANSWER   CHIEF COMPLAINT: Unconsciousness

12-LEAD ECG INTERPRETATION

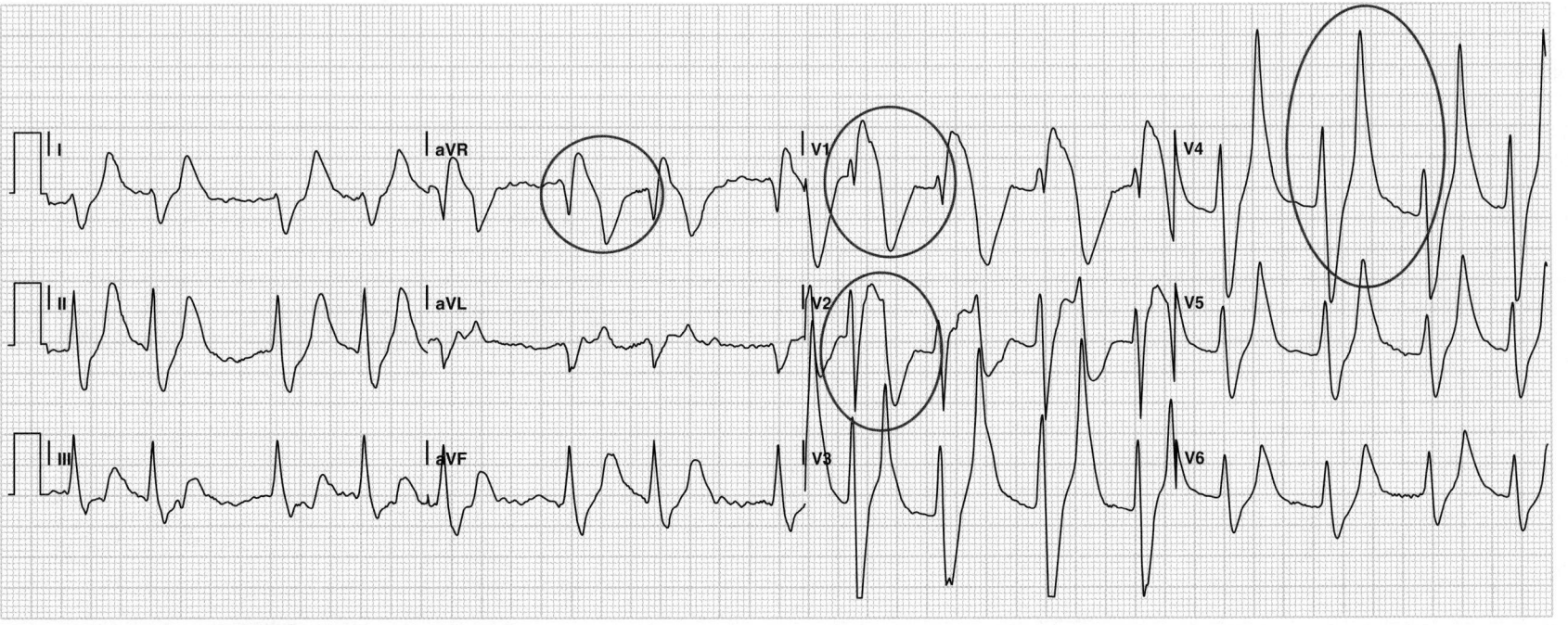

CLINICAL PEARL

To treat patients with hyperkalemia:

- Stabilize the cardiac muscle cell membranes by administering intravenous calcium chloride.
- Hydrate and administer a bolus of isotonic crystalloid. Patients with diabetic ketoacidosis are profoundly dehydrated.
- Shift K+ back into cells: consider administration of inhaled albuterol and 10 units of regular insulin.
- Mnemonic for treatment of hyperkalemia:
  - C: Intravenous calcium
  - BIG: Beta-agonist, intravenous insulin and glucose
  - K: Kayexelate®/potassium-binding resin
  - DIE: Dialysis

Atrial fibrillation, heart rate: approximately 90 beats/min., ST elevation in leads V₁ and V₂, widened QRS complex and diffusely peaked T waves in limb and precordial leads consistent with hyperkalemia. Several troubling findings are present on this ECG. Clear, definitive P waves are not present. The irregular R-to-R intervals suggest either atrial flutter or fibrillation. The QRS complexes are prolonged and ST segment changes persist throughout the ECG. The T waves are abnormally tall and peaked (*large red oval*). "Hyperacute" T waves are present in the early stages of cardiac ischemia, but this patient's clinical history is consistent with life-threatening hyperkalemia. His ECG shows the classic findings of this imbalance: peaked, tented, asymmetric T waves; wide QRS complexes; and absent P waves (see the appendix "Comparison of T Wave Morphology in Hyperkalemia and in AMI"). Note the ST elevation in leads aVR, V₁, and V₂, which is characteristic of hyperkalemia caused by diabetic ketoacidosis (DKA) (*small red ovals*).

The evolution of hyperkalemia on the ECG begins with peaked, hyperacute T waves, continues with the disappearance of P waves, and finally produces widening of the QRS complex. As the serum potassium (K+) level continues to rise, ventricular dysrhythmias eventually appear. A sinusoidal-type ventricular rhythm is a lethal and late finding on the ECG.

You establish large-bore intravenous access and prepare the patient for rapid transport. Medical control protocols authorize empiric treatment for hyperkalemia based on the electrocardiographic findings. You administer a bolus of normal saline and 1 g of intravenous calcium chloride. At the hospital, the patient's potassium level is measured at 8.2 mEq/L (3.5–5.0 mEq/L is considered normal).

12-LEAD ECG INTERPRETATION

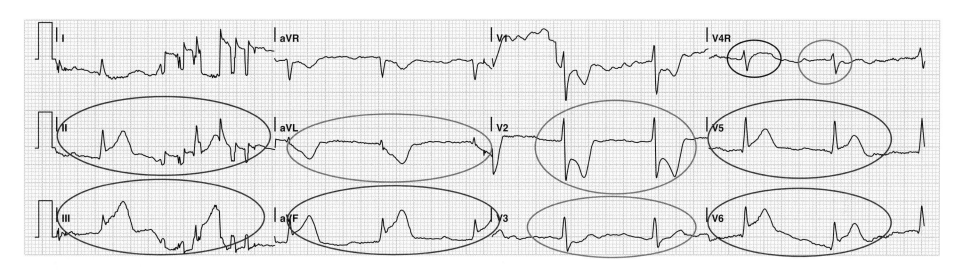

Sinus rhythm with first-degree AV block, heart rate: 50–59 beats/min., inferior lateral right ventricular STEMI.

This ECG demonstrates an acute inferior lateral right ventricular myocardial infarction (MI). It reveals ST elevation in the inferior and lateral leads (*red ovals*) and evidence of reciprocal ST depression (*green ovals*). ST elevation is demonstrated in the right chest lead V$_4$R (*black oval*), confirming right ventricular extension of the infarct. First-degree atrioventricular (AV) block (*green circle*) is diagnosed based on a P-R interval of > 200 ms. AV blocks are common in patients with acute inferior MIs.

Up to one-third of patients with inferior wall ST elevation myocardial infarction (STEMI) will have an infarction that extends to the right ventricle. The right ventricle is largely responsible for providing preload to the left ventricle. Consequently, when the right ventricle has been compromised, patients can easily lose systemic and coronary perfusion if preload is not maintained by systemic volume. The use of nitrates or other preload-reducing medications can further decrease preload and produce persistent hypotension.

You astutely obtain a right-sided ECG to assess for right ventricular involvement. ST elevations in the right precordial lead (V$_4$R) confirm the diagnosis. You then discontinue administration of nitrates and administer additional intravenous fluid boluses. Many patients with hypotension caused by right ventricular infarction respond well to aggressive intravenous hydration alone. In this case, however, evidence of heart failure had already started to emerge, so inotropic agents were needed to maintain BP.

CASE 37 ANSWER

CHIEF COMPLAINT: Respiratory distress

12-LEAD ECG INTERPRETATION

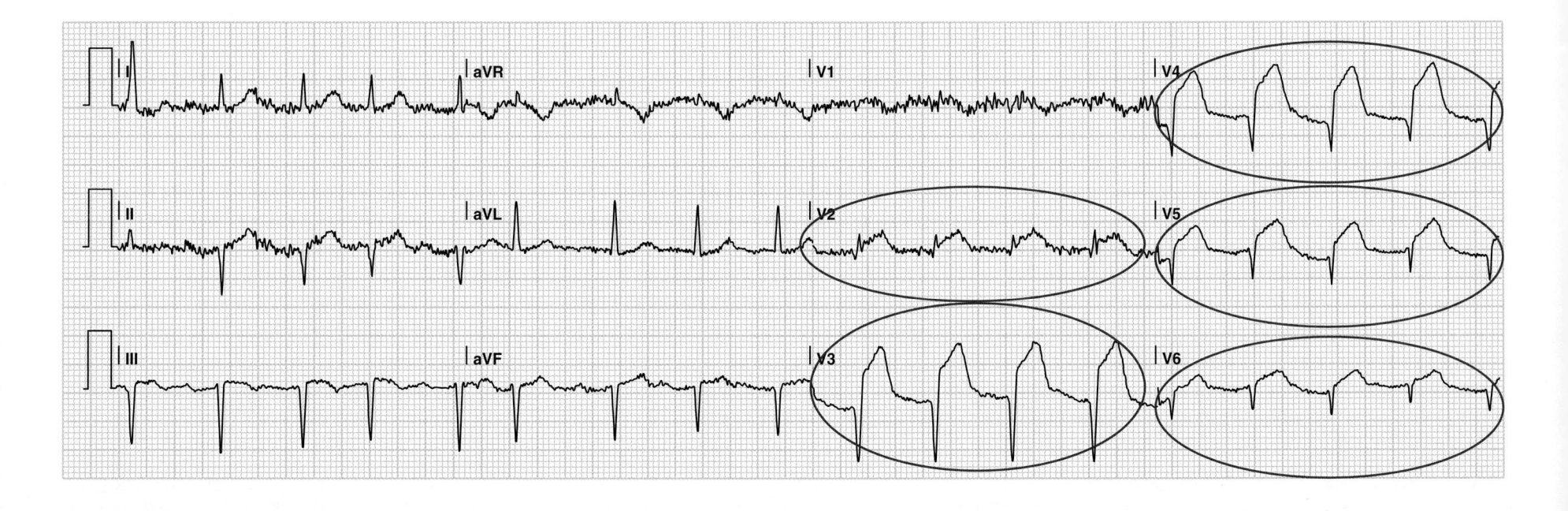

CLINICAL PEARL

In the setting of acute pulmonary edema, morphine sulfate administration has been linked to adverse patient outcomes including intubation, increased intensive care unit length of stay, and mortality. Avoid morphine in patients with congestive heart failure exacerbations.

Sinus tachycardia, heart rate: 100 beats/min., anterior wall STEMI.

The ECG shows ST elevation in leads V_2 through V_6 (*red ovals*). This patient is having a large anterior wall myocardial infarction and is experiencing acute pulmonary edema. He requires rapid prehospital treatment, transport, and emergent cardiac catheterization. The advanced providers attempt to apply continuous positive airway pressure, but the patient does not tolerate the mask. Chewable aspirin is administered, and the provider gives 0.8 mg of sublingual nitroglycerin (NTG), in accordance with established pulmonary edema protocol. A peripheral intravenous line is started. While awaiting the arrival of the transport unit, the patient experiences a 10-beat run of ventricular tachycardia.

After the ambulance has arrived and the patient is loaded, he is given an additional 0.4 mg of NTG, and 1 inch of NTG paste is applied to his chest. A student provider asks about morphine sulfate, but the advanced provider decides against morphine administration and explains that in patients with acute pulmonary edema, the drug has been associated with increased mortality, increased risk of intubation, and increased likelihood for ICU admission.

The presence of an artifact interferes with interpretation of the underlying rhythm. However, the regular R to R interval in the precordial leads indicates that the rhythm is likely sinus in origin. The artifact underscores the importance of a rhythm strip in the process of ECG interpretation.

12-LEAD ECG INTERPRETATION

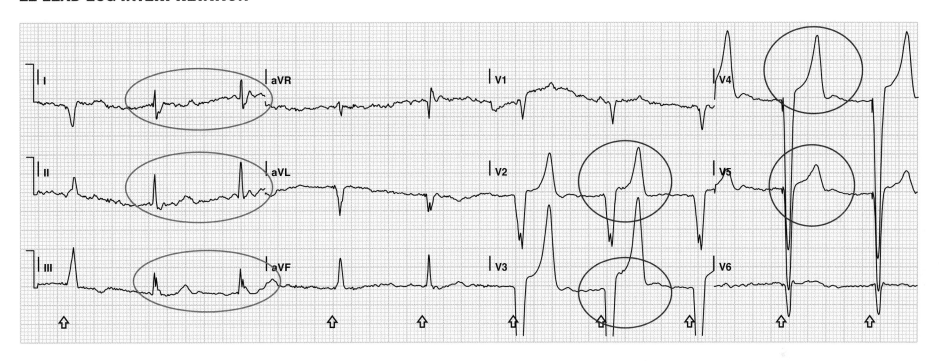

Demand ventricular pacemaker, heart rate: 60 beats/min.

The ECG reveals a demand ventricular pacemaker rhythm. The classic findings of QRS concordance (i.e., all QRS complexes in precordial leads point in the same direction) and QRS complex/ST discordance in the precordial leads, high-voltage complexes, and ST elevation are seen in this case (*red circles*). Both paced rhythms and left bundle branch blocks can cause ST elevation. However, ST elevation that exceeds 5 mm is suggestive of an ischemic event. Concave ST segments in the precordial leads favor benign ST elevation versus acute myocardial infarction. The second and third QRS complexes in leads I through III are the patient's own and have not been artificially initiated (*green ovals*). The lack of clearly discernible P waves preceding these complexes and longer duration of ventricular depolarization suggests that they originated near the atrioventricular junction or bundle of His.

The patient remains without complaint. An old ECG is retrieved for comparison and indicates no change. No emergent intervention is required.

CASE 39 ANSWER   CHIEF COMPLAINT: Weakness

12-LEAD ECG INTERPRETATION

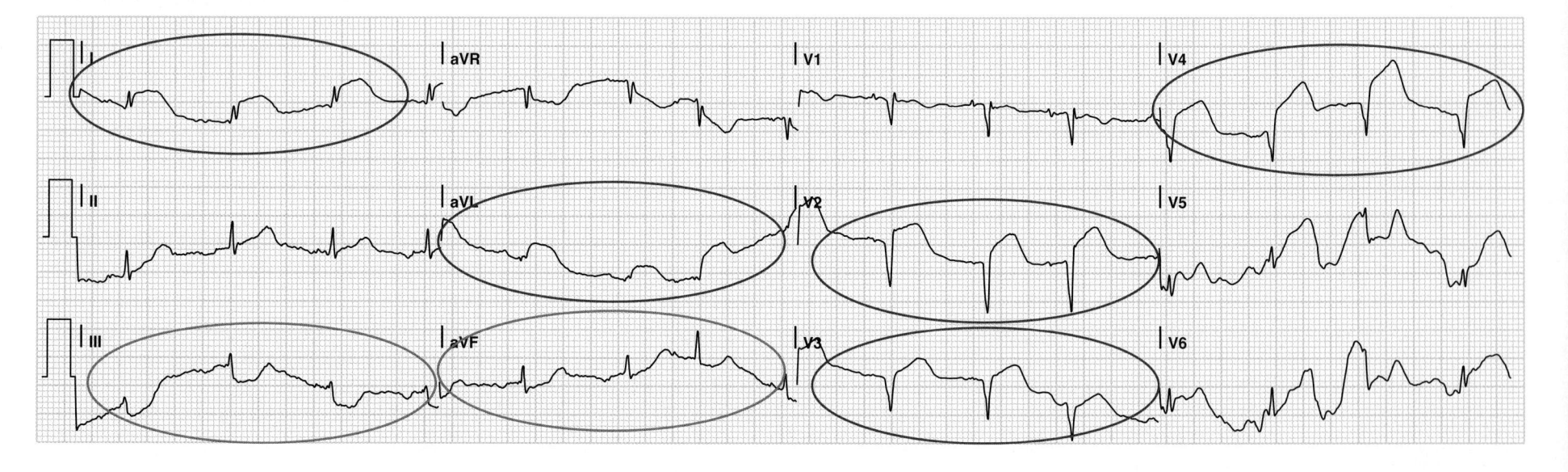

Sinus rhythm, heart rate: 90 beats/min., anterolateral wall STEMI.

Obvious ST elevation is present in leads V_2 through V_4, and in leads I and aVL (*red ovals*). Reciprocal ST depression is noted in leads III and aVF (*green ovals*). These findings are consistent with extensive anterolateral wall myocardial infarction.

You recognize that the ECG changes are suggestive of myocardial infarction and immediately bring the patient into the treatment area. The chest pain protocol is initiated and the emergency department nurses order laboratory studies, a chest X ray, and administration of aspirin. The attending physician concurs with the findings of anterolateral wall ST elevation myocardial infarction (STEMI) and activates the cardiac catheterization team.

12-LEAD ECG INTERPRETATION

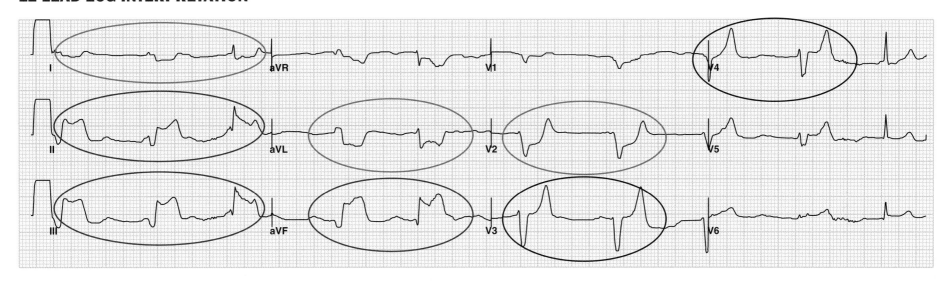

Complete heart block, ventricular rate: 50 beats/min., inferior wall STEMI.

This patient is critically ill. Massive ST elevations appear in the inferior limb leads (*red ovals*). Expected reciprocal ST depressions are present in the lateral leads and in lead V_2 (*green ovals*). Unusually large (or hyperacute) T waves are present in leads V_3 and V_4 (*black ovals*), which is indicative of early ischemia. Most concerning is the presence of a third-degree (complete) heart block: the P-P interval is fixed (i.e., the atrium is beating regularly), but there does not seem to be a constant P-R interval, indicating that the atrium and ventricle are beating independently. This patient requires expeditious transport to a facility that can perform a percutaneous cardiac intervention. En route to the receiving facility, you initiate large-bore peripheral intravenous access and take a blood glucose reading by fingerstick. The patient may require endotracheal intubation and blood pressure support. While you are administering intravenous fluids, consider emergent external cardiac pacing. If cardiac pacing fails to improve perfusion, inotropes and vasopressors may be needed. C-spine precautions are appropriate, given the patient's history of falling and loss of consciousness.

Myocardial infarction may actually present without pain, and such symptoms as weakness, syncope, fatigue, and dyspnea may be the advanced provider's only clues to underlying ischemia.

You have difficulty establishing peripheral intravenous access. High-flow oxygen is continued by bag-valve-mask, and another advanced life support provider places a 16-gauge intravenous line in the right external jugular vein. You begin external cardiac pacing according to protocol. Medical command authorizes an intravenous dopamine infusion at 5 µg/kg/min. The patient's condition rapidly deteriorates during transport, and she subsequently goes into cardiac arrest. At the destination hospital, a Level I cardiac receiving center, the patient is taken to a catheterization laboratory. Multiple stents are placed during the catheterization, and therapeutic hypothermia is initiated in the intensive care unit.

CASE 41 ANSWER   CHIEF COMPLAINT: Chest pain

12-LEAD ECG INTERPRETATION

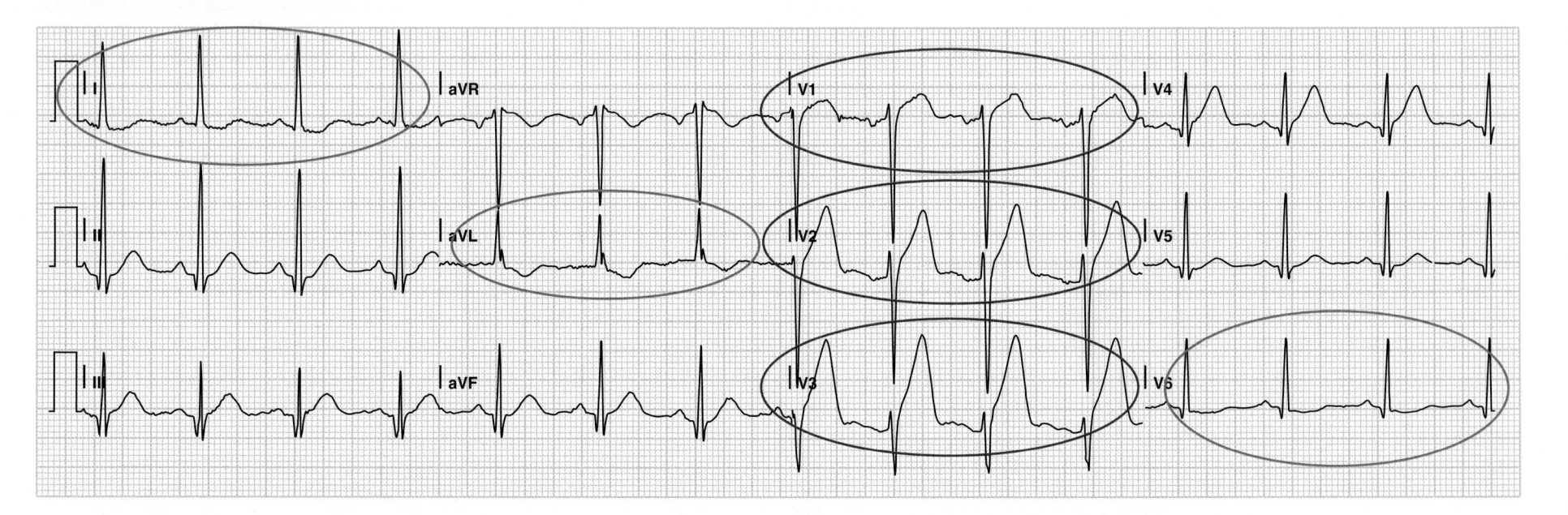

Sinus rhythm, heart rate: 70–80 beats/min., anterior wall STEMI.

Tall, broad-based T waves (hyperacute T waves), which are typical of early ischemia, are noted in leads V_2 and V_3. Concurrent ST elevation (*red ovals*) in leads V_1 through V_3 confirms a diagnosis of an anterior wall myocardial infarction. Hyperkalemia can also be a cause of tall T waves and should certainly be considered in the differential; however, the T waves of hyperkalemia are more narrow-based, and tend to appear in more leads. Additionally, the reciprocal ST depression and inverted T waves in lateral leads I, aVL, and V_6 (*green ovals*) weigh heavily in favor of acute myocardial infarction rather than hyperkalemia. T wave changes associated with electrolyte derangements are not typically found in an anatomic distribution. This patient's ECG should trigger activation of the cardiac catheterization laboratory.

In this case, advanced providers alerted medical control and administered nitroglycerin and aspirin. The patient's blood pressure remained stable, and an additional 4 mg of morphine sulfate was administered for ongoing pain. On arrival at the hospital, a second ECG revealed persistent ST elevation. A second large-bore intravenous line was started. A chest film showed a normal mediastinum, and a bolus of heparin was given in the emergency department. The patient was expeditiously transported to the cardiac catheterization laboratory, where interventional cardiologists diagnosed an acute occlusion of the diagonal branch of the left anterior descending artery.

12-LEAD ECG INTERPRETATION

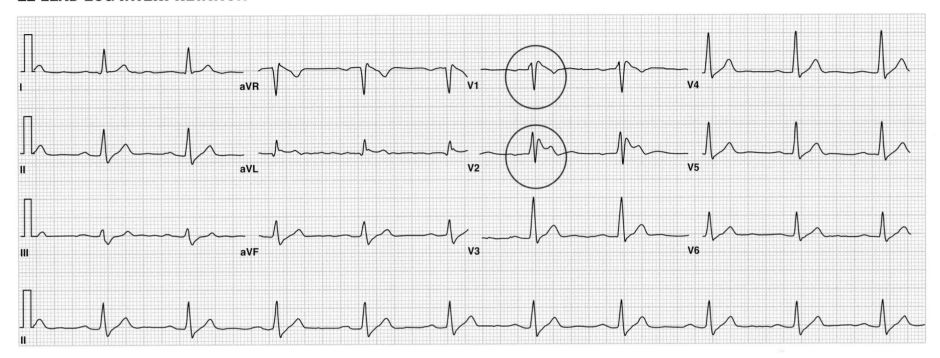

CLINICAL PEARL

Obtain a 12-lead ECG on patients presenting with syncope. A 12-lead ECG may contain important clues to an underlying dysrhythmia, disorder, or structural problem involving the heart.

Sinus rhythm, heart rate: 80 beats/min., Brugada syndrome.

The ECG reveals sinus rhythm. Note the incomplete right bundle branch block pattern (rSr') and ST elevations in leads V_1 and V_2. The T waves are inverted in V_1 and V_2, and upright in V_3. These are the classic electrocardiographic findings of Brugada syndrome (see the appendix "Brugada Syndrome"). Brugada syndrome is a genetic disorder involving an abnormality of sodium channels found within the heart's muscle cells. The exact mechanism is incompletely understood, but this disorder renders the heart more vulnerable to electrical disturbances. The disease can cause ventricular dysrhythmias (ventricular tachycardia and ventricular fibrillation) resulting in syncope (if the arrhythmia terminates spontaneously) or sudden death. Patients are usually diagnosed after a syncopal episode, often between 30 and 40 years of age. However, the syndrome can also manifest in the very young or the elderly. The only effective treatment is placement of an automatic internal cardioverter-defibrillator. Although Brugada syndrome is not an ischemic heart disorder, always err on the side of caution and transport to a facility capable of percutaneous coronary intervention when the ECG shows ST elevation. Brugada syndrome is a "mimic" of ischemia in that it is characterized by ST elevation in the precordial leads. Reciprocal changes, such as ST depression or T wave inversion, are absent in this particular ECG.

Advanced providers recognized the ST segment abnormalities found in the ECG's precordial leads and transported the patient to the hospital for confirmatory testing.

CASE 43 ANSWER   CHIEF COMPLAINT: Syncope

12-LEAD ECG INTERPRETATION

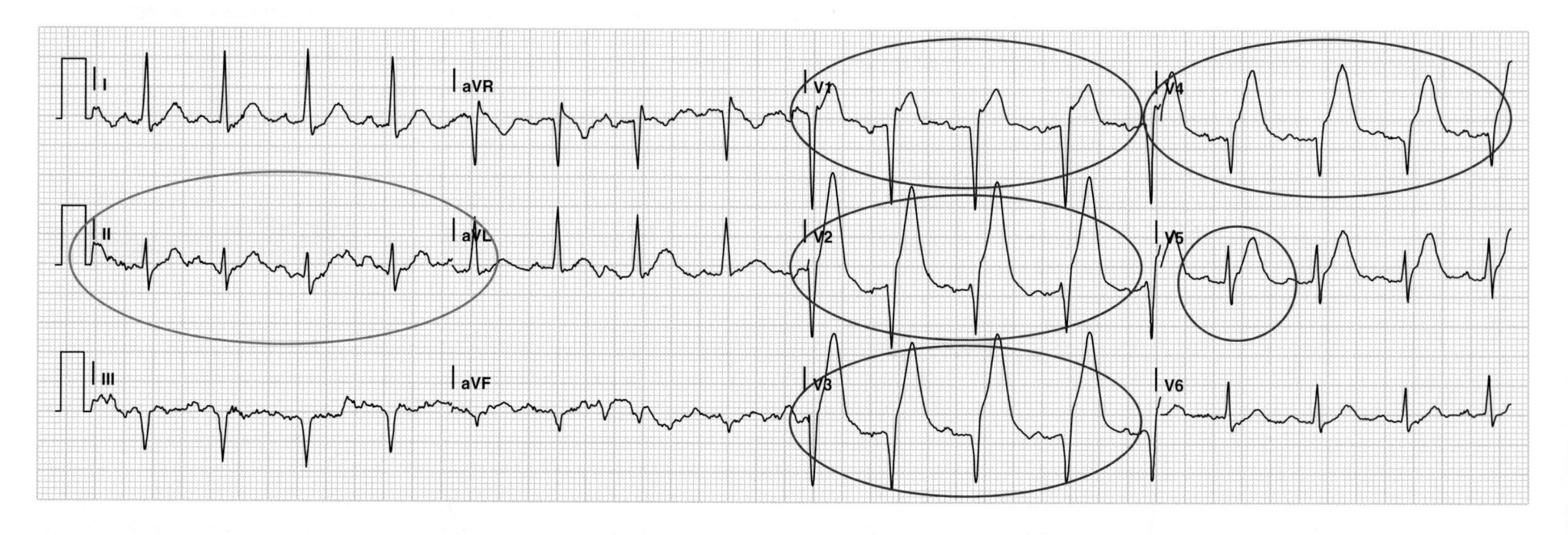

Sinus tachycardia, heart rate: 100 beats/min., anterior wall STEMI.

This ECG demonstrates ST elevation across the precordial leads in V_1 through V_4 (*red ovals*). Lead V_5 shows some hyperacute (tall and peaked) T waves (*red circle*). This finding is consistent with anterior wall injury. Typical reciprocal changes are not immediately evident in the patient's limb leads, although there is slight ST depression in lead II (*green oval*). It is imperative to obtain 12-lead ECGs in patients who recover from a syncopal episode, even in the absence of any symptoms suggestive of an acute coronary syndrome. Congestive heart failure and dysrhythmias are frequently encountered in patients with anterior wall myocardial infarction. It is possible that the syncope resulted from a brief episode of ventricular tachycardia. The widespread elevation across the entire precordium (*red ovals*) suggests left main or left anterior descending artery occlusion.

The patient received aspirin and nitroglycerin en route to the hospital. Paramedics also administered oxygen at 2 L/min. The patient was transported to the local emergency department and underwent successful angioplasty of the left anterior descending artery.

RHYTHM STRIP INTERPRETATION

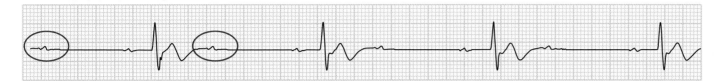

Second-degree atrioventricular block with 2:1 conduction, ventricular rate in the 30s.
Second-degree atrioventricular (AV) block is characterized by nonconducted atrial beats (*red circles*) and a regular relationship between the P waves and the QRS complexes (see the appendix "Heart Blocks Made Simple"). In this ECG, for example, the R-R intervals remain constant. By contrast, in complete heart block the PR intervals change randomly. Causes of second-degree AV heart block include myocardial infarction; drugs (e.g., digoxin, beta blockers, calcium channel blockers, amiodarone); and Lyme disease, which was the cause in this patient. Cardiac involvement is rare but bacterial invasion of heart tissue may manifest itself as AV nodal block. Second-degree type II heart block is usually associated with pathology below the level of the AV node. QRS complexes may appear slightly wider, even though they originate above the ventricles.

CASE 45 ANSWER   CHIEF COMPLAINT: Weakness

12-LEAD ECG INTERPRETATION

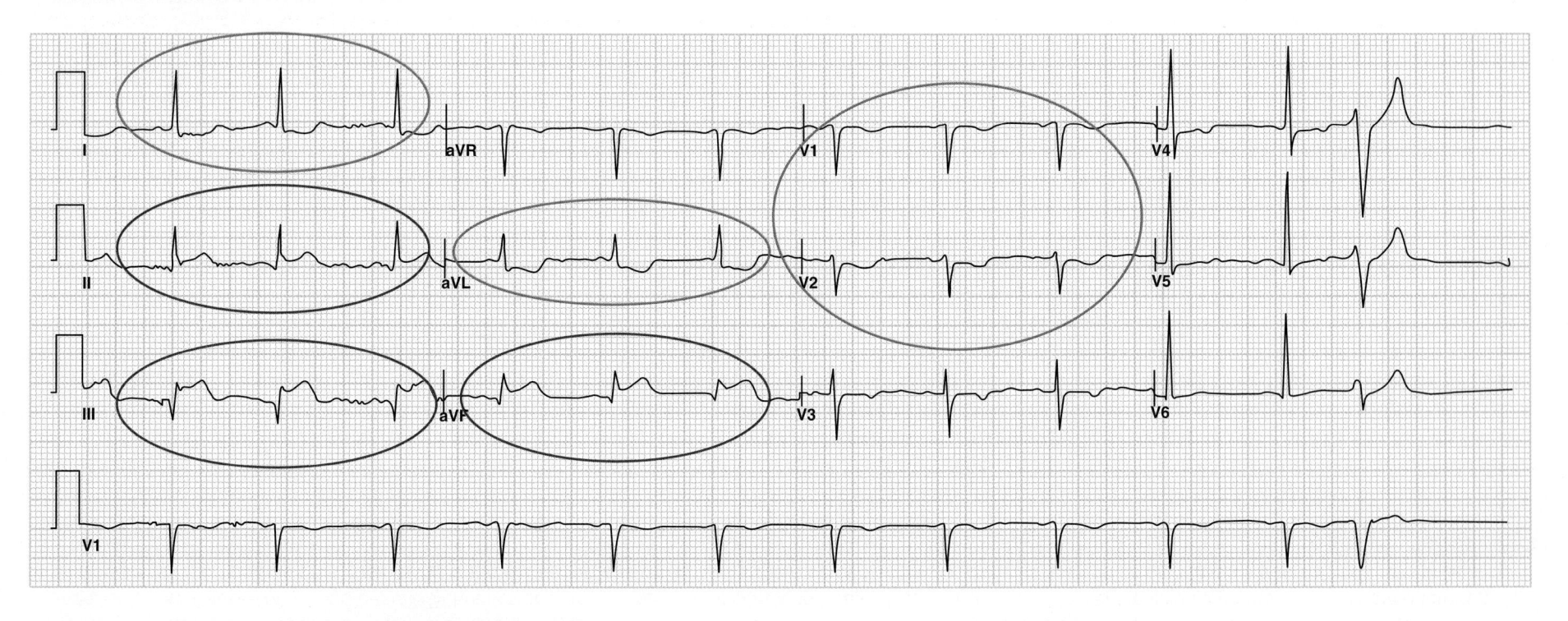

CLINICAL PEARL

- Elderly patients, people with diabetes, and women might have atypical signs and symptoms of cardiac ischemia; have a low threshold for 12-lead electrocardiography in these patients.
- Shortness of breath and weakness are common "anginal equivalents" in the elderly.
- Q waves do not always indicate irreversible ischemia. Although commonly interpreted as evidence of necrosis, Q waves may be present in acute ischemia and should always prompt consideration of transport to a facility with resources for percutaneous cardiac intervention.

Sinus rhythm, heart rate: 82 beats/min., inferior wall STEMI.
This patient's ECG reveals an inferior wall injury pattern. The presence of ST depression in leads V$_1$ and V$_2$ (*green ovals*) raises the possibility of posterior wall involvement. ST elevation is present in leads II, III, and aVF (*red ovals*). Reciprocal changes in the form of ST depression are evident in leads I and aVL (*green ovals*). You also note a pathologic Q wave (>0.04 ms, or more than one-third the height of the R wave) in lead III. You establish intravenous access and administer aspirin according to protocol. The patient remains stable while en route to the local STEMI center.

12-LEAD ECG INTERPRETATION

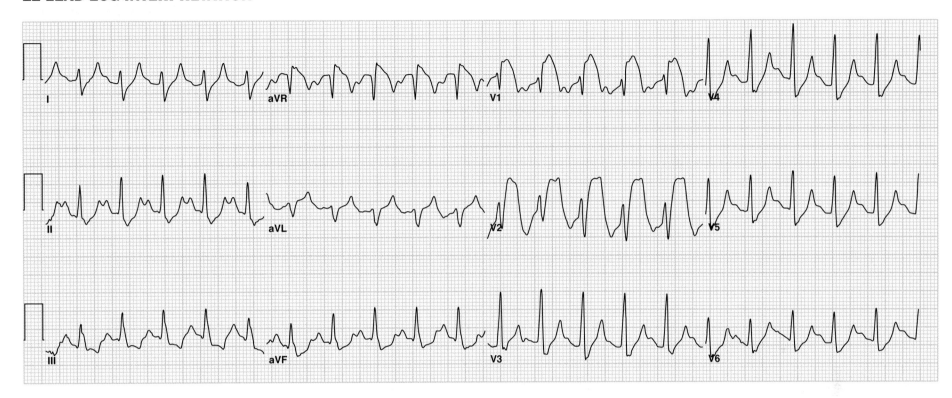

Sinus tachycardia, heart rate: 145–155 beats/min., ST elevation in leads V₁ and V₂, widened QRS complex, and diffusely peaked T waves in limb and precordial leads consistent with hyperkalemia.

The ECG reveals sinus tachycardia; hyperacute, peaked, narrow-based, and asymmetric T waves; and wide QRS complexes. Potassium is necessary for muscle contraction but, in excess, it causes myocardial irritation and leads to ventricular dysrhythmias. This patient had a K+ level of 8.7 mEq/L (3.5–5.0 mEq/L is normal).

The following electrocardiographic changes are associated with hyperkalemia: dysrhythmia (ventricular flutter is a late finding); diffusely peaked T waves; ST elevation; small or absent P waves; and widening of the QRS complex.

You recognize ECG changes consistent with hyperkalemia and administer 1 ampule of calcium gluconate to stabilize the myocardial membranes. You transport the patient to the emergency department for further testing and stabilization.

CASE 47 ANSWER   CHIEF COMPLAINT: Stomach burning

12-LEAD ECG INTERPRETATION

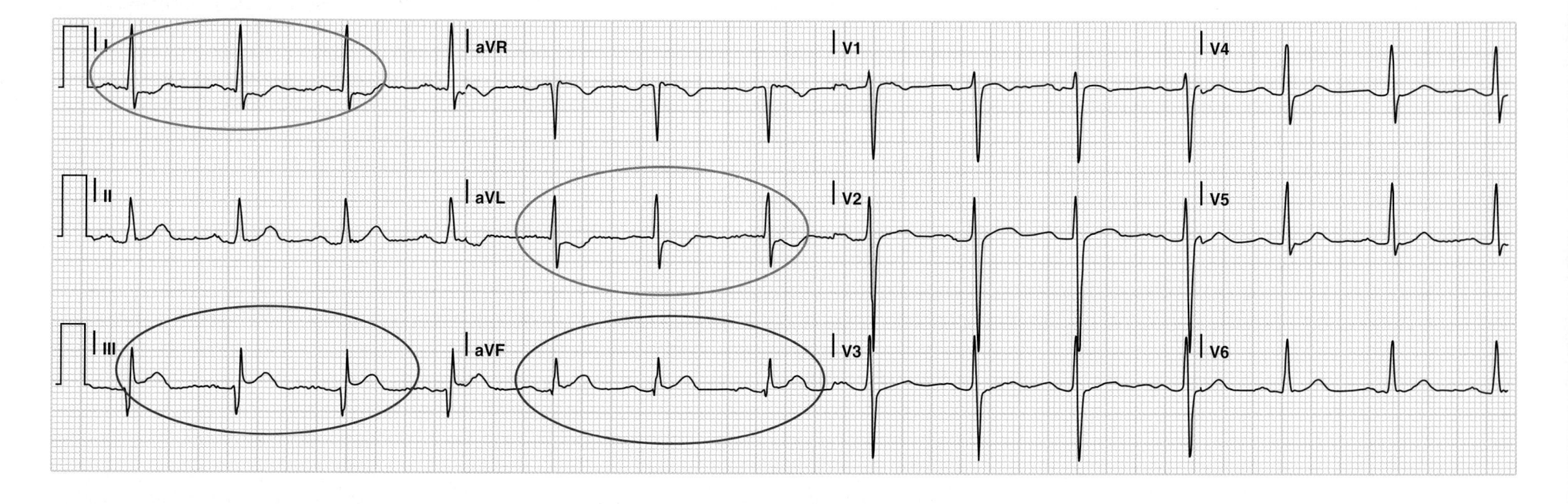

Sinus rhythm, heart rate: 80 beats/min., inferior wall STEMI.

This patient's ECG indicates ST elevation in leads III and aVF (*red ovals*). Lead III shows a developing pathologic Q wave (i.e., more than one-third the height of the R wave; see the appendix "Pathologic Q wave"). ST and T segment changes in the inferior leads (II, III, and aVF) indicate active injury. Another indication of ischemia is the presence of reciprocal changes. Leads I and aVL indicate reciprocal ST depression (*green ovals*). The presence of such reciprocal changes increases the likelihood that a patient with ST elevation is experiencing a true ST elevation myocardial infarction (STEMI).

Infarcts of the right ventricle often coexist with inferior wall myocardial injury. Right ventricular extension of an inferior infarct is important to diagnose because patients with this condition often require liberal intravenous fluid administration to maintain the blood pressure. The presence of ST elevation on a right-sided ECG indicates a right ventricular myocardial infarction (MI). Be prepared to administer intravenous fluids. Patients with a right ventricular MI are preload dependent, so preload-reducing medications, such as nitrates, should be avoided because they can induce a precipitous fall in blood pressure.

Gastrointestinal symptoms are common with inferior wall infarcts. These patients are often misdiagnosed as having gastro-esophageal reflux disease or peptic ulcer disease. Always consider the possibility of an inferior wall MI or ischemia for a patient with chest pain or upper abdominal pain before assigning a diagnosis of "reflux."

This patient should be transported expeditiously and treated with aspirin. Nitrates can be administered according to protocol if there is no evidence of right ventricular MI. A second large-bore intravenous line should be established if protocol permits.

CLINICAL PEARL

Do not be too quick to dismiss abdominal pain in the prehospital environment, and be sure to consider myocardial ischemia in patients that present with gastrointestinal symptoms.

CLINICAL PEARL

Obtain a right-sided ECG in patients presenting with ST elevation in the heart's inferior wall.

CHIEF COMPLAINT: Sharp chest pain

12-LEAD ECG INTERPRETATION

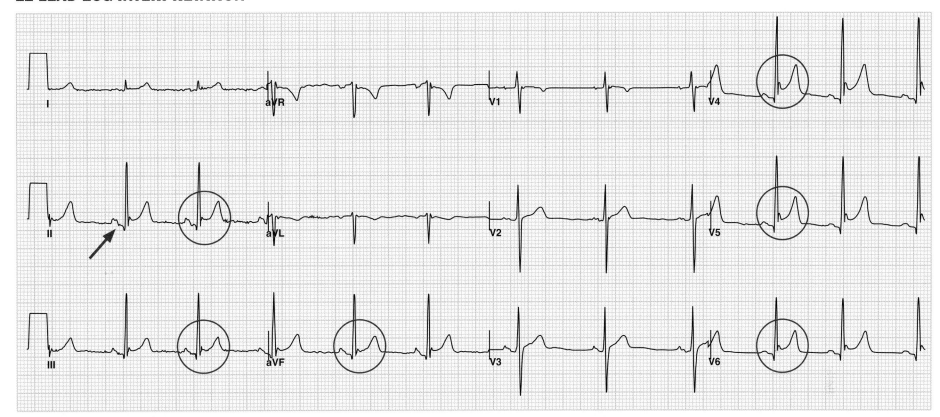

CLINICAL PEARL

Always err on the side of caution when you encounter ST elevation on the ECG! When in doubt, assume that any ST elevation is ST elevation myocardial infarction until you can prove otherwise. Obtain medical direction when unsure about the ECG findings and transmit the tracing to the receiving facility when possible.

Sinus rhythm, heart rate: 60–70 beats/min., diffuse ST elevation consistent with pericarditis.

The ECG demonstrates evidence of acute pericarditis. Note the diffuse ST elevation (*red circles*); the characteristic PR segment depression (*red arrow*) throughout the ECG (except in aVR, where the PR segment is elevated); and the lack of reciprocal changes. The ST segment in pericarditis is generally concave upward. Together with the patient's history of recent illness, these electrocardiographic findings are diagnostic of pericarditis rather than acute myocardial infarction.

You consult with the base station physician. Based on the patient's age and clinical presentation, the physician agrees that this patient should be transported to the closest hospital.

CASE 49 ANSWER   CHIEF COMPLAINT: Unconsciousness

RHYTHM STRIP INTERPRETATION, ECG #1

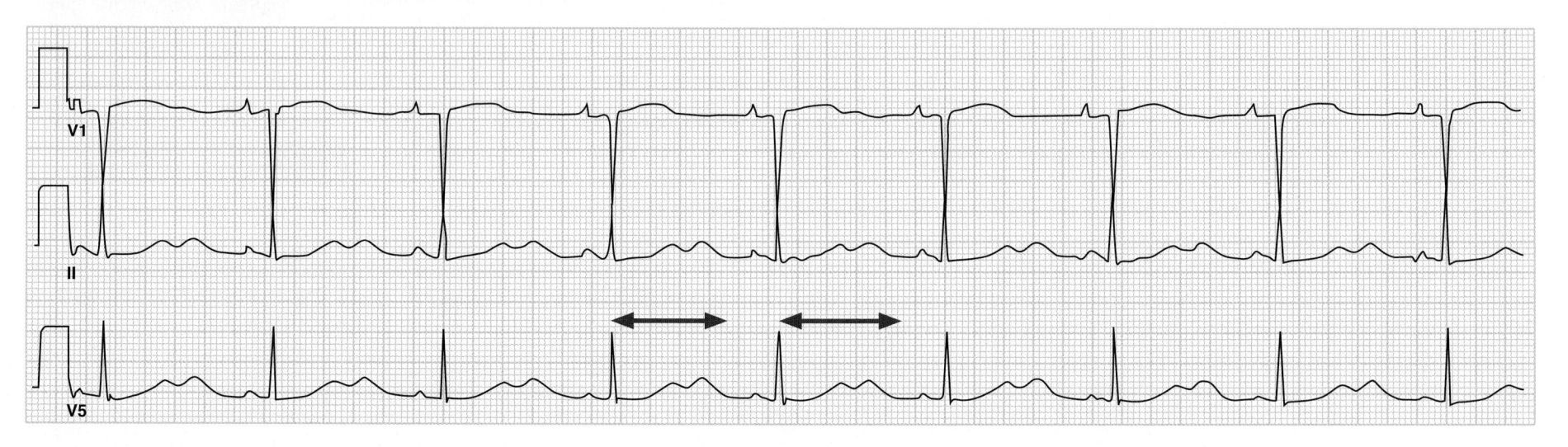

Sinus rhythm; prolonged QT interval.

The first tracing reveals a baseline sinus rhythm. T waves are generally upright, and prominent "U" waves are present in leads II and V$_5$. Although U waves are a normal variant found during routine ECG testing, their presence may indicate an underlying electrolyte imbalance. T waves are present in electrolyte disturbances, such as hypokalemia and hypocalcemia. The differential diagnosis related to U waves is quite broad; their appearance on an ECG should prompt astute clinicians to more closely scrutinize the QT segment for abnormalities, such as prolongation. The QT interval in this particular ECG (*red arrows*) is dangerously prolonged. Inverted U waves might appear in the setting of myocardial ischemia.

Measuring the QT interval is the first step in determining if its duration is normal. However, the raw QT interval measurement does not take into consideration the effects of the heart rate on the duration of the interval. For example, a patient with a heart rate of 40 has a longer QT interval than a patient with a heart rate of 180. To decide if the QT interval is prolonged, clinicians use several mathematical formulas to calculate a new value known as the "QT corrected" (QTc). The QTc is the predicted value of the measured QT interval at a standard heart rate of 60 beats/min. QT and QTc are only equal when the actual heart rate is 60 beats/min. If the actual heart rate is < 60, the QTc is less than the measured QT; if it is > 60, the QTc is more than the measured QT interval. A detailed discussion of these methods is beyond the scope of this textbook. Generally speaking, the QTc is considered prolonged when it is > 460 milliseconds. A QTc interval > 550 milliseconds increases the patient's risk of malignant dysrhythmia, such as torsades de pointes (TdP). A quick glance at this tracing's QT interval reveals that the measurement exceeds three large boxes, or 600 milliseconds. A large U wave (> 1 mm in amplitude) that is fused to the T wave should be included in a formal calculation of the QT interval. A field expedient method for determining if the QT interval is prolonged is to find the halfway point between two R waves and evaluate the location of the T or U wave in relation to that point. If the T or U wave extends beyond half the distance between R waves, the QT interval is prolonged; if not, the QT interval is normal.

(Continued)

CHIEF COMPLAINT: Unconsciousness

RHYTHM STRIP INTERPRETATION, ECG #2

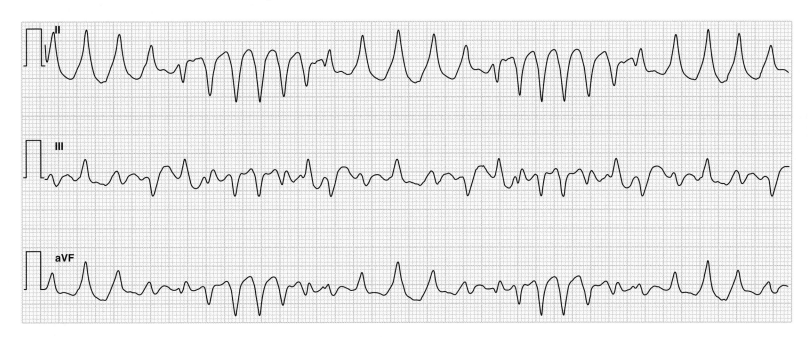

Polymorphic ventricular tachycardia; torsades de pointes.

Polymorphic ventricular tachycardia (PMVT) is a type of ventricular tachycardia characterized by variations in QRS morphologies. In this case, it is also notable that the axis changes and there is a pattern of increasing-decreasing-increasing QRS complex amplitude. This is a specific type of PMVT often called torsades de pointes (TdP), which is French for "twisting of the points." It is important to note that not all PMVT is TdP. A diagnosis of TdP is also defined by the presence of a long QT interval, measured before or after the arrest period. The presence of a normal-duration QT interval favors the diagnosis of generic PMVT. The initial tracing reveals a QT interval of 800 ms, well above the upper normal limit of 460 ms.

Treatment is started in accordance with standard advanced cardiac life support protocols. The cornerstones of management include uninterrupted, high-quality compressions and the delivery of prompt defibrillation. Intravenous magnesium sulfate, if available, is considered first-line treatment for PMVT. Such drugs as amiodarone are associated with prolongation of the QT interval and should be avoided in suspected cases of TdP.

CASE 50 ANSWER   CHIEF COMPLAINT: Weakness

12-LEAD ECG INTERPRETATION

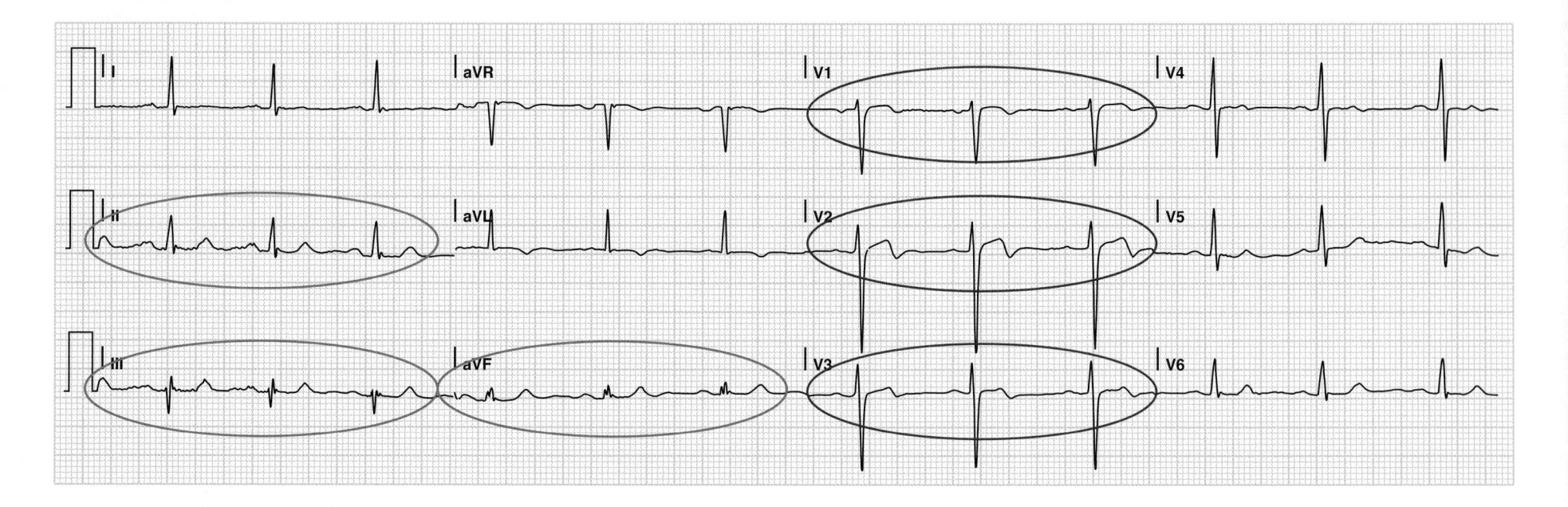

Sinus rhythm, heart rate: 90 beats/min., anterior wall ischemia.

The ECG reveals terminal T wave inversion in leads V_1 through V_3 (*red ovals*). Downsloping ST segments are observed in the inferior leads (*green ovals*). The presence of terminal T wave inversion in the right precordial leads is consistent with Wellens' syndrome. Wellens' is associated with blockage of the left anterior descending artery. Downsloping ST segments are typically associated with myocardial ischemia. The attending physician alerts the on-call cardiology team and the patient is transferred to a coronary care unit.

Close inspection of the anterior precordial leads (V_1 through V_4) is key to the electrocardiographic diagnosis of Wellens' syndrome. Manifestations of Wellens' syndrome include deep T wave inversions in the precordial leads or biphasic T waves in same distribution (*red ovals*). Wellens' syndrome is linked to occlusion of the left anterior descending artery and benefits from percutaneous coronary intervention as opposed to medical management.

12-LEAD ECG INTERPRETATION

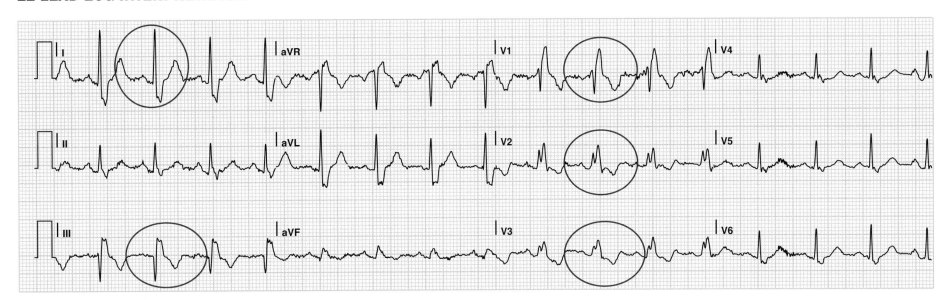

Sinus rhythm, heart rate: 100 beats/min., right bundle branch block.

The ECG reveals sinus rhythm. Note the following findings: large S wave in lead I, deep Q wave in lead III, and T wave inversion in lead III. The "S1Q3T3" pattern (*red circles*) is present in approximately 15% of patients with pulmonary embolism (PE). The ECG also reveals a right bundle branch block and inverted T waves in the precordial leads. These electrocardiographic findings suggest PE. The pattern is the result of right ventricular strain secondary to a large increase in pulmonary artery pressure. A large embolism or numerous small ones have caused pressure to build in the pulmonary circuit, and the right ventricle has become dilated and strained. Although tachycardia is a classic finding in PE, it might not always be present.

PE is diagnosed through physical examination findings in conjunction with the patient's medical history and perhaps diagnostic imaging. Prehospital treatment includes supportive therapy with oxygen. Notify the receiving facility early and transport the patient rapidly.

The diagnosis of PE was confirmed with contrast-enhanced computed chest tomography. Elevated troponin and unstable vital signs are markers of a grave prognosis. In-hospital treatment consists of anticoagulation and further diagnostic testing directed at discovering an underlying cause, such as a lower leg venous thrombosis or a blood-clotting disorder.

CASE 52 ANSWER   CHIEF COMPLAINT: Syncope

12-LEAD ECG INTERPRETATION

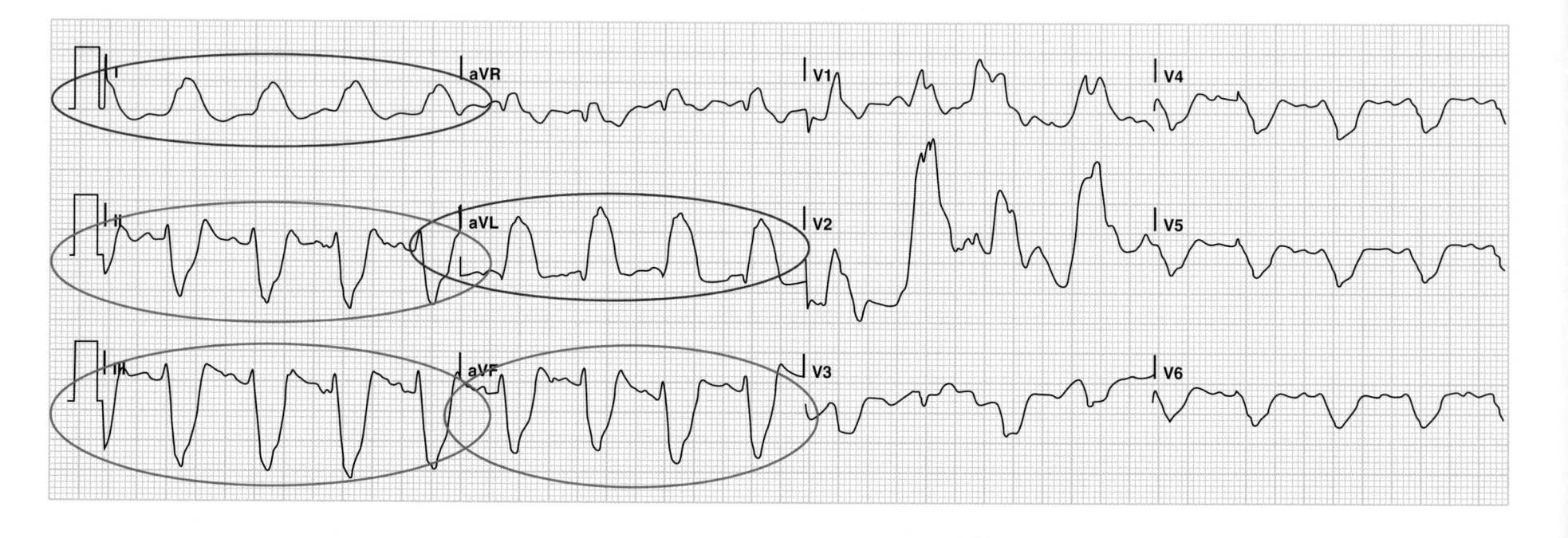

Sinus tachycardia, heart rate: 150 beats/min., anterior/lateral STEMI.

This patient's syncopal episode was the first sign of a critical lesion. Syncope, hypotension, and diaphoresis support the diagnosis of a significant cardiac event. Syncope and hypotension can also signal critical disasters, such as aortic dissection or internal bleeding. The patient's ECG shows prominent ST elevations in leads I and aVL (*red ovals*). Furthermore, deep reciprocal depressions are evident in leads II, III, and aVF (*green ovals*). This patient is best managed with immediate percutaneous coronary intervention (PCI). He is hemodynamically unstable and in cardiogenic shock. The S_3 is an additional heart sound that may indicate impaired ventricular filling. Auscultation of an S_3 that resembles a "galloping" sound suggests heart failure. You notify the responding advanced life support unit of a "priority 1 patient." You establish two large-bore intravenous lines and begin administering a fluid bolus. The patient chews four baby aspirin tablets. While transferring him to the stretcher, you note occasional ventricular ectopy. The patient is taken to the closest PCI facility, which is an additional 10 minutes away by ground. Medical control supports this decision, given the electrocardiographic findings and clinical picture suggestive of active ischemia.

The patient is taken directly to the catheterization laboratory. He is diagnosed with a large circumflex artery lesion not amenable to stenting. The patient is prepared for emergency cardiac bypass and is transferred to the cardiac care unit in critical condition. The interventional cardiologist places an intra-aortic balloon pump as a temporizing measure until the cardiac operating suite is ready.

CHIEF COMPLAINT: Chest pain, fever, cough

12-LEAD ECG INTERPRETATION

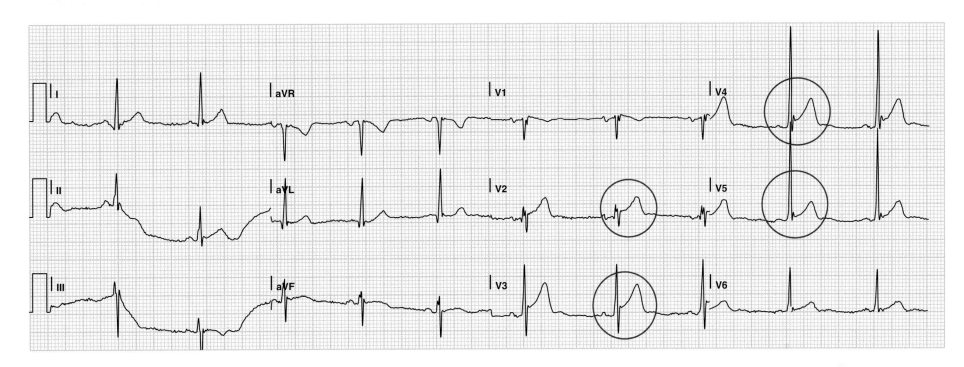

Sinus rhythm, heart rate: 60 beats/min., J point elevation consistent with benign early repolarization.

Sinus rhythm with benign early repolarization is evident on the ECG. ST elevation is present in leads V₂ through V₅ (*red circles*). The concave-upward ST segment morphology, early departure from the QRS complex, and "fishhook" appearance of the J point strongly favor benign early repolarization versus acute myocardial infarction. After you discuss the findings with on-line medical control and transmit the 12-lead ECG, the physician concurs that the ECG and clinical picture are inconsistent with ischemia. You establish intravenous access, administer oxygen, and transport the patient to the local emergency department.

One other note of interest is that the ECG shows relative bradycardia, a relatively low heart rate considering the presence of a fever. We normally anticipate a faster heart rate in patients with fever (it is commonly held that the heart rate increases by 10 beats/min. for every 1° rise in temperature above normal). In this case, the absence of tachycardia is likely caused by the beta-adrenergic blocking effects of atenolol.

CLINICAL PEARL

Benign early repolarization is not associated with ST depression or T wave inversion (reciprocal changes)!

CASE 54 ANSWER   CHIEF COMPLAINT: Syncope

12-LEAD ECG INTERPRETATION

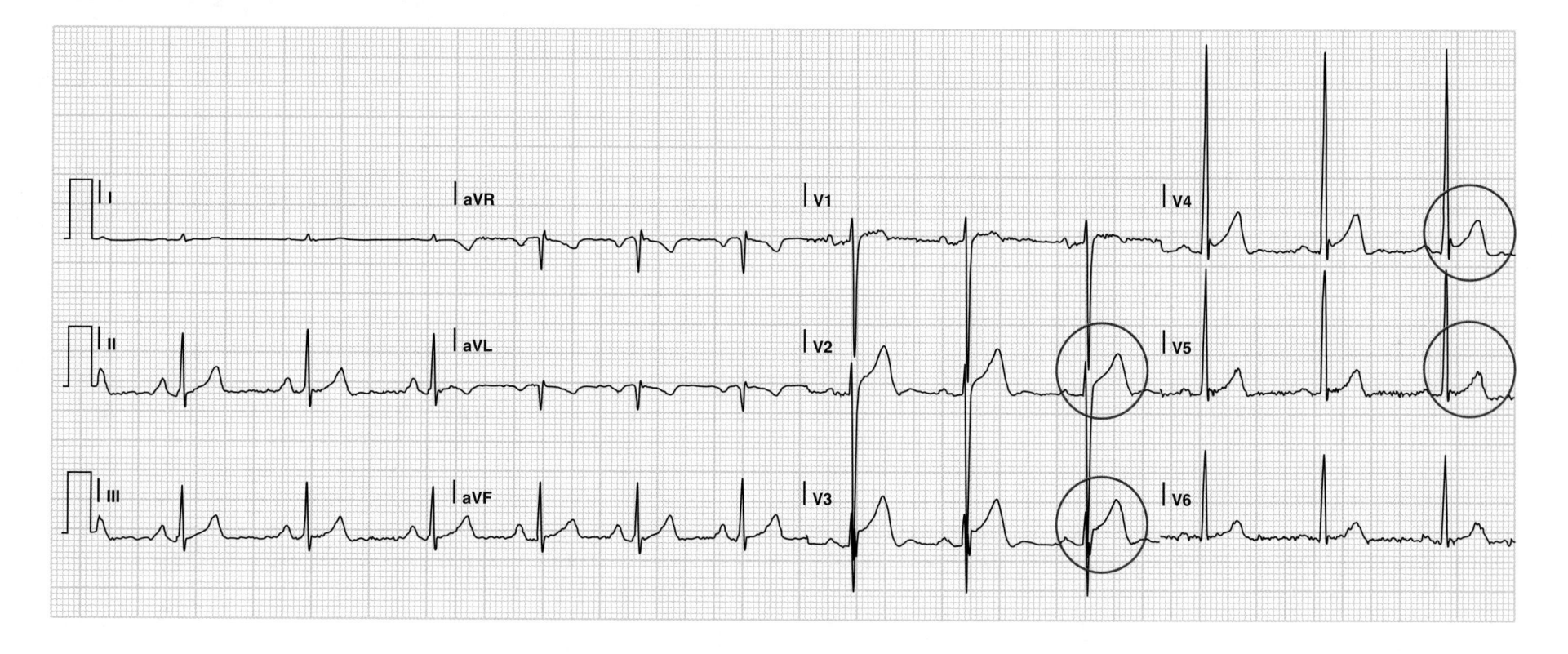

Sinus dysrhythmia, heart rate: 80 beats/min., benign early repolarization.

The slight irregularity of the heart rate is a normal variant referred to as "sinus dysrhythmia." Benign early repolarization is indicated by the concave-upward ST segment morphology (*red circles*), large T waves, early departure from the QRS complex, and "fishhook" appearance of the J point. The absence of reciprocal ST depressions also strongly favors a benign cause of the ST elevation. Large-amplitude QRS complexes are present, suggesting left ventricular hypertrophy (LVH) ; however, LVH should generally not be diagnosed in patients younger than 45 years of age based on electrocardiographic findings. Instead, this finding is simply referred to as "high left ventricular voltage," a common normal variant in young patients. It is likely that this patient experienced vasovagal syncope associated with pressure applied to the eye during the procedure.

A chief complaint of syncope should prompt emergency responders to consider underlying causes. Twelve-lead electrocardiography, measurement of blood glucose, vital signs, and transport to an emergency department are all appropriate prehospital interventions.

CLINICAL PEARL

Concave ST segments are typically associated with benign conditions, whereas convex ST segments indicate pathology, such as ischemia.

12-LEAD ECG INTERPRETATION

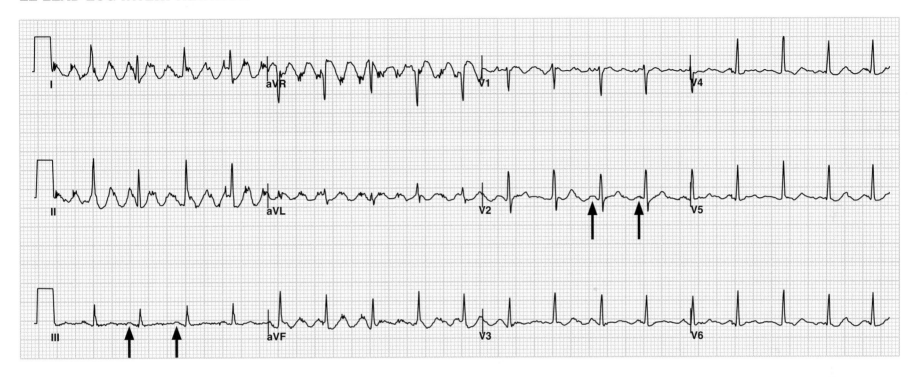

Sinus tachycardia, heart rate: 110 beats/min., somatic tremor resembling atrial flutter.

At first glance, the rhythm seems to be atrial flutter with 2:1 conduction. Closer inspection of leads III and V$_2$ (*black arrows*) reveals the presence of normal P waves and the absence of flutter wave morphology. In this case, the source of the interference was determined to be patient tremor. You should challenge ECG findings if they do not make sense in the clinical context. If you suspect interference, eliminate common sources of artifacts, such as cellular phones and patient tremor.

CLINICAL PEARL

You should challenge ECG findings if they do not make sense in the clinical context.

CASE 56 ANSWER   **CHIEF COMPLAINT:** Chest pain

12-LEAD ECG INTERPRETATION

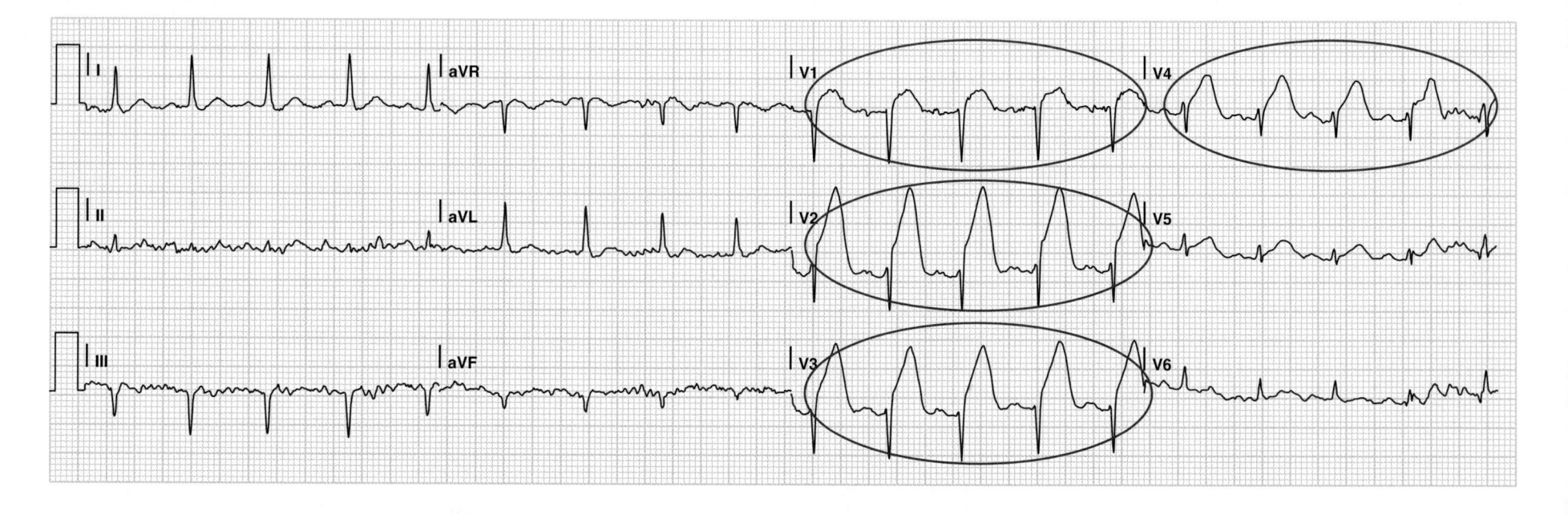

Sinus rhythm, heart rate: 110 beats/min., anterior wall STEMI.

ST elevations are illustrated in leads V_1 through V_4 (*red ovals*). No obvious reciprocal changes are noted in the limb leads. This ECG is consistent with an anterior wall ST elevation myocardial infarction.

En route to the referral center, the patient develops pulmonary edema. His blood pressure increases to 180/100 and his oxygen saturation level falls to 91%, despite receiving oxygen by nasal cannula. The patient is switched to high-flow oxygen by non-rebreather mask. Your CCT paramedic partner suggests continuous positive airway pressure (CPAP), and the patient is transitioned from the non-rebreather to noninvasive positive-pressure ventilation starting at 10 cm H_2O. In accordance with protocol, you administer 0.5 mg of lorazepam for anxiolysis. The nitroglycerin infusion is titrated upward every 10 minutes in increments of 10 μg to treat the developing pulmonary edema. You advise the receiving center about the change in the patient's condition. A cardiac specialist at the receiving center advises you to continue CPAP and nitroglycerin, and authorizes direct transport to the catheterization lab.

3-LEAD ECG INTERPRETATION

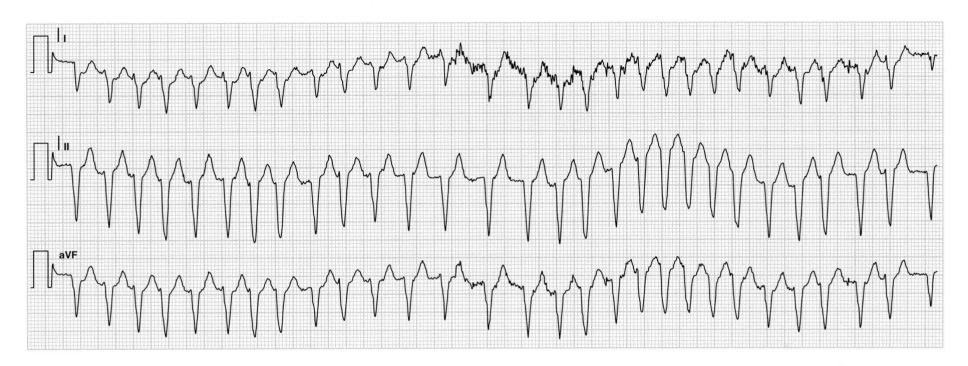

Atrial fibrillation with rapid ventricular response, variable ventricular rate of 170–280 beats/min., Wolff-Parkinson-White syndrome.

The 3-lead ECG reveals an irregularly irregular wide-complex rhythm with no discernible P waves. The rhythm is atrial fibrillation. The ventricular rate ranges from 170 to near 280 beats/min. This patient is stable and symptomatic, and requires rate control. How should this be achieved? Prehospital medications for rate control include calcium channel blockers, such as verapamil and diltiazem. Any hemodynamically compromised patient warrants urgent direct-current cardioversion. Wide complex tachycardias in an unstable or symptomatic patient should be considered ventricular tachycardia (VT) until proved otherwise. This patient's rhythm strip is concerning, but the irregular R-R intervals are not typical of VT. Ventricular trachycardia manifests as a regular, wide-complex tachycardia at a rate > 150 beats/min. This ECG reveals an irregular R-R interval, which is more typical of atrial fibrillation.

A layer of connective tissue separates atrial and ventricular tissue. The only communication between the two is by way of the atrioventricular (AV) node. The AV node receives a signal from the internodal pathways and delays conduction to the ventricles for 120–200 milliseconds, allowing them time to fill completely. The node then allows the impulse to continue, causing ventricular depolarization.

(Continued)

CASE 57 ANSWER

CHIEF COMPLAINT: Shortness of breath

CLINICAL PEARL

Wide-complex tachycardia in an unstable patient should be considered ventricular in origin until proved otherwise. Unstable patients warrant rapid assessment and urgent electrical cardioversion.

Several minutes later, a 12-lead ECG (shown below) was obtained from the same patient. He remained symptomatic and stable. What is the goal of your treatment?

In this patient's ECG, delta waves, indicating pre-excitation of ventricular tissue, are visible in leads II, III, V_5, and aVF (*red circles*). This is a subtle but crucial finding. This patient has atrial fibrillation and Wolff-Parkinson-White syndrome. Administration of a calcium channel blocker to achieve rate control in this patient could produce a lethal dysrhythmia. This category of drugs blocks conduction through the AV node and, in the presence of an accessory pathway (the bundle of Kent), promotes transport of electrical stimuli through that pathway. The "delay" mechanism of the accessory pathway is thus eliminated; therefore, if 300–600 impulses reach the pathway, then 300–600 impulses make it to ventricular tissue. This rate is not sustainable and the rhythm quickly deteriorates to ventricular fibrillation and asystole.

Tips for spotting electrocardiographic findings indicative of Wolff-Parkinson-White syndrome include the following: any atrial fibrillation with ventricular rate > 170–180 beats/min. should prompt consideration of an accessory pathway; any wide-complex atrial fibrillation should prompt consideration of an accessory pathway or bundle branch block; and the presence of delta waves confirms the presence of an accessory pathway (their absence favors bundle branch block).

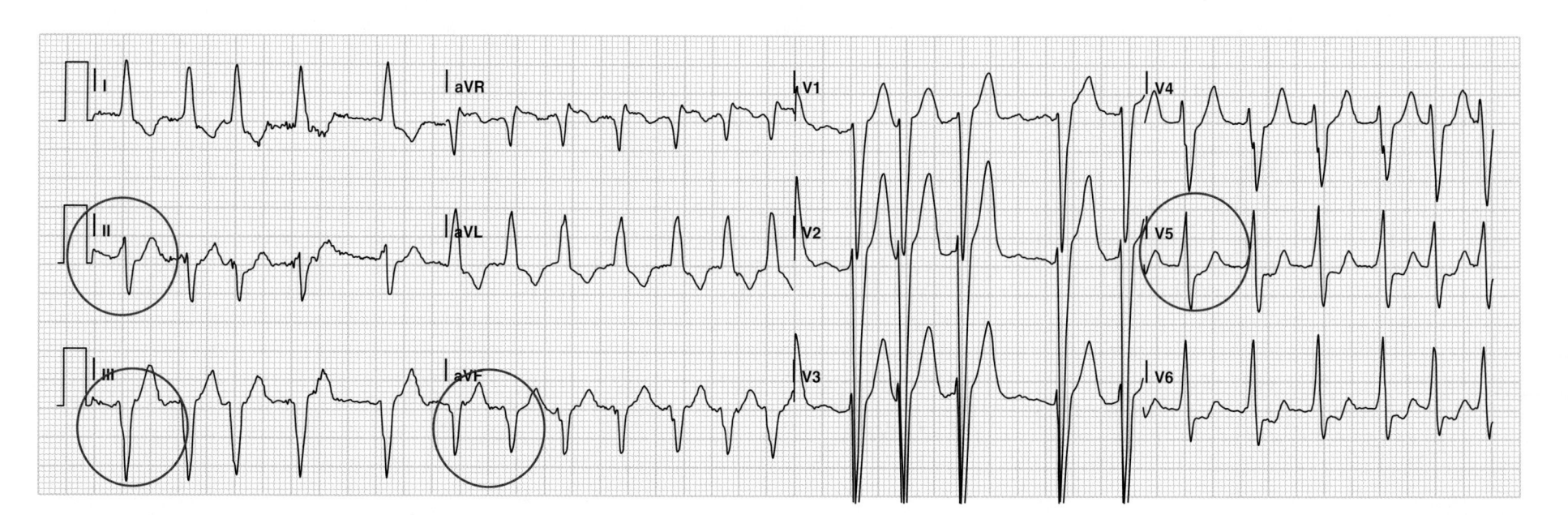

(Continued)

CHIEF COMPLAINT: Shortness of breath

The patient received procainamide in the emergency department, and rate control was achieved. An ECG obtained 1 week after the initial event is shown below. Delta waves are clearly visible across the entire tracing. On the 12-lead ECG, a delta wave appears as a "slurring" of the R wave, or the upstroke of the QRS complex (*red arrows*). Several days later, the patient was scheduled for ablation therapy.

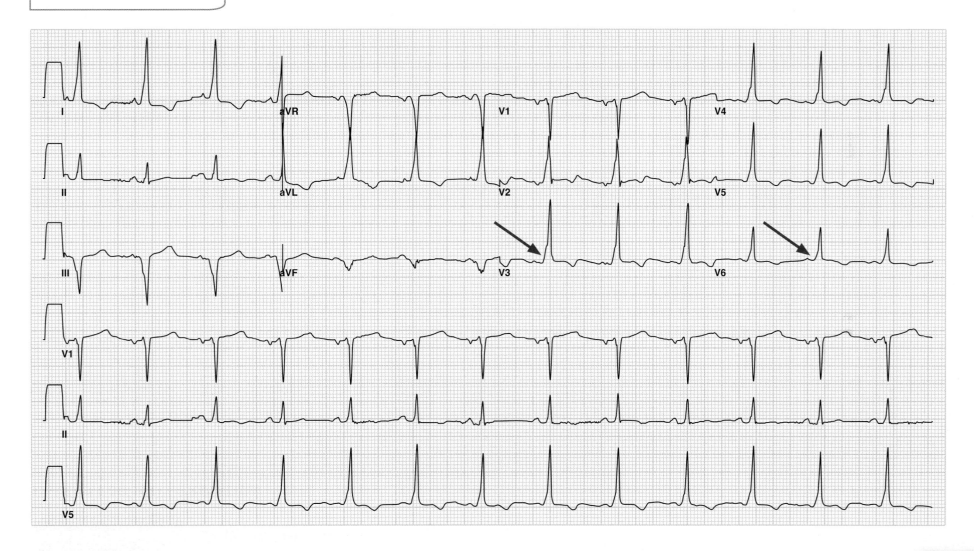

CASE 58 ANSWER   CHIEF COMPLAINT: Chest pain

12-LEAD ECG INTERPRETATION

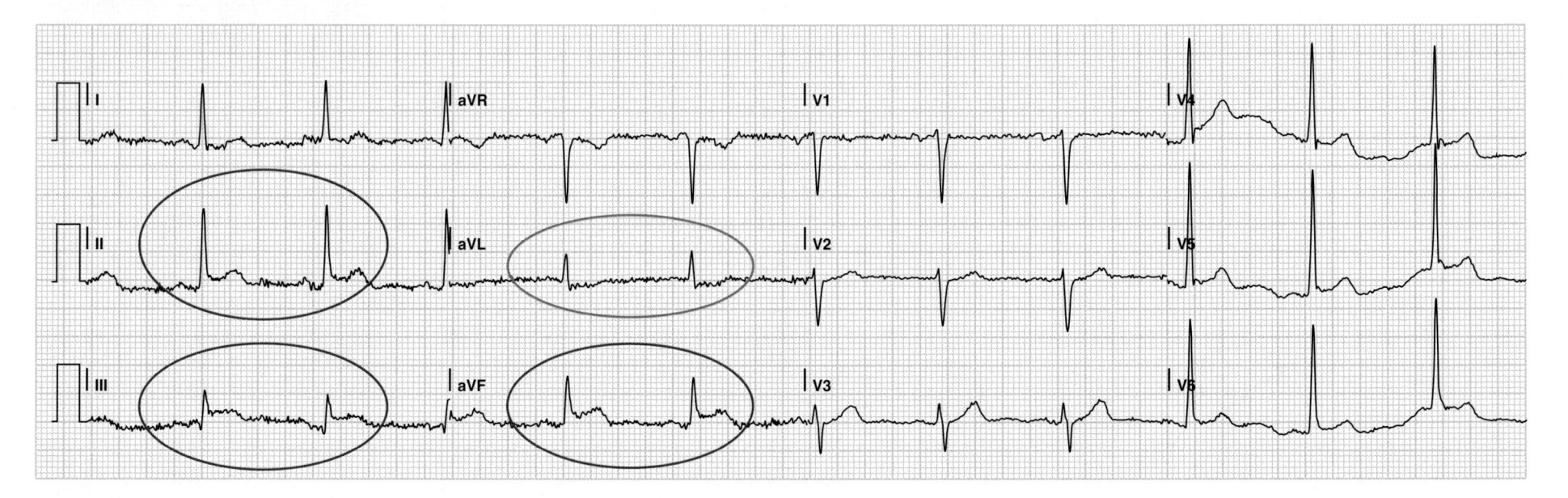

CLINICAL PEARL

Remember to always acquire a right-sided ECG (lead V$_4$R) when the ECG reveals ST elevation in the inferior leads. Withhold nitrates when the ECG demonstrates ST elevation in right-sided chest leads.

Sinus rhythm, heart rate: 60–70 beats/min., inferior wall STEMI.

ST elevations are present in inferior leads II, III, and aVF (*red ovals*), and reciprocal ST depression is noted in lead aVL (*green oval*). Advanced providers must remain alert for right ventricular involvement whenever an inferior wall ST elevation myocardial infarction (STEMI) is present. In this case, repeating the ECG with right-sided leads to evaluate right ventricular involvement is advisable. These patients should be treated with aspirin. If hypotension develops, aggressive fluid resuscitation is indicated. Nitroglycerin is routinely administered for ischemic chest pain, but in the case of right ventricular involvement, it is prudent to establish large-bore intravenous access before its administration. As always, bear local protocols in mind. This patient requires transport to a facility with the resources for percutaneous cardiac intervention.

12-LEAD ECG INTERPRETATION

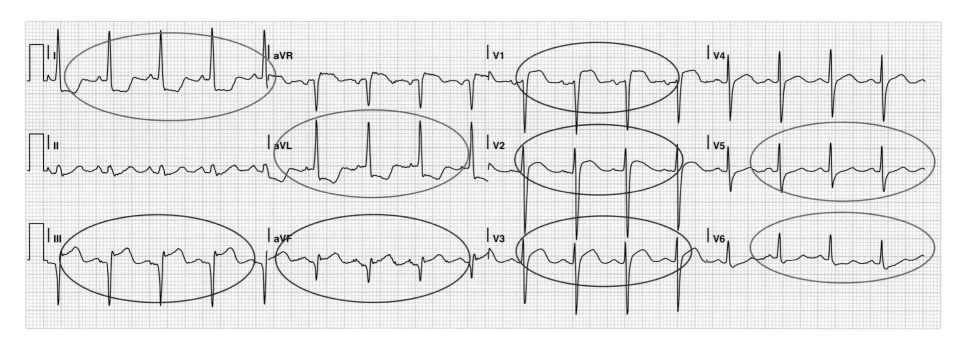

CLINICAL PEARL

Patients experiencing right ventricular infarction are preload dependent and often require administration of intravenous fluid to maintain an adequate blood pressure.

Sinus rhythm, heart rate: 100 beats/min., anterior inferior wall STEMI.

ST elevations are seen in the inferior leads (*red ovals*), which are indicative of an acute inferior wall infarction. In addition, ST elevation is revealed by leads V_1 through V_3 (*red ovals*), which also indicates anterior wall infarction. Note the morphology of the ST segments in these leads: they are convex upward ("tombstones"), which is highly specific for acute infarction and almost certainly rules out other causes of ST elevation, such as early repolarization or acute pericarditis. ST elevation in lead V_1 might suggest right ventricular infarction, which is certainly an important consideration in a patient with an inferior wall ST elevation myocardial infarction (STEMI). Reciprocal ST depression is present in the lateral leads (*green ovals*). This patient's marginal blood pressure further raises suspicion for right ventricular myocardial infarction. A provider should consider discontinuing the nitroglycerin drip, and give the patient an intravenous fluid bolus.

In this case, the medevac crew administered an intravenous fluid bolus and the patient responded well. After a thorough review of her medical history and referral paperwork, the advanced provider also administered a bolus dose of unfractionated heparin followed by a heparin infusion. The patient was successfully transferred to a cardiac catheterization laboratory.

CASE 60 ANSWER

CHIEF COMPLAINT: Interfacility transport

12-LEAD ECG INTERPRETATION

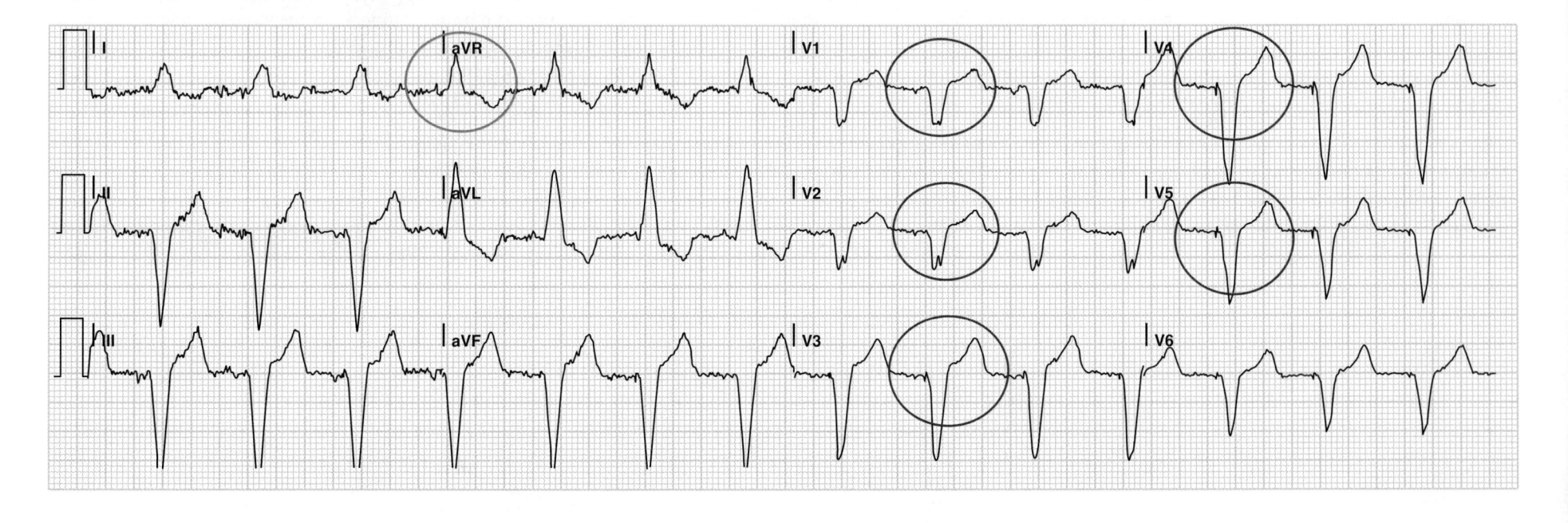

Sinus rhythm, heart rate: 80–90 beats/min., ventricular pacemaker.

The tracing reveals the classic findings associated with ventricular pacemakers: ST elevation in the inferior leads and across the precordium, QRS concordance, QRS complex/ST segment discordance, and prolonged QRS duration in the precordial leads (*red circles*). An additional finding consistent with a ventricular pacemaker is the presence of a large R wave in lead aVR (*green circle*). P waves are seen best in lead V_1. Direct trauma to the myocardium can cause physical damage to the conduction system connecting the atria to the ventricles, as in this case. The sinoatrial node is still fully functional, but the impulse is unable to travel through to the ventricles, making implantation of a pacemaker necessary. This particular patient has no acute complaint, and the electrocardiographic findings are consistent with the presence of a ventricular pacemaker. No further intervention is required.

CLINICAL PEARL

Ventricular pacemakers rarely cause ST elevation >5 mm.

12-LEAD ECG INTERPRETATION

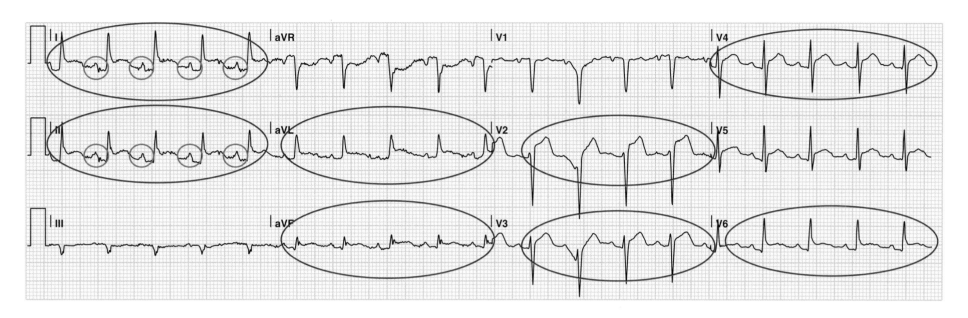

Sinus tachycardia, heart rate: 115 beats/min., acute pericarditis.

This patient's clinical picture causes less concern than the ECG. Almost all leads show ST elevation (*red ovals*).

ST elevation in the inferior, lateral, and precordial leads can certainly indicate a massive myocardial infarction. However, in the absence of diaphoresis or abnormal vital signs, that life-threatening diagnosis is less likely. This patient's ECG reveals a finding that is highly specific for acute pericarditis: P-R segment depression (*green circles*). Pericarditis is an inflammation of the connective tissue sac that surrounds the heart. Causes include systemic inflammatory disorders, viral infections, and trauma. Acute pericarditis itself is usually not a life-threatening condition, but its diagnosis is critical because of the potential complications of pericardial effusion and subsequent tamponade.

Patients with acute pericarditis should be transported in a comfortable position and oxygen should be administered according to protocol. A patient who displays this ECG and hypotension or respiratory distress should be transported expeditiously and given intravenous fluid boluses. Hypotension combined with widespread ST elevation is an ominous clinical picture suggesting cardiac tamponade or massive myocardial infarction with cardiogenic shock.

CLINICAL PEARL

ST elevation in the inferior, lateral, and precordial leads can certainly indicate a massive myocardial infarction. However, in the absence of diaphoresis or abnormal vital signs, that life-threatening diagnosis is less likely.

CASE 62 ANSWER   CHIEF COMPLAINT: Weakness

12-LEAD ECG INTERPRETATION

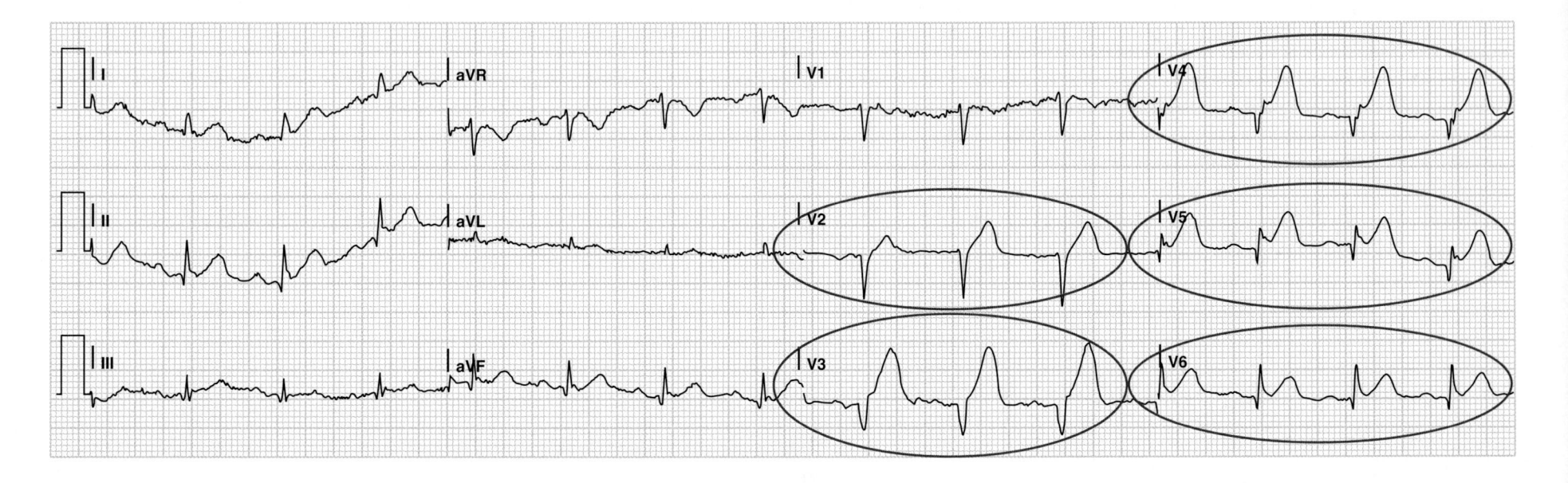

Sinus rhythm, heart rate: 90 beats/min., anterior wall STEMI.

Leads V_2 through V_6 show ST elevation (*red ovals*) consistent with anterior wall injury. Q waves have already developed in these precordial leads, suggesting that myocardial infarction has already occurred, but the presence of the ST elevation indicates ongoing ischemia of viable myocardium. The lack of R wave progression across the precordial leads substantiates that some degree of myocardial necrosis, or death, has already occurred. Recall that R waves should generally appear as positive deflections in leads V_3 through V_6.

You recognize the electrocardiographic changes suggestive of acute myocardial infarction and immediately bring the patient into the treatment area. The chest pain protocol is initiated. The emergency department nurses order laboratory studies and a chest film, and they administer aspirin. The attending physician concurs with the findings of anterior wall ST elevation myocardial infarction (STEMI) and alerts the on-call cardiology team.

Pathologic Q waves can develop within hours of acute coronary syndrome symptom onset. Patients presenting with pathologic Q waves and ST elevation on the ECG demonstrate ongoing ischemia and are candidates for urgent reperfusion therapy.

CLINICAL PEARL

Pathologic Q waves are > 0.03 seconds in duration and 0.1 mV in amplitude. Isolated Q waves in lead III are generally NOT pathologic provided that they are not found in other contiguous leads, such as II and aVF.

12-LEAD ECG INTERPRETATION

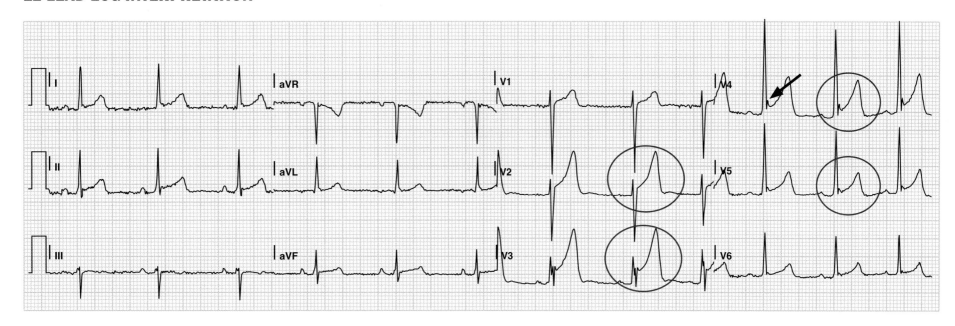

Sinus rhythm, heart rate: 70–80 beats/min., J point elevation consistent with benign early repolarization.

The ECG shows sinus rhythm with benign early repolarization. ST elevation is present in leads V_2 through V_5 (*red circles*). The absence of reciprocal ST depression along with concave upward ST segment morphology, early departure from the QRS complex, and a "fishhook" appearance of the J point (*black arrow*) favor benign early repolarization (BER) rather than acute myocardial infarction. Large T waves are often seen in BER; they are also seen in association with hyperkalemia and acute myocardial infarction (see the appendix "Comparison of T Wave Morphology in Hyperkalemia and in AMI"). In this case, the patient's age is another factor indicative of BER, which occurs more often in younger patients than in elderly patients. However, emergency care providers must always consider the most life-threatening diagnosis. Do not hesitate to consult medical control when confronted with troubling electrocardiographic findings.

CASE 64 ANSWER   CHIEF COMPLAINT: Respiratory distress

12-LEAD ECG INTERPRETATION

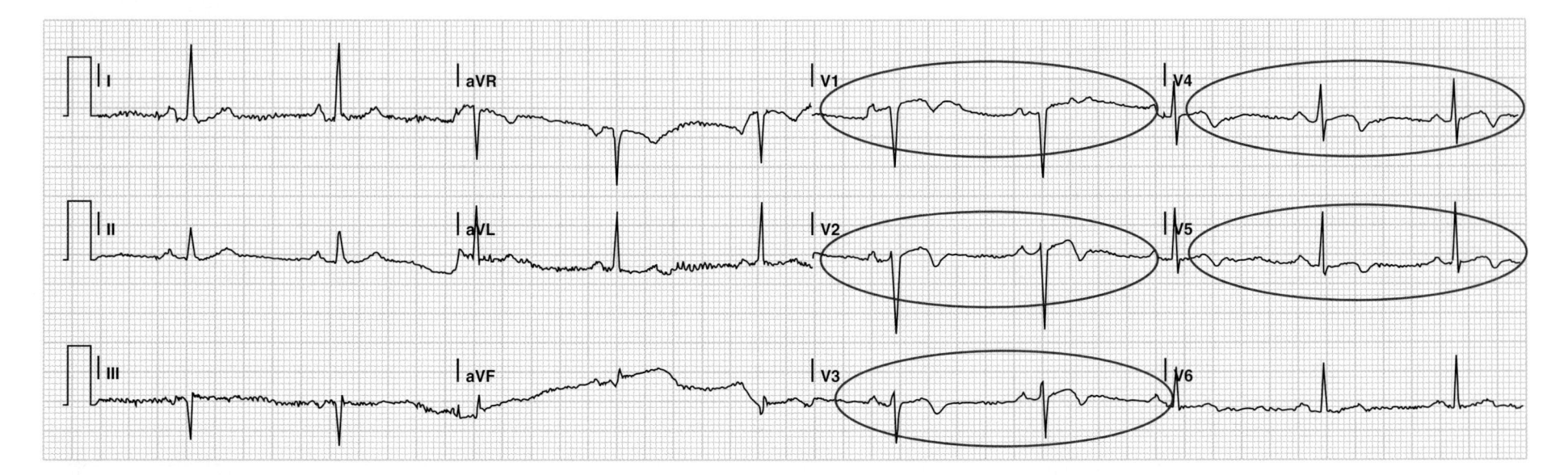

CLINICAL PEARL

Wellens' syndrome, also referred to as "LAD coronary T wave syndrome," is evidenced by symmetric or deep T wave inversions and biphasic T waves in the precordial leads. This pattern typically presents during chest pain-free periods.

Sinus rhythm, heart rate: 60 beats/min., anterior wall ischemia.

The ECG demonstrates terminal T wave inversion in leads V_1 through V_5 (*red ovals*). No reciprocal changes are noted in the inferior leads. The changes are consistent with anterior wall ischemia. In the absence of chest pain, the ECG abnormality is known as Wellens' syndrome. Wellens' syndrome is the electrocardiographic manifestation of left anterior descending artery occlusion. The T wave changes on this 12-lead ECG are subtle but critical findings!

You administer 162 mg of aspirin and two doses of 0.4 mg of sublingual nitroglycerin. The patient also received oxygen by nasal cannula at 2 L/min. You transmit the ECG to the receiving facility and transport the patient expeditiously to the hospital.

12-LEAD ECG INTERPRETATION

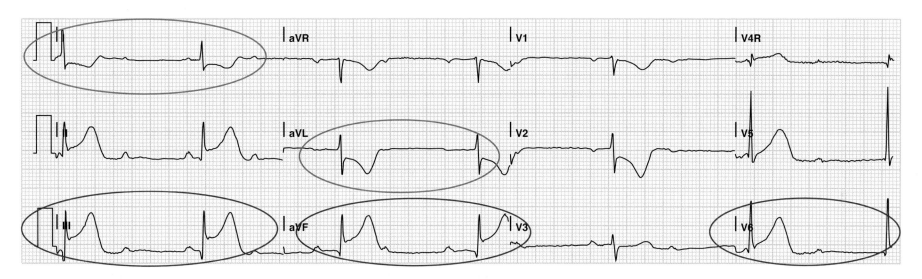

Third-degree heart block, ventricular rate: 40 beats/min., acute inferolateral STEMI.

The sinus node is firing at a rate of 90 beats/min. The ventricular rate is 40 beats/min. Third-degree heart block is characterized by variable P-R intervals, constant R-R intervals, and multiple P waves per QRS complex. This ECG also reveals ST elevation (*red ovals*) in leads II, III, aVF, and V_6, with reciprocal ST depression and T wave inversions in leads I and aVL (*green ovals*). A right-sided lead was recorded (V_4R) and demonstrates ST elevation, confirming right ventricular infarction. Nitrates and other preload-lowering agents should be avoided in this setting. Patients with right ventricular infarction are very preload-dependent and can become hypotensive if preload reducers are administered. Patients who are hypotensive with evidence of a right ventricular myocardial infarction should be treated with boluses of intravenous fluid.

However, the presence of crackles on physical examination and the patient's history of heart failure should make providers think twice before administering fluid boluses. This patient's relative hypotension likely results from the third-degree heart block. This patient would benefit from transcutaneous pacing and rapid transport to a facility capable of cardiac intervention.

CASE 66 ANSWER   CHIEF COMPLAINT: Weakness

12-LEAD ECG INTERPRETATION

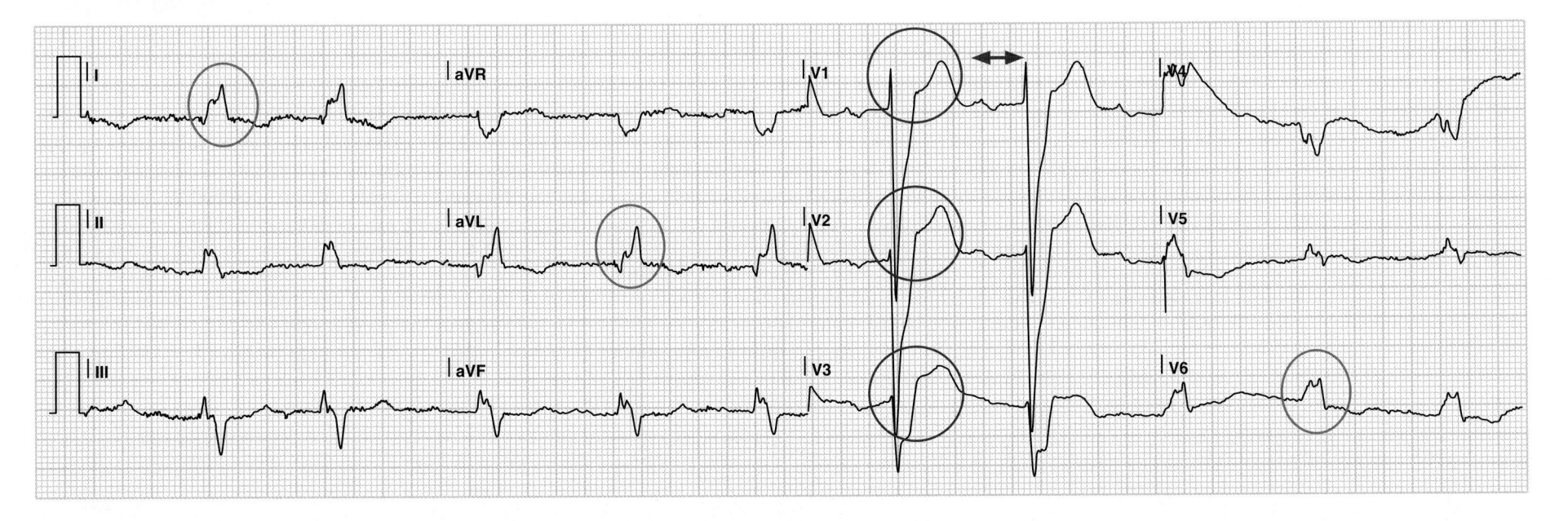

Sinus rhythm with first-degree heart block, heart rate: 60 beats/min., nonspecific intraventricular conduction delay.
Sinus rhythm with a nonspecific intraventricular conduction delay is present on the ECG. A first-degree heart block (*red arrow*) is demonstrated by a PR interval >0.2 seconds. ST elevation is present in leads V_1 through V_3 (*red circles*). The QRS complex is >120 ms, but a small Q wave is present in lead I. The electrocardiographic diagnosis of left bundle branch block (LBBB) requires the presence of monophasic R waves in the lateral leads. A true LBBB presents with a QRS complex >120 ms (three small boxes); QRS-ST discordance; a terminal S wave (or "downwardly deflected" QRS complex) in V_1; and terminal R waves in leads I, aVL, and V_6 (*green circles*). The presence of Q waves in the lateral leads is diagnostic of intraventricular conduction delay, not LBBB.

You obtain a 12-lead ECG and administer aspirin according to local protocol. Given the patient's initial report of weakness and demonstrated conduction delay on the ECG, medical control concurs with your decision to transport the patient to the local emergency department for further evaluation.

CLINICAL PEARL

Weakness and shortness of breath are "anginal equivalents" in elderly patients. Consider their presence as indicators of ischemia until proved otherwise.

12-LEAD ECG INTERPRETATION

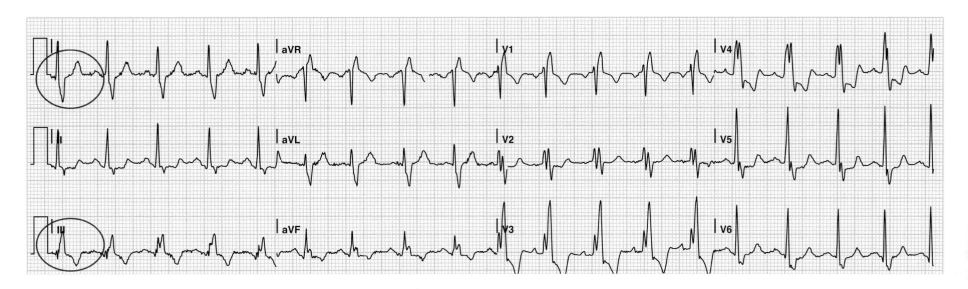

Sinus rhythm, heart rate: 110 beats/min., right bundle branch block, no evidence of STEMI.
Sinus tachycardia is present on the ECG. The ECG also displays the S1Q3T3 pattern suggestive of pulmonary embolism: a deep S wave in lead I, a small Q wave in lead III, and T wave inversion in lead III (*red ovals*). Furthermore, the presence of right bundle branch block and T wave inversion in the right precordial leads indicates right heart strain. Right bundle branch block is characterized by a positively deflected, wide QRS complex (>0.12 seconds) in lead V1. Classically, the QRS shape in RBBB follows an rSR' pattern. The classic triad of dyspnea, chest pain, and hemoptysis, along with the findings of right heart strain, suggests the presence of a pulmonary embolism. Other concerning symptoms consistent with the diagnosis of pulmonary embolism include tachypnea, tachycardia, and a pleural friction rub. Fewer than 20% of patients present with classic symptoms, but almost all elderly patients with pulmonary embolism have tachycardia.

CASE 68 ANSWER   CHIEF COMPLAINT: Weakness

12-LEAD ECG INTERPRETATION

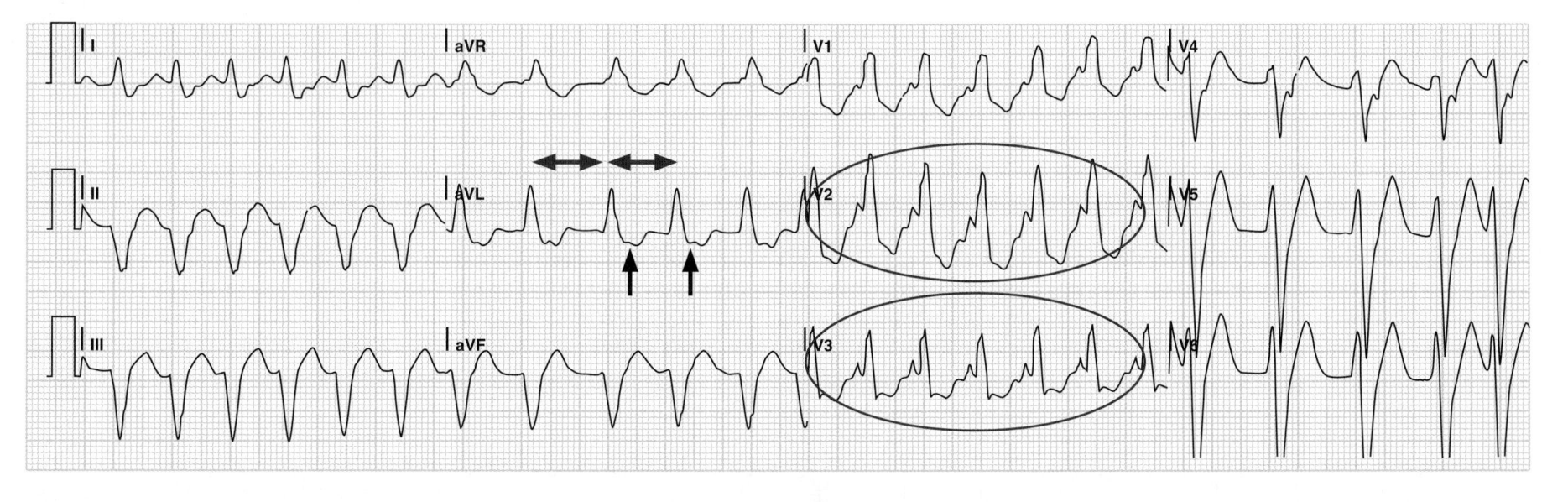

Supraventricular tachycardia with aberrantly conducted ventricular complexes (wide QRS); heart rate: 150 beats/min.

Your first impression should be one of a troubling dysrhythmia, specifically ventricular tachycardia (VT). Although there is no doubt that the ECG shows a wide-complex tachycardia, a closer look reveals that retrograde P waves are present in several leads (*black arrows*). The retrograde P waves and wide QRS complex suggest that the origin of this rhythm lies somewhere near the atrioventricular node. Furthermore, VT is almost always a regular rhythm. The R-R interval (*red arrows*) in this case is variable, suggesting the presence of underlying atrial flutter or fibrillation. The patient's clinical picture is somewhat reassuring in that he has a measurable blood pressure, is speaking in full sentences, and has no chest discomfort. However, weakness is considered an "anginal equivalent" in patients older than 50. You should have an extremely low threshold for transporting such patients for further diagnostics. Always treat unstable wide complex tachycardia as VT until proven otherwise.

The patient's blood glucose reading is 48 mg/dL, and he states that he has not been eating well. You establish an intravenous line and administer 25 g of dextrose according to standing order. The patient becomes slightly more comfortable, but his heart rhythm remains unchanged. At the emergency department, blood samples are drawn for measurement of cardiac enzymes and electrolytes. The patient is rehydrated with intravenous normal saline. After he receives 1 L of saline, his heart rate comes down to 100 beats/min. The emergency department work-up is negative for any obvious evidence of infection, and the patient is admitted to the hospital for further diagnostics. A prior ECG on file at the hospital reveals QRS complexes of similar morphology.

CLINICAL PEARL

Remember the following:
- Always err on the side of treating wide-complex tachycardia as VT until proved otherwise.
- VT demonstrates regular R-R intervals and usually appears at heart rates >150 beats/min.
- Look for P waves in leads II, V_1, and V_2.
- The diagnosis of sinus tachycardia with aberrancy or aberrantly conducted beats is complex and should be left to a cardiologist. Misdiagnosis of VT for sinus tachycardia with aberrancy can result in poor patient outcome and possibly death.
- Unstable, wide-complex tachycardias warrant urgent cardioversion. Treat an unstable, wide-complex tachycardia as VT.

RHYTHYM STRIP INTERPRETATION

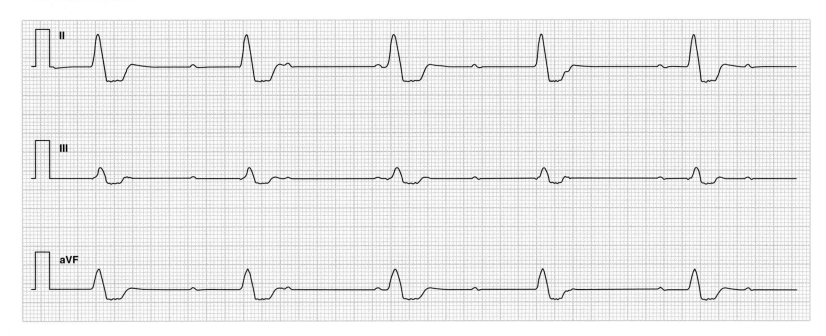

Third-degree heart block, ventricular escape rhythm, heart rate in the 30s.

The sinus node is firing at a rate of 60 beats/min. (P waves). The ventricular rate is 40 beats/min. The QRS complexes are wide, suggesting a ventricular escape rhythm. Third-degree heart block is characterized by variable P-R intervals, constant R-R intervals, and multiple P waves per QRS complex as seen in the tracing above (see the appendix "Heart Blocks Made Simple"). Remember that heart block indicates a degree of disconnect between the atria and ventricles. In this case, when the rate of atrial impulses reaching the ventricles dropped below the intrinsic firing rate of the ventricular tissue, a ventricular escape rhythm developed. New-onset third-degree heart block is a cardiologic emergency. The wide-complex ventricular escape rhythm is not likely to respond to atropine. Symptomatic patients may benefit from transcutaneous pacing. Vasoactive agents, such as dopamine, might be required to maintain blood pressure.

CASE 70 ANSWER   CHIEF COMPLAINT: Respiratory distress

12-LEAD ECG INTERPRETATION

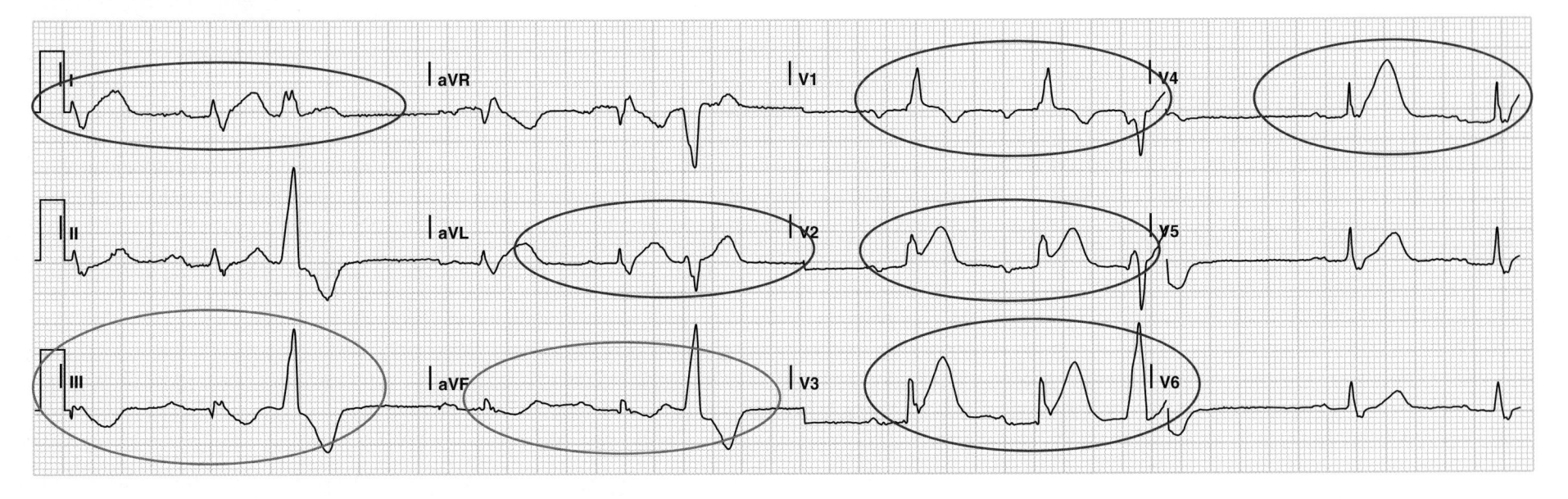

Sinus rhythm with premature ventricular complexes, heart rate: 60 beats/min., anterolateral wall STEMI.

This ECG demonstrates ST elevation in leads V_1 through V_4, and in leads I and aVL (*red ovals*). Reciprocal ST depression and T wave inversion are present in leads III and aVF (*green ovals*). This patient is having a large anterolateral wall myocardial infarction and a concurrent acute pulmonary edema. This patient requires rapid prehospital treatment, transport, and emergent cardiac catheterization.

Prehospital treatment includes aggressive management of pulmonary edema with high doses of nitroglycerin and continuous positive airway pressure. Chewable aspirin should also be administered. Paramedics rapidly transported the patient to a cardiac catheterization–capable facility.

12-LEAD ECG INTERPRETATION

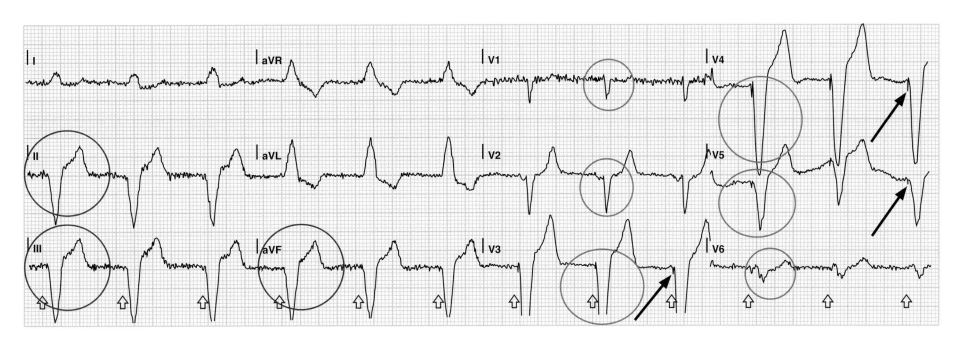

Paced ventricular rhythm, heart rate: 70 beats/min.

A paced ventricular rhythm is seen on this ECG. Pacemaker "spikes" are often difficult to see or are absent altogether, but they are easily found in this tracing in leads V_3 through V_5 (*black arrows*). Also note the direction of the QRS complexes in the precordial leads (*green circles*): all six leads exhibit a pattern of QRS concordance (i.e., all QRS complexes point in the same direction). Note the ST elevation in the inferior leads (*red circles*) and anterolateral leads. This is a common finding in paced ventricular rhythms. Similar to the effects of left bundle branch block, pacemakers produce discordance between the QRS complex and the ST segment, so it is perfectly normal to have a few millimeters of ST elevation in leads in which the QRS points primarily downward. ST elevation of >5 mm in patients with paced rhythms or bundle branch blocks is more likely to indicate underlying cardiac ischemia.

You establish an intravenous line and administer antiemetics according to local medical protocols. You give the patient a bolus of isotonic crystalloid, and he reports improvement during transport to the local emergency department.

CASE 72 ANSWER   CHIEF COMPLAINT: Unresponsiveness

12-LEAD ECG INTERPRETATION

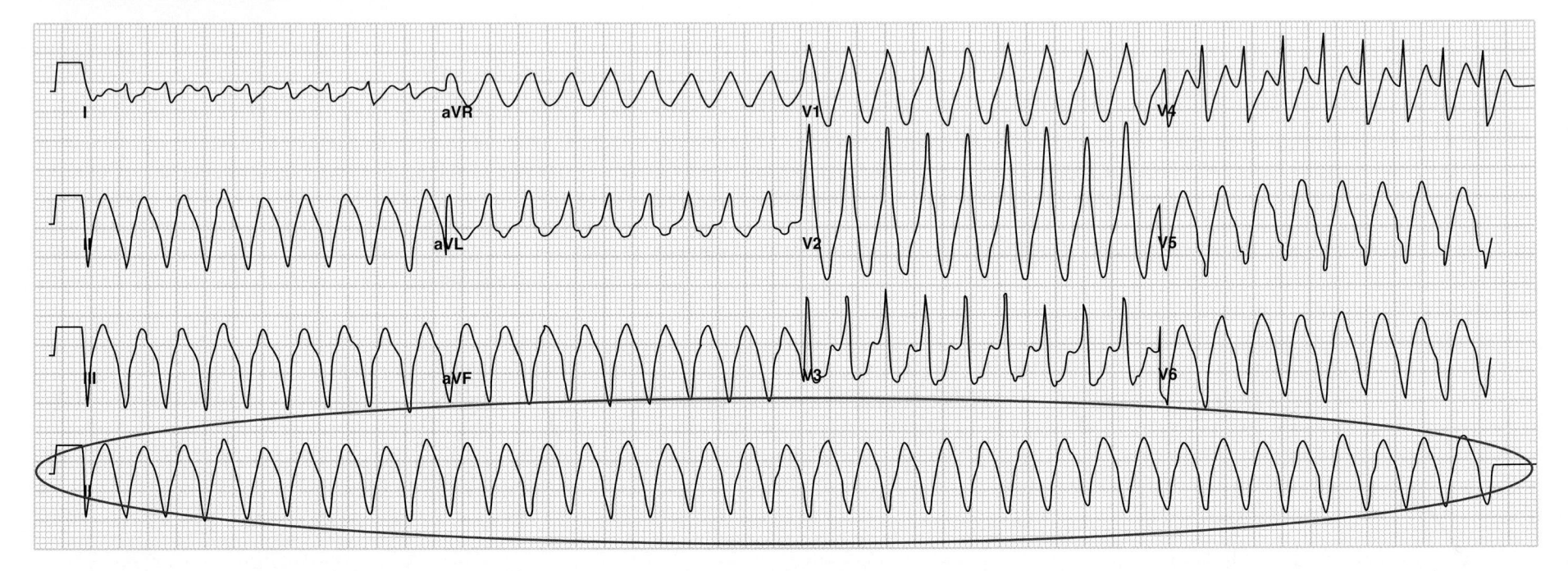

Ventricular tachycardia, heart rate: 180 beats/min.

The rapid rate, regular R-R intervals, and wide QRS complexes (*red oval*) are consistent with a diagnosis of ventricular tachycardia. Never assume alternative diagnoses, such as supraventricular tachycardia or sinus tachycardia with aberrant conduction, in patients with signs of hemodynamic instability. Your partner shuts off the dopamine drip and administers lidocaine. The patient's radial pulse is still thready. You prepare the patient's chest and apply the defibrillator pads. Because the patient is semiconscious, you opt for immediate synchronized cardioversion with 100 J. The patient screams and arouses almost instantly. The rhythm converts to sinus rhythm at a rate of 100 beats/min., and your partner initiates a lidocaine infusion at 2 mg/min. A repeat systolic blood pressure measurement reads 90 mm Hg, so you initiate gentle fluid hydration to raise it.

A wide complex tachycardia in an unstable patient is best treated with electrical countershock. Resist the temptation to treat these dysrhythmias with adenosine.

CLINICAL PEARL

Adenosine is not an appropriate diagnostic tool in symptomatic and unstable patients. Unstable patients are candidates for electrical therapy!

CHIEF COMPLAINT: Shortness of breath

12-LEAD ECG INTERPRETATION

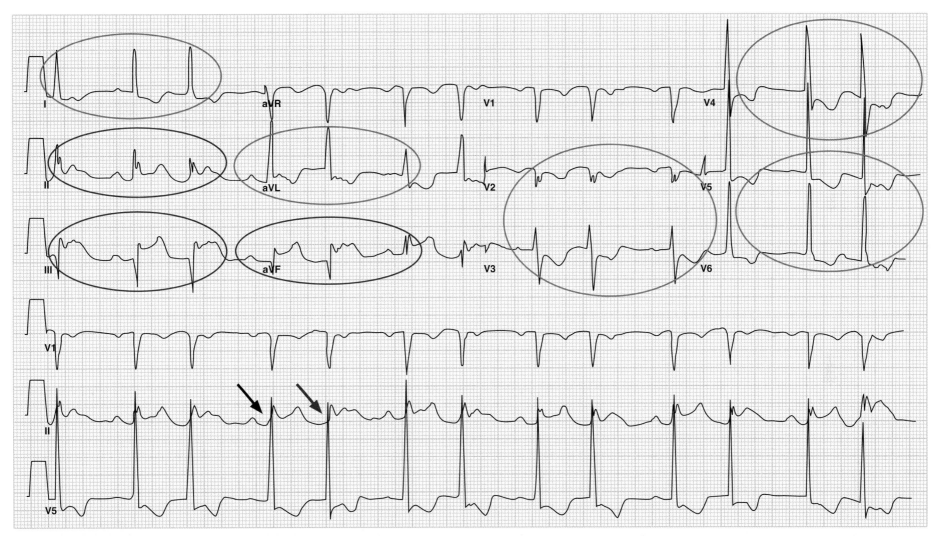

(Continued)

CASE 73 ANSWER   CHIEF COMPLAINT: Shortness of breath

Sinus rhythm, first-degree heart block with premature atrial complexes in a pattern of bigeminy, ventricular rate between 80 and 100 beats/min, inferior wall STEMI.

ST elevations appear in the inferior leads II, III, and aVF (*red ovals*). ST depressions across the entire precordium (*green ovals*) raise the possibility of a posterior myocardial infarction, although the absence of tall R waves or upright T waves in the right precordial leads suggests that these ST depressions are simply reciprocal changes. Reciprocal ST depressions are also present in leads I and aVL (*green ovals*). You should also consider the possibility of right ventricular infarction in any patient with inferior wall infarction; therefore, any medications that may decrease preload (e.g., sublingual nitroglycerin) should be administered with caution. The *black arrow* indicates complexes originating from the sinus node, and the *red arrow* indicates premature beats. The premature beats account for the variable pulse felt.

You administer aspirin according to protocol, initiate intravenous access, and transport with lights and sirens to the emergency department. You transmit the ECG to the receiving physician by cellular telephone picture messaging. It is interpreted as possibly being consistent with near total occlusion of the right coronary artery. The patient is transported rapidly to the cardiac catheterization lab for further diagnostics and possible intervention.

12-LEAD ECG INTERPRETATION

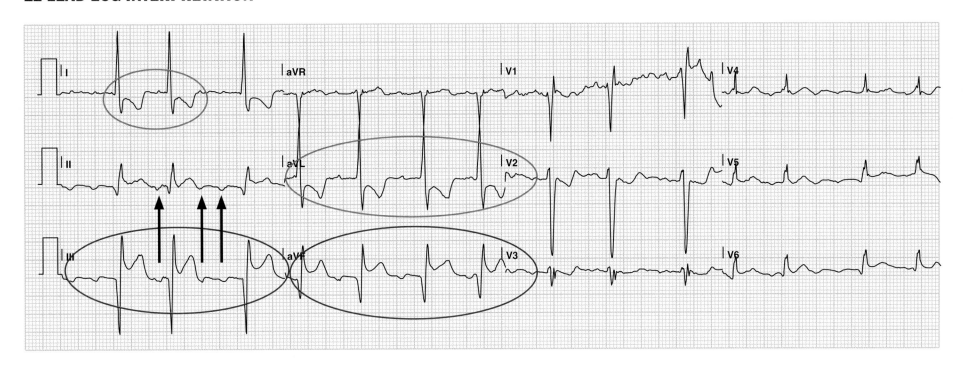

Atrial flutter with variable conduction, heart rate in the 80s, inferior wall STEMI.

The differential diagnosis for irregularly irregular narrow complex rhythms includes atrial fibrillation, atrial flutter with variable conduction, second-degree heart block with variable conduction, and wandering atrial pacemaker. Close inspection of the tracing reveals atrial beats at a rate of >250 (*arrows*), consistent with the diagnosis of atrial flutter. The ventricular response is irregular (i.e., there is variable conduction rather than a fixed ratio of atrial/ventricular beats). Deep, wide Q waves and ST elevation (*red ovals*) are present in the inferior leads. Reciprocal ST depression and T wave inversion are seen in the high lateral leads (*green ovals*), confirming the diagnosis of inferior wall ST elevation myocardial infarction (STEMI). Although uncommon, atrial flutter and STEMI can occur simultaneously, as seen in this case.

CASE 75 ANSWER   **CHIEF COMPLAINT:** Syncope

RHYTHM STRIP INTERPRETATION

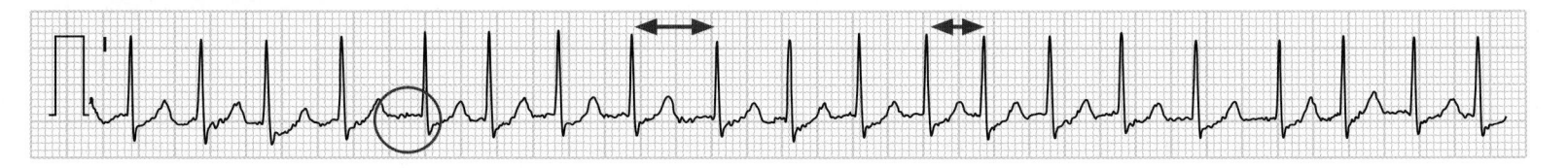

CLINICAL PEARL

It is sometimes difficult to identify rhythm irregularity when the ventricular rate is > 150 beats/min. It is important to use calipers or a paper and pencil to carefully measure the R-R intervals and determine whether the rhythm is regular or irregular. A-fib with rapid ventricular response is often misdiagnosed as supraventricular tachycardia. Careful assessment of the R-R intervals and recognition of rhythm irregularity help to make the correct diagnosis.

Atrial fibrillation with rapid ventricular response, heart rate: 150–160 beats/min.
This ECG indicates atrial fibrillation (a-fib). "Rapid ventricular response" refers to a ventricular rate >120 beats/min. A-fib should be considered whenever a patient presents with an irregular pulse. The irregular and rapid contraction of the atria puts the patient at risk for syncope. Syncope can occur because of reduced cardiac output. The loss of this "atrial kick" represents a decrease in cardiac output of almost 30%. Patients in persistent a-fib are also at risk for thrombotic and embolic events, such as stroke and pulmonary embolism. Hemodynamically unstable patients are candidates for electrical cardioversion. Calcium-channel blockers, beta blocking agents, and occasionally magnesium sulfate are used in cases where rate control (ventricular rate <120 beats/min.) is desired.

The *red arrows* illustrate the unequal distance between the R waves. An irregular R-R interval is characteristic of a-fib. The *red oval* illustrates the "fibrillatory" baseline. In cases of a-fib, the atria often contract at a rate >300 beats/min. Note the lack of discernible P waves throughout the tracing.

CHIEF COMPLAINT: Chest pain

12-LEAD ECG INTERPRETATION

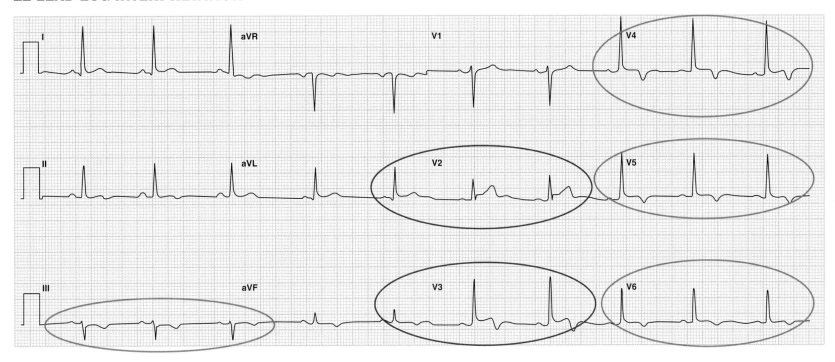

Sinus rhythm; heart rate: 60 beats/min.; ST elevation in leads V_2 and V_3; T wave inversions in inferior and lateral leads.

CLINICAL PEARL

- Isolated, physiologic ST elevation might be present in V_1 and V_2. In symptomatic patients, always consider the presence of ST elevation as pathologic and indicative of ischemia.
- In patients with changing or ongoing symptoms, obtain a repeat 12-lead ECG. A change in ST segments over time or resolution of ECG changes provides the receiving hospital with valuable information.

The ECG reveals ST elevation in leads V_2 through V_3 (*red ovals*). Furthermore, T wave inversions are present in the inferior and lateral lead of V_6 (*green ovals*). Although this ECG does not meet strict criteria for activation of the catheterization lab (i.e., >2 mm of ST elevation in the precordial leads), you recognize T wave inversions and reciprocal changes as findings consistent with ischemia. Ischemia can present with peaked T waves, inverted T waves, ST depression, and ST elevation.

You advise the charge nurse that the patient requires a monitored bed. You establish an intravenous line and administer 162 mg of chewable baby aspirin according to protocol. Your patient's chest pain abates spontaneously and a repeat ECG is obtained. A patient care technician retrieves the patient's ECG from a previous visit to the emergency department, which demonstrated upright T waves across the precordial leads. The patient is admitted to the hospital for further testing and formal cardiology consultation.

CASE 77 ANSWER

CHIEF COMPLAINT: Unresponsiveness

12-LEAD ECG INTERPRETATION

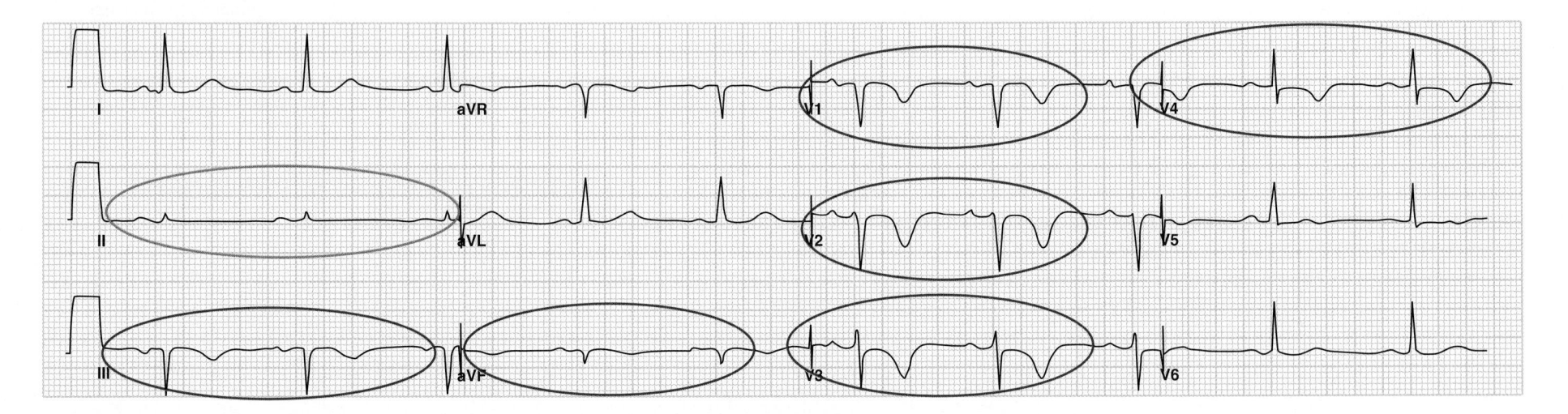

Sinus rhythm, heart rate: 60 beats/min., T wave inversions and ST depression noted in inferior and anteroseptal leads, nonspecific T wave changes.

The diffuse ischemia indicated by this ECG is cause for concern. T wave inversions are present in inferior and anteroseptal leads (*red ovals*). Slight ST depression is present in leads V_3 and V_4. Despite these findings, this patient's initial presentation is not consistent with myocardial ischemia, and 12-lead ECGs are not a routine part of prehospital care for trauma patients. This ECG was obtained as a routine part of the initial evaluation.

While establishing in-line stabilization, you perform a jaw thrust. The patient's airway is maintained with noninvasive measures, and an intravenous line is placed while awaiting the arrival of the transport unit. En route to the hospital, the patient suffers a generalized tonic-clonic seizure with subsequent desaturation and extensor posturing. The patient is intubated with rapid-sequence technique on arrival in the emergency department. Emergency CT scanning reveals an epidural hematoma.

CLINICAL PEARL

- T wave inversion, ST depression, and positive cardiac troponins have all been reported in patients with stroke and intracranial hemorrhage.
- The relationship between electrocardiographic changes and intracranial pathology is unclear.
- Abnormal ECGs should prompt a thorough investigation of the patient's chief complaint.

12-LEAD ECG INTERPRETATION

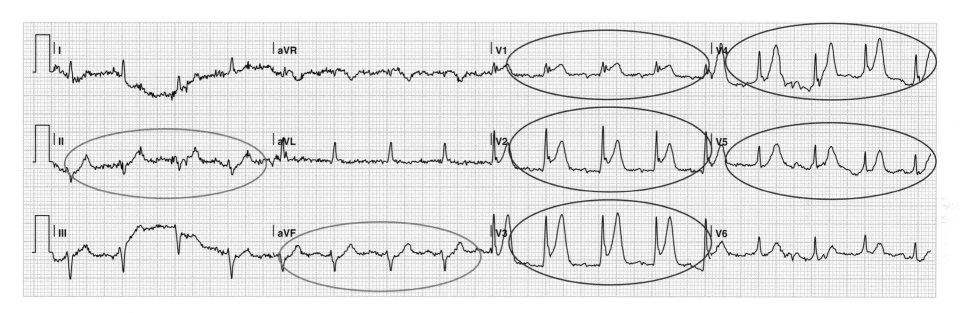

Sinus rhythm, heart rate: 90–100 beats/min., anterior wall STEMI.

This ECG demonstrates ST elevation in leads V_1 through V_5 (*red ovals*). Reciprocal ST depression is seen in the inferior leads (*green ovals*). The presence of ST elevation, hyperacute, peaked/tented, and symmetric T waves with reciprocal changes is virtually diagnostic of acute myocardial infarction. A sizeable portion of the heart's anterior wall is supplied by the left anterior descending (LAD) artery (see the appendix "Coronary Artery Anatomy"). Acute occlusion of this blood vessel results in a large territorial infarct; this is why the LAD is commonly referred to as "the widow-maker." Maintain a low threshold for applying defibrillation pads in patients experiencing acute anterior wall myocardial infarction, and be prepared to deliver electrical therapy if ventricular tachycardia or fibrillation develops.

    The advanced providers administer 162 mg of aspirin, 0.4 mg of nitroglycerin, and oxygen at 2 L/min., and they transmit the ECG to the receiving facility. After reviewing the prehospital ECG, the emergency department physician immediately activates the cardiac catheterization team.

CASE 79 ANSWER   CHIEF COMPLAINT: Syncope

12-LEAD ECG INTERPRETATION

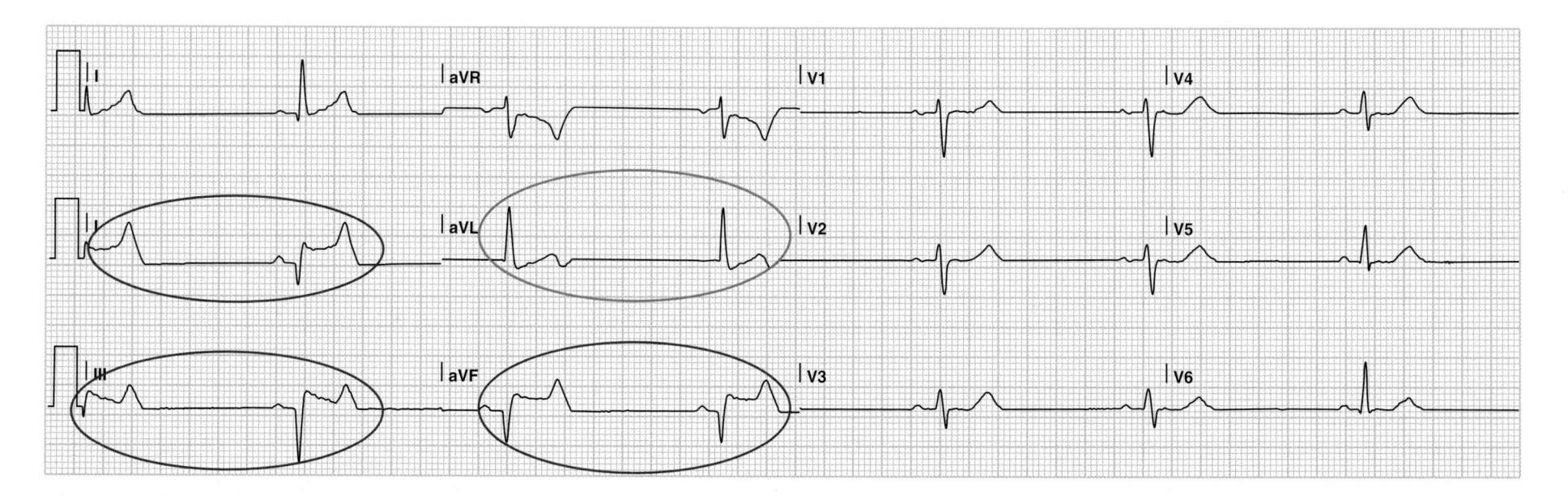

Sinus bradycardia, heart rate: 40 beats/min., inferior wall STEMI.

This ECG demonstrates ST elevation in leads II, III, and aVF (*red ovals*). Very subtle reciprocal ST depression is apparent in lead aVL (*green oval*). This patient is having an inferior wall myocardial infarction (MI). Acute MI of the inferior wall involves the right ventricle and posterior wall up to 40% of the time. The ECG should be repeated with right-sided chest leads to evaluate the patient for right ventricular infarction. If these right-sided chest leads show ST elevation, preload reducing medications, such as nitrates, should be withheld so as to avoid precipitous decreases in blood pressure. Note that this patient did not present with chest pain, but reported indigestion. Inferior wall myocardial infarction often presents with indigestion or epigastric discomfort. Remain vigilant for these atypical presentations of acute coronary syndrome.

The advanced providers explain the ECG findings to the patient and convince him of the need for emergent treatment. They administer 162 mg of chewable aspirin and initiate oxygen via nasal cannula. A peripheral intravenous line is started. While awaiting the arrival of the transport unit, the providers transmit the ECG to the local emergency department.

12-LEAD ECG INTERPRETATION

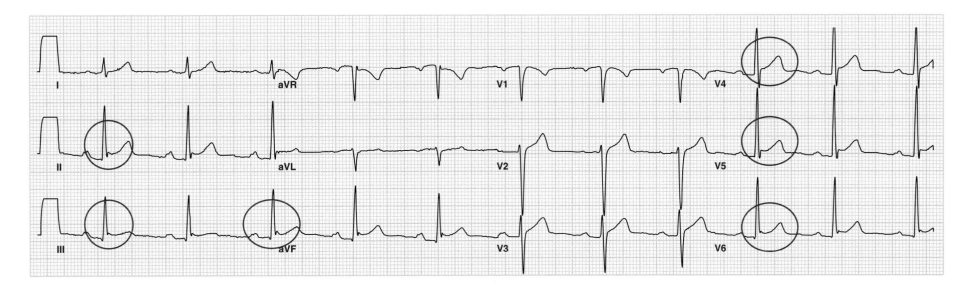

Sinus rhythm, heart rate: 60 beats/min., diffuse ST elevation consistent with pericarditis.

Indications of pericarditis are present on the ECG. Diffuse concave-upward ST elevation (*red circles*), slightly depressed PR segments in some leads, and absence of reciprocal ST depression are classic findings of the disease. These findings on the ECG, coupled with the patient's medical history and physical examination findings, strongly suggest pericarditis.

You establish an intravenous line and administer analgesics according to regional protocol. At the receiving facility, a bedside echocardiogram demonstrates a small pericardial effusion. Given the presence of comorbidities and fever, the patient is admitted to an overnight observation unit. He is treated with analgesics and nonsteroidal anti-inflammatory medications.

Patients with HIV may be at increased risk for adverse events from various cardiac diseases. An impaired immune response may contribute to atypical presentations of disease and confound the recognition of acute pathology. Maintain a low threshold for treatment and transport of patients with known HIV/AIDS who have cardiac-type complaints, regardless of their age or the absence of other more traditional risk factors.

CLINICAL PEARL

Immunocompromised patients, such as those with HIV, diabetes, and autoimmune disease, are also at risk for atypical presentations of acute coronary syndromes.

CASE 81 ANSWER   CHIEF COMPLAINT: Chest pain, nausea

12-LEAD ECG INTERPRETATION

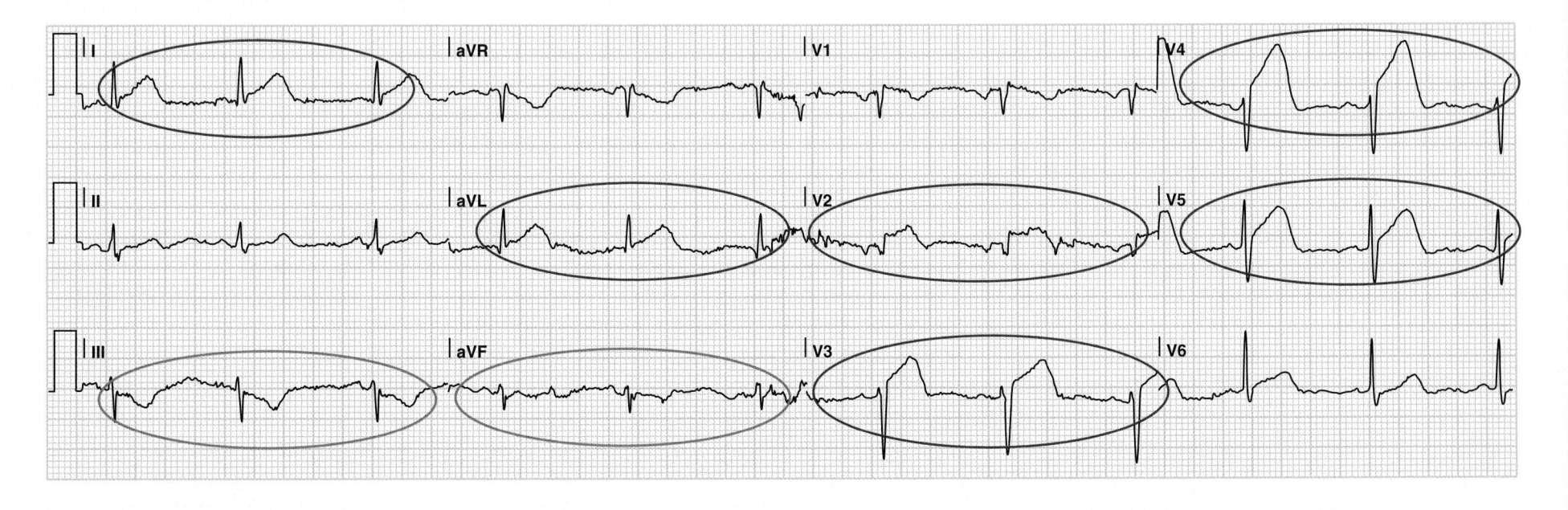

Sinus rhythm, heart rate: 60–70 beats/min., anterior and lateral wall STEMI.

ST elevations are demonstrated in leads V_2 through V_5, and in I and aVL (*red ovals*). Mild reciprocal ST depression and T wave inversion are seen in the inferior leads (*green ovals*). The changes on this ECG strongly favor the diagnosis of anterolateral wall ST elevation myocardial infarction (STEMI). This patient is also developing pulmonary edema. Acute myocardial infarction can cause left ventricular failure and pulmonary edema. The hypotension seen in this patient may be an early sign of cardiogenic shock. Typically, the body's response to hypotension is to increase the heart rate to maintain cardiac output. In this case, however, the patient's heart rate remains virtually unchanged at 60–70 beats/min. Always consider the patient's medications and their impact on the body. This patient is taking a beta adrenergic blocker (atenolol), which is likely preventing the reflexive tachycardia normally seen during episodes of hypotension.

Prehospital treatment of this patient is centered on aggressive blood pressure and airway management. Paramedics initiated continuous positive airway pressure therapy and monitored the patient's blood pressure closely. The patient received 162 mg of aspirin and was rapidly transported to an awaiting cardiac care team.

CHIEF COMPLAINT: Sharp chest pain

12-LEAD ECG INTERPRETATION

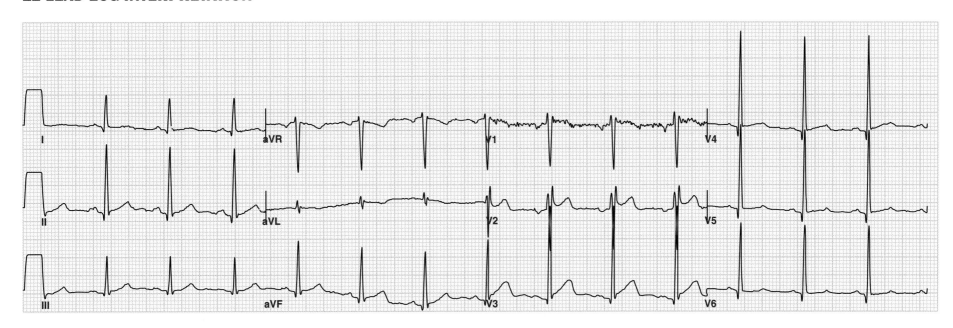

Sinus rhythm, heart rate: 70–80 beats/min.

Large-amplitude QRS complexes are common and normal in young people. In an older person, these would be considered diagnostic of left ventricular hypertrophy (LVH), a pathologic condition. In patients younger than 45 years of age, the term "high left ventricular voltage" (HLVV) is used, instead, to avoid implying the presence of under-lying pathology. Regardless of whether a patient truly has LVH or simply HLVV, large-amplitude QRS complexes are associated with ST elevation. The absence of recipro-cal ST depression and the concave upward ST elevation are also reassuring—although not definitive—findings that the ST elevation is benign. Additionally, the patient's presentation is consistent with muscular pain.

Although this patient was eventually diagnosed with musculoskeletal chest pain, it is prudent to be aware that ischemia often is associated with presentations that do not seem cardiac related. Women, elderly patients, diabetics, and immunocompromised patients especially may present with fatigue, weakness, or dyspnea. Some patients with ischemia describe chest pain that is worse with movement and palpation. It is imperative for prehospital providers to obtain a detailed history of the pres-ent illness, perform a thorough physical examination, and obtain medical consultation to reduce the possibility of missing a cardiac event. Simply stated, it is impossible to definitively "rule out" a myocardial infarction that occurs outside the hospital environment. Even when armed with sophisticated imaging technologies and highly sensi-tive cardiac enzyme assays, emergency physicians miss approximately 2% of myocardial infarctions.

CASE 83 ANSWER   CHIEF COMPLAINT: Stomach burning

12-LEAD ECG INTERPRETATION

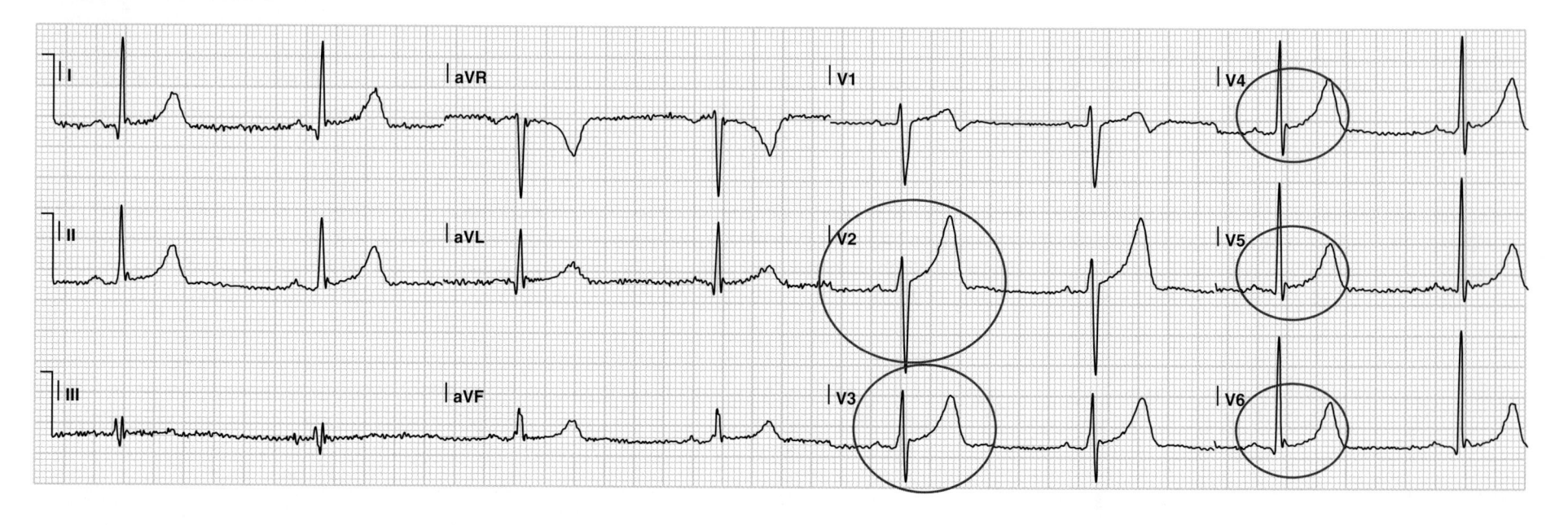

Sinus bradycardia, heart rate: approximately 50 beats/min., benign early repolarization.

Sinus bradycardia with benign early repolarization (BER) is present on the ECG. ST elevation is present in V_2 though V_6 (*red circles*). The bradycardia is attributed to beta blockade from atenolol. The concave-upward ST segment morphology, large T waves, absence of reciprocal ST depression, and "fishhook" appearance of the J point are classic findings of BER. This is an incidental finding in this patient and requires no acute intervention.

Procedural sedation is well tolerated, and the patient undergoes an uneventful manual reduction of his left shoulder. He is discharged from the emergency department in stable condition.

CLINICAL PEARL

The concave-upward ST segment morphology, large T waves, absence of reciprocal ST depression, and "fishhook" appearance of the J point are classic findings of benign early repolarization.

12-LEAD ECG INTERPRETATION

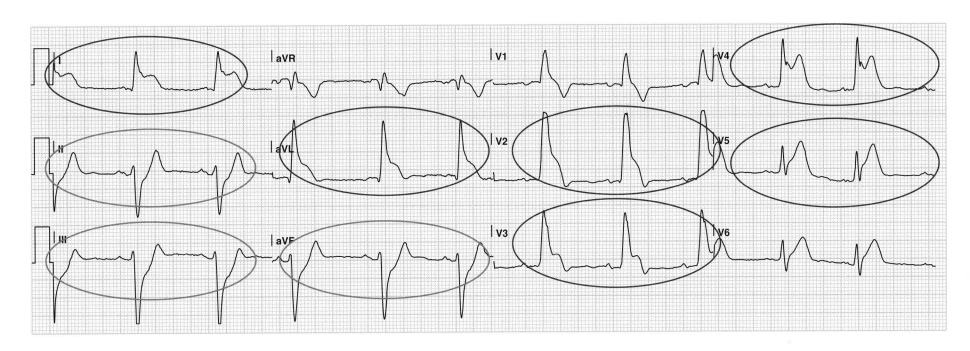

Sinus rhythm, heart rate: 60 beats/min., anterior and lateral wall STEMI.

This ECG demonstrates clear ST elevation in leads V_2 through V_5, I, and aVL (*red ovals*). Reciprocal ST depression is present in the inferior leads (*green ovals*). Anterior wall ST elevation myocardial infarction (STEMI) is associated with a high mortality rate. The ischemic myocardium is often extremely irritable, and ventricular tachycardia or fibrillation can occur spontaneously. Maintain a low threshold for applying defibrillation pads, and be prepared to defibrillate the patient if necessary.

The advanced providers notify the receiving facility of the STEMI, and they administer aspirin and start a large-bore peripheral intravenous line. Nitroglycerin is administered as per protocol. The patient is transported directly to a cardiac catheterization lab.

CASE 85 ANSWER   CHIEF COMPLAINT: Syncope

12-LEAD ECG INTERPRETATION

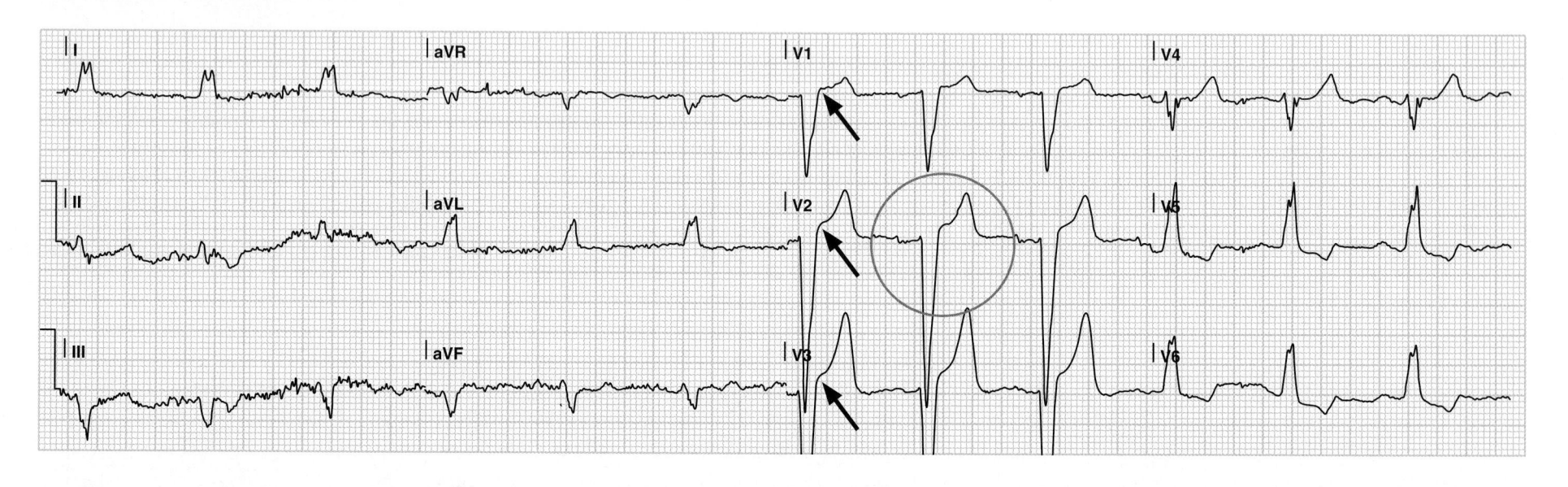

Sinus rhythm, heart rate: 70 beats/min., left bundle branch block.

CLINICAL PEARL

The repolarization changes that accompany left bundle branch block (QRS-T discordance and ST elevation) might mimic the electrocardiographic appearance of ischemia. Syncope in an elderly patient mandates a thorough medical evaluation.

The ECG reveals a sinus rhythm with the left bundle branch block (LBBB) pattern. LBBB is demonstrated by a wide QRS complex (>120 ms); large R waves in leads I, aVL, V_5, and V_6; and the absence of Q waves in these same lateral leads. Left bundle branch block may also produce ST elevation, as seen in leads V_1 through V_3 (*black arrows*). QRS complex/T wave discordance (*green circle*) is also evident across the precordium. The repolarization changes that accompany LBBB (i.e., QRS-T discordance and ST elevation) might mimic the electrocardiographic appearance of ischemia. For example, the QRS points "downward" in leads V_1 through V_3 while the T wave is upright in the same leads. This phenomenon, called discordance, is expected in the setting of LBBB. Also note that the J point (loosely defined as the intersection of the QRS complex and the T wave) is elevated above the isoeletric line. Syncope in an elderly patient mandates a thorough medical evaluation. The LBBB might be a preexisting condition in this patient, but it is usually impossible to verify such a relationship in the out-of-hospital setting.

You establish intravenous access and measure the patient's blood glucose concentration. The reading is 76 mg/dL. Given the presence of a presumably new LBBB in the setting of a syncopal episode, you transport to a hospital capable of performing percutaneous coronary intervention and transmit the ECG to the receiving facility. The patient is admitted to a telemetry unit for further diagnostics and testing.

12-LEAD ECG INTERPRETATION

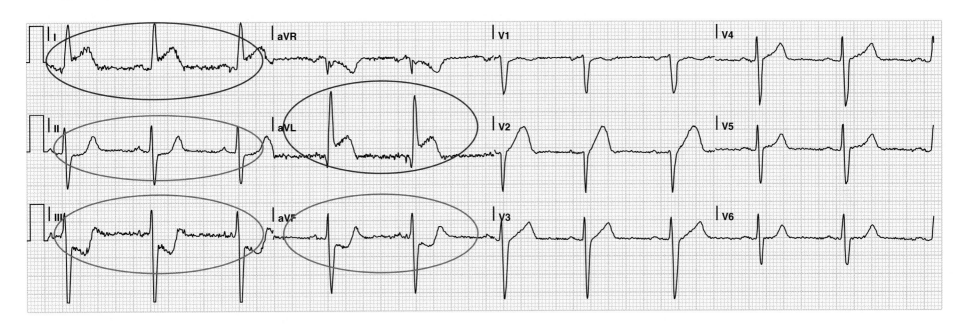

CLINICAL PEARL

The presence of reciprocal ST depression and T wave inversion is highly confirmatory that the ST elevation seen on the ECG is caused by acute myocardial infarction. The absence of reciprocal changes does **not** rule out acute myocardial infarction.

Sinus rhythm, heart rate: 60 beats/min., high lateral wall STEMI.

The ECG reveals ST elevations in leads I and aVL (*red ovals*). Reciprocal ST depressions are demonstrated in the inferior leads (*green ovals*). These ECG changes strongly favor the diagnosis of acute lateral wall ST elevation myocardial infarction (STEMI).

You recognize ECG changes suggestive of myocardial infarction. The patient is immediately brought back into the triage area. The emergency department physician is notified and alerts the on-duty cardiology team. You administer aspirin and initiate a peripheral intravenous line. The patient is prepared for emergent transfer to the cardiac catheterization lab.

CASE 87 ANSWER   **CHIEF COMPLAINT:** Difficulty breathing

RHYTHM STRIP INTERPRETATION

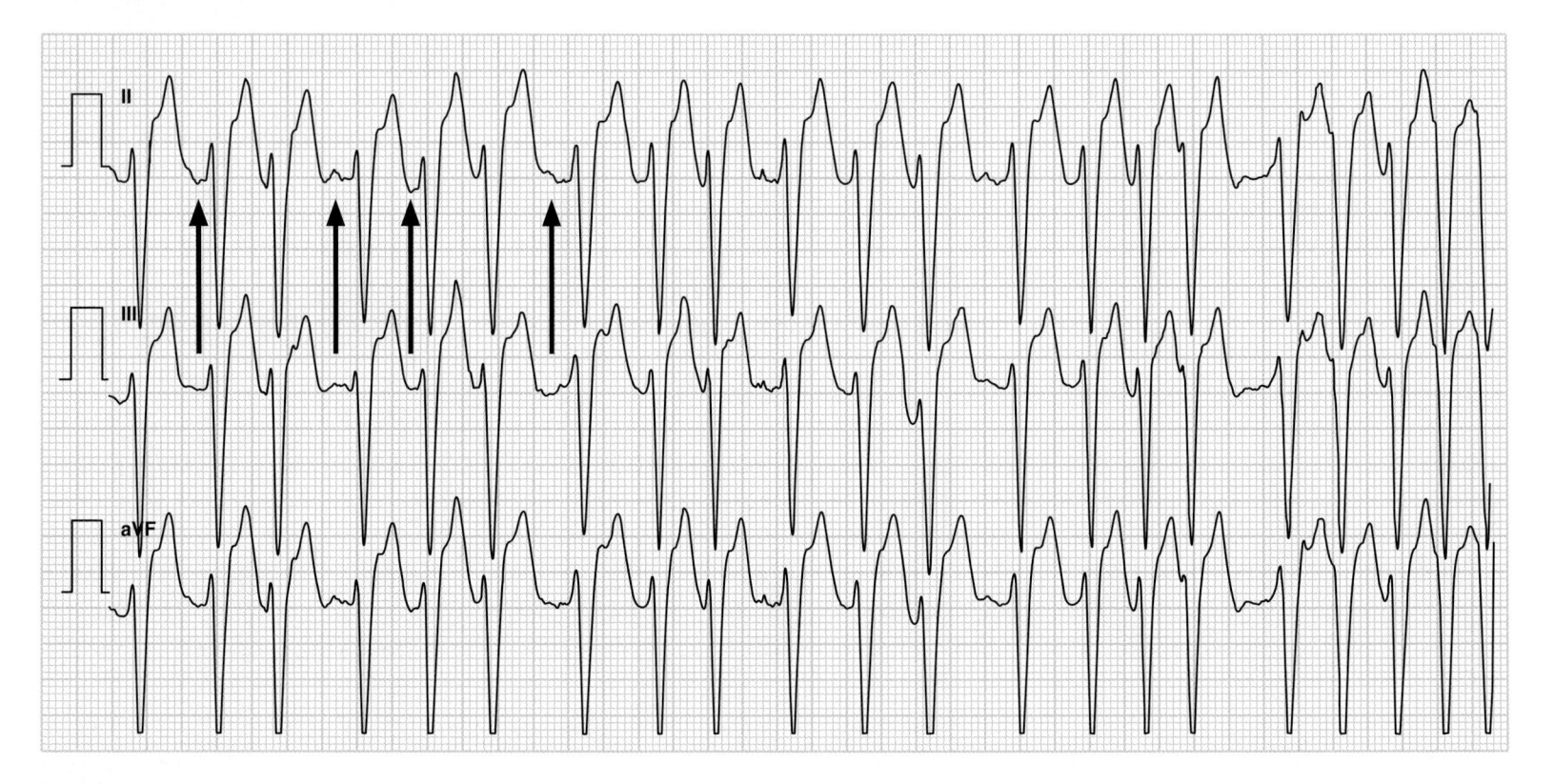

Multifocal atrial tachycardia, heart rate in the 150s.

The differential diagnosis of irregularly irregular narrow complex tachycardia includes atrial fibrillation with rapid ventricular response (AF RVR), atrial flutter with variable conduction, and multifocal atrial tachycardia. P waves can be seen throughout the ECG (*black arrows*), a finding that rules out the possibility of AF RVR. A diagnosis of atrial flutter is also eliminated because the atrial rate is not fast enough. Multifocal atrial tachycardia is characterized by an irregularly irregular rhythm, three or more P wave morphologies, and three or more P-R interval variations. This particular dysrhythmia is associated with lung pathology, such as chronic obstructive pulmonary disease. Treatment should attempt to correct the underlying cause. In this case, the patient might benefit from bronchodilators, corticosteroids, and intravenous fluids.

CLINICAL PEARL

Multifocal atrial tachycardia is almost exclusively seen in patients with a history of chronic pulmonary disease.

12-LEAD INTERPRETATION

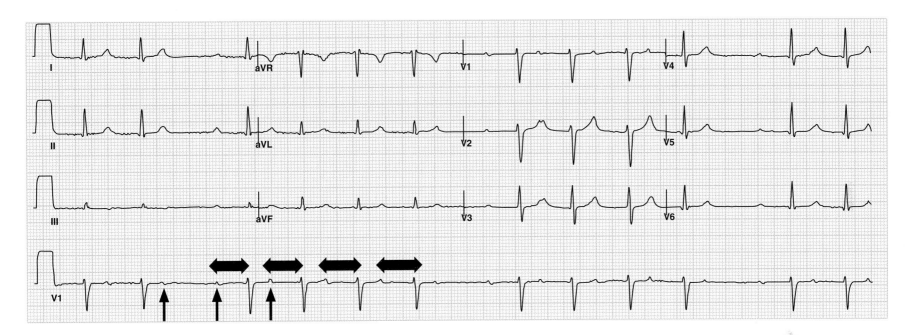

CLINICAL PEARL

Always consider premature beats (i.e., premature atrial complexes in patterns of bi/trigeminy) and second-degree type I atrioventricular block when confronted with a regularly irregular rhythm.

Sinus rhythm, ventricular rate: approximately 70, regularly irregular rhythm consistent with type 1, second-degree AV block.

This ECG shows a regularly irregular rhythm, manifested by "cousins" of grouped QRS complexes. P waves are subtle but visible in lead V_1 (*thin black arrows*). The differential diagnosis for a regularly irregular rhythm includes atrioventricular (AV) block and premature beats. The P-R interval prolongs (*thick black arrows*) and the R-R interval shortens, which is visible across the V_1 rhythm strip. The P-R prolongation is subtle, and can be best seen by comparing the P-R interval after the dropped beat to the P-R interval preceding the dropped beat. The differential diagnosis of AV block in a young patient should include medications or drug effects; Lyme disease; and autoimmune disease, such as systemic lupus erythematosis and sarcoidosis. In general, type I second-degree AV block does not require pacing. However, this patient should be transported to the emergency department for further evaluation. Prehospital treatment for dysrhythmias with a narrow QRS complex and present P waves includes intravenous atropine, fluid boluses, and transcutaneous pacing.

CASE 89 ANSWER   CHIEF COMPLAINT: Chest pain

12-LEAD ECG INTERPREATION

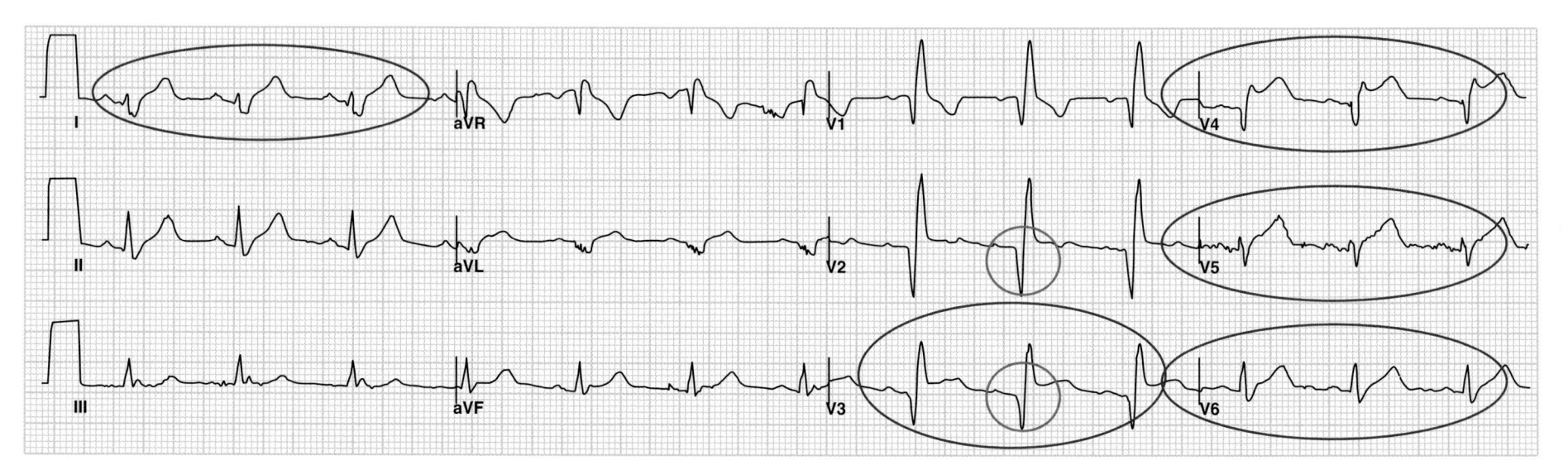

CLINICAL PEARL

ST elevation and upright T waves are not expected in leads V_1 through V_3 in uncomplicated right bundle branch block and are referred to as "inappropriate concordance." When present, inappropriate concordance indicates acute myocardial ischemia. Unlike left bundle branch block, right bundle branch block does not interfere with the diagnosis of acute myocardial infarction.

Sinus rhythm, heart rate: 80, right bundle branch block, anterior wall STEMI.

ST elevations (*red ovals*) of ≥2 mm are present in leads V_3 and V_4. The remaining precordial leads demonstrate broad-based, hyperacute T waves. The presence of deep Q waves (*green circles*) across the early precordial leads (V_2 and V_3) is a concerning finding. Recall that abnormal Q waves are ≥0.03 seconds and >0.1 mV in amplitude (see the appendix "Pathologic Q Wave"). Right bundle branch block is characterized by a positively deflected, wide QRS complex (>0.12 seconds) in lead V_1. Classically, the QRS shape in RBBB follows an rSR′ pattern. Collectively, these findings are consistent with ischemia of the heart's anterior wall. Minimal (i.e., <1 mm) ST elevation is present in lead I, but elevation is not observed in the contiguous lead of aVL. It is the constellation of findings (Q waves, ST elevation, and broad-based T waves) that alerts the advanced provider to the diagnosis of infarction.

You prepare the patient for transport to a cardiac interventional center. Monitor leads are left in place so that serial ECGs can be obtained. You administer 324 mg of chewable aspirin and establish a large-bore intravenous line. Sublingual nitroglycerin should be considered for active chest pain. Your crew transmits the 12-lead ECG, and the patient is taken to a waiting catheterization laboratory immediately on arrival. Two stents are deployed within the left anterior descending artery and the patient is admitted to the hospital for recovery.

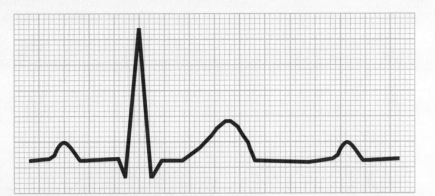

Appendices

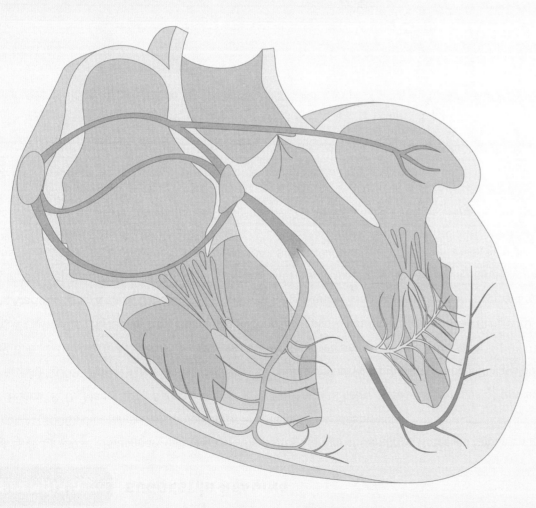

APPENDIX A   SUGGESTED READING

Beers, M. H. (Ed.). (2010). Pulmonary embolism. In *The Merck Manual of Geriatrics*. Retrieved from www.merck.com/mkgr/mmg/sec10/ch77/ch77a.jsp.

Goldberger, A. (2006). *Clinical electrocardiography*. Philadelphia, PA: Mosby.

Libby, P., Bonow, R. O., Mann, D. L., & Zipes, D. P. (2007). *Braunwald's heart disease: A textbook of cardiovascular medicine.* Philadelphia, PA: WB Saunders.

Marx, J. A. (Ed.) (2009). *Rosen's emergency medicine: Concepts and clinical practice* (7th ed.). Philadelphia, PA: Mosby.

Mattingly, B. B., & Gentile, K. M. (2010). *Wellens syndrome.* Retrieved from www.Emedicine.com.

Mattu, A., & Lawner, B. (2009). Prehospital management of congestive heart failure. *Heart Fail Clin, 5,* 19–24.

Mattu, A., Martinez, J. P., & Kelly, B. S. (2005). Modern management of cardiogenic pulmonary edema. *Emerg Med Clin North Am, 23,* 1104–1125.

Nable, J. V., & Brady, W. (2009). The evolution of electrocardiographic changes in ST-segment elevation myocardial infarction. *Am J Emerg Med, 27,* 734–746.

Thuresson, M. T., Jarlov, M. B., & Lindahl, B., et al. (2004). Symptoms and type of symptom onset in acute coronary syndrome in relation to ST elevation, sex, age, and a history of diabetes. *Am Heart J, 150*(2), 234–242.

Yanowitz, F. (2006). *Lesson VIII: left ventricular hypertrophy. The Alan E. Lindsey ECG Learning Center.* Retrieved from http://library.med.utah.edu/kw/ecg/ecg_outline/Lesson8/index.html.

Zevitz, M. (2010). *Cardiomyopathy, hypertrophic.* Retrieved from www.Emedicine.com.

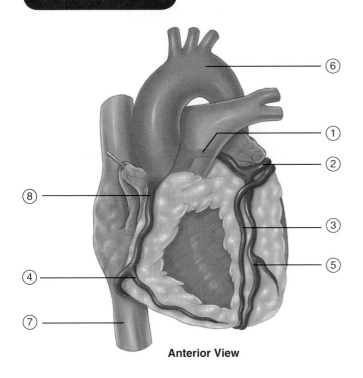

Anterior View

NUMBER	DESCRIPTION/ANATOMY	BLOOD SUPPLY/FUNCTION
1	Left main coronary artery	Left ventricle, interventricular septum
2	Left circumflex coronary artery	Left atrium, left ventricle
3	Left anterior descending coronary artery	Left ventricle, interventricular septum
4	Right marginal coronary artery	Inferior wall, cardiac apex
5	Posterior descending coronary artery	Both ventricles, posterior wall
6	Aorta	Great vessel, supplies major organs
7	Vena cava	Great vessel, returns blood to heart via superior and inferior portions
8	Right main coronary artery	Inferior wall, sinoatrial node in 60% of patients

APPENDIX C   ECG LOCALIZATION OF ISCHEMIC CHANGE

ECG Leads	Expected Reciprocal Leads	Location	Anatomy*
I, aVL	II, III, aVF	High lateral or anterior	Left anterior descending
II, III, aVF	I, aVL	Inferior wall	Right coronary artery
V_1, V_2	ST depression in V_1 and V_2 might actually represent ST elevation in posteriorly placed leads	Posterior or septal wall	Variable, septal perforators from the left coronary artery can supply septum Posterior wall can be supplied from right coronary artery or left circumflex artery
V_2–V_6	Might show reciprocal changes in inferior leads	Anterior	Left coronary artery or its branches, left anterior descending
V_5–V_6	Might show reciprocal changes in inferior leads	Anterior lateral	Left coronary artery or its branches, left anterior descending

* Anatomy and corresponding blood supply can be variable. Definitive coronary artery anatomy and its relationship to ischemia is established at the time of coronary artery catheterization. For example, 60% of patients have right-side dominant circulation in which the sinus node is supplied by the right coronary artery. In some individuals, the blood supply to the sinoatrial node originates from the left circumflex artery. The septal wall usually receives blood from perforator branches that originate from the left anterior descending coronary artery.

(**1 small box = 1 mm**)

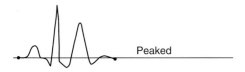

Peaked

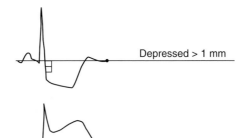

Depressed > 1 mm

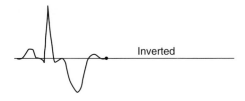

Inverted

Elevated > 1 mm

APPENDIX E   THE MANY FACES OF ISCHEMIA

The following tracings represent common electrocardiographic findings suggestive of myocardial ischemia.

The "J" Point

J-point depression	J-point elevation
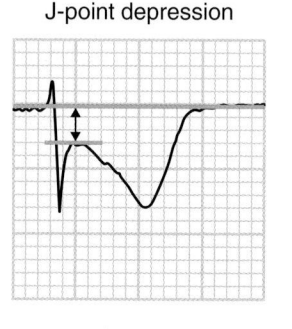	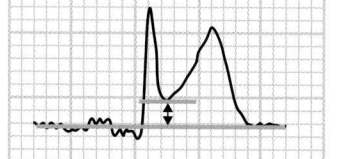

ST Segment Morphology

Convex–A convex ST segment favors ischemia. Test for this by drawing a line from the J point to the peak of the T wave. If the line superimposes or if the T wave is above the line, the segment is convex.

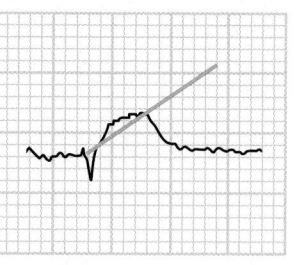 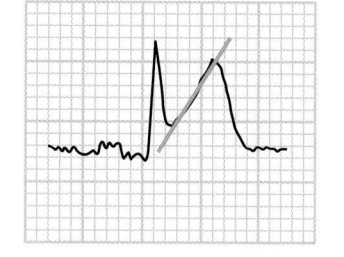

Concave – A concave ST segment favors benign conditions. But beware, ischemia can *also* manifest with this pattern, as seen in this STEMI.

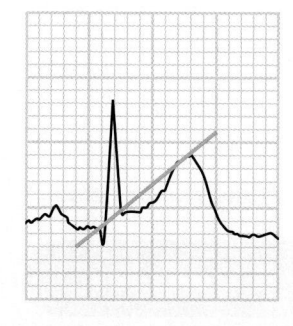

Direction of Slope

Up-sloping	Horizontal	Down-sloping

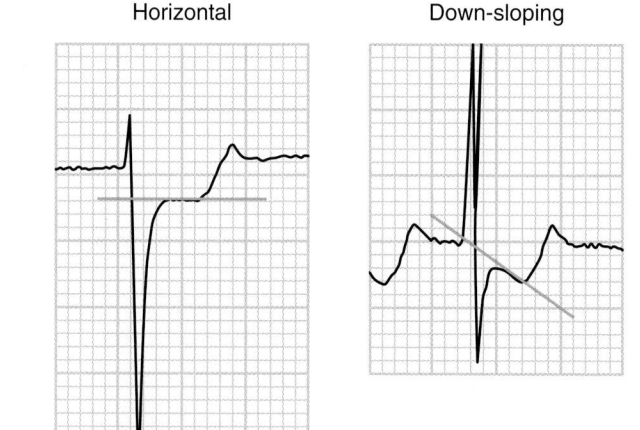

All of the examples above illustrate myocardial ischemia. The horizontal and down-sloping ST segments are always pathologic findings. A "slow" up-slope is most often a pathologic finding. A rapidly up-sloping ST segment is generally a normal electrocardiographic change, as demonstrated during exercise stress testing.

(Continued)

T Wave Morphology

Peaked / tented – The apex of the T wave elevates and forms a "peaked" appearance

Hyperacute – The height of the T wave exceeds ½ the overall height of the QRS

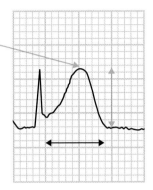

Symmetry – The T wave becomes symmetrical with respect to the Y axis

Broad base – The base of the T wave elongates during ischemia

Inversion

Without ST segment depression

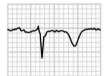

With ST segment depression

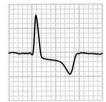

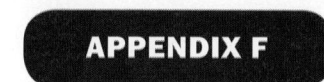

PATHOLOGIC Q WAVE

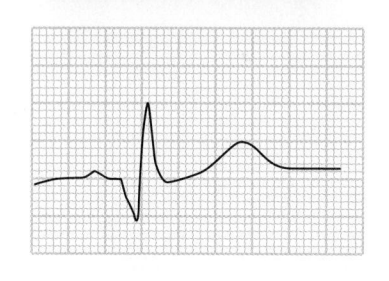

Criteria for "pathologic Q waves":

- Duration > 0.03 seconds in at least two contiguous leads (I, II, aVL, aVF, or V_4 through V_6)
- Amplitude > 1 mm

HEART BLOCKS MADE SIMPLE

The atrioventricular (AV) node is sometimes unable to transmit impulses to the ventricles because of hypoxia or disease. The sinus node continues to function, causing P waves to appear on the ECG. If the number of atrial impulses reaching the ventricles falls below the intrinsic firing rate of the junction because of AV node blockage, a junctional escape rhythm develops. Essentially, three distinct elements are taking place: (1) sinus node activity, (2) AV junctional activity, and (3) ventricular response. To accurately classify a heart block, you must identify each of the three elements. Think of it as breaking down a complex process into simpler parts:

1. Determine the sinus node activity (i.e., sinus bradycardia if P waves occur <60 times/min., sinus rhythm if P waves occur 60–100 times/min., or sinus tachycardia if P waves occur > 100 times/min.).
2. Identify the type of ventricular activity. If the QRS complex is <120 ms in duration and the rate is 40–60 beats/min., a junctional escape rhythm is present. If the QRS complex is >120 ms in duration and the rate is <40 beats/min., a ventricular escape rhythm is present.
3. Identify the level of AV nodal blockage. Second-degree type I AV block is characterized by progressively lengthening P-R intervals until a nonconducted P wave occurs. Second-degree type II AV block is characterized by constant P-R intervals and nonconducted P waves. Complete, or third-degree, heart block is characterized by variable P-R intervals, constant R-R intervals, and more P waves than QRS complexes.

If you find more P waves than QRS complexes, evaluate the following:

1. Measure the R-R interval
2. Measure the P-R interval

If the R-R interval is CONSTANT, you are seeing a second-degree type II or a third-degree block. The one caveat here is that when second-degree AV block is associated with 2:1 conduction (i.e., two P waves for every QRS complex), it is not possible to definitely identify the block as type I or type II; by convention, we simply refer to it as second-degree AV block with 2:1 conduction.

Does the P-R interval vary?

1. If it elongates, the block must be a second-degree type I.
2. If it is random, you are seeing a third-degree block.

Types of Heart Blocks and Associated P-R/R-R Intervals			
	Second-Degree Type I	Second-Degree Type II	Third-Degree
P-R Interval	Elongates	Constant	Variable
R-R Interval	Variable, dropped QRS complexes	Constant	Constant

APPENDIX H   DIAGNOSTIC CRITERIA FOR SGARBOSSA, LVH, AND LBBB

Sgarbossa criteria for diagnosis of STEMI in presence of LBBB

1. ST elevation ≥ 5mm that is in the opposite direction of a predominantly negative QRS complex.

2. ST depression ≥ 1 mm in leads V_1, V_2, or V_3.

3. ST elevation ≥ 1 mm that is in the same *direction* of a predominantly positive QRS complex.

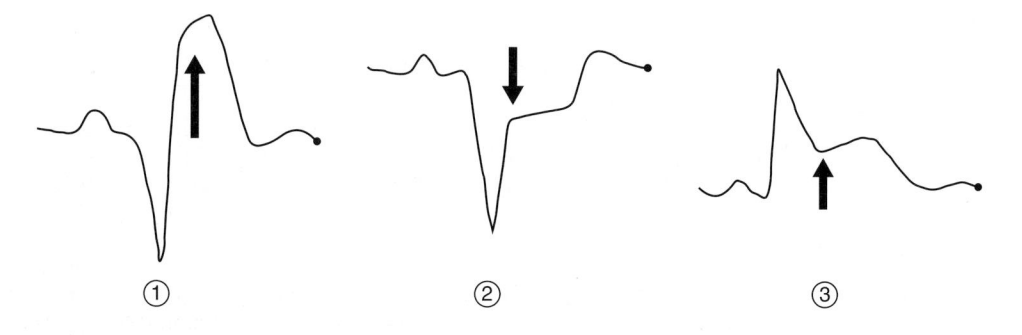

Voltage criteria seen in left ventricular hypertrophy (LVH)

Left ventricular hypertrophy can cause numerous changes to the ECG. Although LVH is diagnosed by echocardiogram, we say that the ECG meets the voltage criteria for LVH. We have chosen to present only a few voltage criteria in this text.

General features of LVH may include:

- Tall R waves in leads V_4–V_6 and deep S waves in leads V_1–V_3.
- QRS complex/T wave are oriented in opposite directions.
- Left axis deviation in the frontal leads.

Voltage criterion 1:
R wave amplitude in lead aVL >11 mm.

Voltage criteria 2:
S wave amplitude (measure in millimeters) in lead V_1 + R wave amplitude in lead V_5 or V_6 > 35 mm.

Criteria for ECG diagnosis of left bundle branch block (LBBB)

- QRS complex duration is >120 milliseconds.
- The QRS complex in lead V_1 ends in an S wave (terminal S wave).
- The QRS complex in leads I, aVL, and V_6 ends in an R wave (terminal R wave).
- The ST-T waves must be oriented opposite to the direction of the terminal wave. For example, in lead V_1, the ST-T waves must be deflected upwards, in leads I, aVL, and V_6, the ST-T waves must be deflected downwards. *Concordant ST-T waves must be considered myocardial ischemia.*

Brugada syndrome is a hereditary disorder involving an abnormality of the sodium channels present within the heart muscle cells, or cardiac myocytes. Brugada syndrome is important to recognize because it can result in sudden cardiac death. It is most commonly discovered in young males, particularly in the third or fourth decade of life. Brugada may present as a syncopal event.

ECG Findings
Incomplete right bundle branch block pattern (rSR')
ST elevation in leads V_1 and V_2
T wave inversion in leads V_1 and V_2

Treatment
Symptomatic patients typically undergo electrophysiologic testing. Patients may also receive an automated implantable cardioverter defibrillator. Currently, no drug therapy has been shown to prevent dysrhythmia or sudden cardiac death in patients with this disorder.

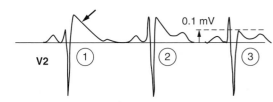

ECG findings associated with Brugada syndrome.

The figure depicts three types of ST segment morphologies that may be evident in the precordial leads, particularly lead V_2. All three types show significant J-point elevation (*black arrow*) and an inverted T wave. The type 2 pattern is described as having a "saddleback" appearance of the ST segment. Type 3 shows less pronounced (<0.1 mV) J-point elevation.

APPENDIX J   COMPARISON OF T WAVE MORPHOLOGY IN HYPERKALEMIA AND IN AMI

T Wave	Hyperkalemia	AMI*
Size	Hyperacute	Hyperacute
Symmetry	Asymmetric	Symmetric
Base	Narrow	Broad
Shape	Peaked/tented	Peaked/tented

*Acute myocardial infarction.